Geriatric Emergencies

Geriatric Emergencies

Iona Murdoch
Specialty Registrar (ST3) Emergency Medicine
East of England Deanery

Sarah Turpin
Specialty Registrar (ST4) Geriatric Medicine and General Internal Medicine
South East Scotland Deanery

Bree Johnston
Director of Palliative Care, St Joseph Hospital at PeaceHealth
Clinical Professor in Geriatrics, University of California, San Francisco

Alasdair MacLullich
Honorary Consultant in General and Geriatric Medicine, Royal Infirmary of Edinburgh
Professor of Geriatric Medicine, University of Edinburgh

Eve Losman
Assistant Professor, Emergency Medicine, University of Michigan Health System

WILEY Blackwell

Library of Congress Cataloging-in-Publication Data

Murdoch, Iona, 1984- , author.
    Geriatric emergencies / Iona Murdoch, Sarah Turpin, Bree Johnston, Alasdair MacLullich, Eve Losman.
        p. ; cm.
    Includes bibliographical references and index.
    ISBN 978-1-118-65557-3 (cloth)
    I. Turpin, Sarah, 1985- , author. II. Johnston, Bree, author. III. MacLullich, Alasdair, author.
IV. Losman, Eve, author. V. Title.
    [DNLM: 1. Aged. 2. Emergencies. 3. Emergency Treatment—methods. WB 105]
    RC86.7
    616.02'5—dc23
                                                                                2014034303

A catalogue record for this book is available from the British Library.

Wiley also publishes its books in a variety of electronic formats. Some content that appears in print may not be available in electronic books.

Cover image: Main front cover image of an emergency service rescuing a victim of an accident: istock © Seanshot; ambulance: istock © Scott Kochsiek; emergency room: istock © Pgiam

Set in 9.5/12pt Meridien by Laserwords Private Limited, Chennai, India
Printed and bound in Singapore by Markono Print Media Pte Ltd

1   2015

Contents

Contents

Preface

some that there is nothing apologetic with frail, and nothing geniar about polypathology. However, good management decisions rely on expert of knowledge, good years of practice, and the experiences, pitfalls and challenges of everyday clinical life. We hope the next editions are influences of those questions and uncertainties as they mature, and to the pinnacle of care of older people.

This book was written after two of the authors were discussing how disastrous it can be for a frail older person to present to hospital unnecessarily. Conversation soon spiralled to why this was the case, and onto the many inadequacies of a health system designed to treat single organ illness now delivering healthcare to a population of older patients with ever-growing polypathology and complex comorbidity.

The changing demographics of our population are an immense tribute to the success of modern medicine. With these changes come new and exciting challenges. How does one deliver care to a frail older patient with multiple comorbidities in an environment designed for single organ illness and rapid discharge? How can a clinician gather the complex but vital information about a patient's medications, social network and care needs when under time pressure with many others waiting to be seen? How can older persons be efficiently but safely assessed when they have so many active and inactive problems? When are these aspects taught during undergraduate training?

The treatment of older patients at the front door of the hospital is now the core business of clinicians working in the emergency department and acute medical unit. These patients constitute the majority, rather than the minority, of clinical work in modern medicine. Clinical outcomes are poor, with increased morbidity and mortality, if good initial care is overlooked; the first few hours in hospital are precious and the stakes are high.

An essential way of improving the care of older patients in the emergency department is through educating and improving the competence of all emergency personnel to deal with the specific needs of this large group of patients. This is the purpose of this book.

This book is aimed primarily at junior doctors, although we hope it will be a useful resource for any health care professional who encounters older patients in acute and emergency situations. There is a strong focus around the emergency department, but many of the presentations covered are frequent occurrences at the acute medical unit and in general medical and surgical wards.

The two introductory chapters place the subject in context and cover the essentials of thorough but concise history taking and clinical examination in older patients, relevant to the emergency setting. Tables and diagrams provide clear and practical information in relation to the work-up and management of each presenting complaint. Chapters include the classic common geriatric presentations including falls, delirium and stroke; the book also covers other emergencies such as head injury, abdominal pain, burns and major trauma, which often require a different approach to management in older patients. Throughout the text, 'key points' are used to highlight particularly relevant pieces of information or useful tips, and 'take home messages' at the end of each chapter provide a brief summary of the areas covered.

This is *not* a general medical textbook: while some emergencies in older patients are managed similarly to the way they would be in a younger patient, others require different approaches and management techniques. The content of this book will reflect these variations by addressing some topics in greater depth than others. This text is designed to cover the particular issues and challenges directly relevant to *frail, older* patients. In some situations, for example, a patient who has cardiac failure and acute kidney injury, there is no single 'right answer'. Instead, good management decisions rely on experiential knowledge, gained from years of practice, and the expert opinion and guidance of respected colleagues. We hope the text reflects the intricacies of these situations and that is serves as a useful aid in the optimal care of older people.

IM, ST, AM, BJ and EL

Acknowledgements

There are many people who made the writing of this book possible and provided support and encouragement during a steep learning curve. Thanks to Wiley for accepting our book proposal in the first place and to Catriona Cooper and James Schultz for answering numerous questions with patience and clarity. Thanks also to Zeshan Qureshi for generous and invaluable advice on how to start writing a book.

Expert review was provided by respected colleagues, of whom particular thanks must go to Dr Catherine Labinjoh (Consultant Cardiologist), Dr Julie Mardon (Consultant in Emergency Medicine), Dr Nolan Arulraj (Consultant in Geriatric and Stroke Medicine), Professor Gillian Mead (Professor of Stroke and Elderly Care Medicine), Dr Katie Marwick (ST4 in General Adult Psychiatry and ECAT Lecturer in Psychiatry), Dr Katherine Beck (CT3 Psychiatry) and Dr Robert McCutcheon (CT2 Psychiatry).

We would also like to thank our friends and families for the hours spent listening to the ups and downs relating to 'The Book'. In particular, thanks to Michael Kowalski and Matthew Coles for their love and support, for time spent listening, for keeping us fed and watered and on solid ground.

We would like to thank our fellow professionals, both known and unknown in the wider world, whose interest and research into the optimal care of older people is a source of huge and ongoing inspiration.

Finally, we must thank all of the older patients we have encountered. Such patients have, at their most vulnerable time, allowed us the privilege of caring for and learning from them as we develop and grow as doctors; without them this book could not exist.

List of Abbreviations

	UK
A-a	Alveolar-arterial
AAA	Abdominal aortic aneurysm
ABCDE	Airway, breathing, circulation, disability, exposure
ABG	Arterial blood gas
ACE	Angiotensin converting enzyme
ACEP	American College of Emergency Physicians
ACS	Acute coronary syndrome
AECOPD	Acute exacerbation of COPD
AF	Atrial fibrillation
AKI	Acute kidney injury
ALS	Advanced life support
AMU	Acute medical unit (US – general floor)
ARF	Acute respiratory failure
ATLS	Advanced trauma life support
AV	Atrio-ventricular
AVPU	Alert, verbal, pain, unresponsive
AXR	Abdominal X-ray
BNP	B-type natiuretic peptide
BP	Blood pressure
BPPV	Benign paroxysmal positional vertigo
CAP	Community acquired pneumonia
CEM	College of Emergency Medicine (UK)
CCU	Coronary care unit
CK	Creatinine kinase
CKD	Chronic kidney disease
CNS	Central nervous system
COPD	Chronic obstructive pulmonary disease
CPR	Cardio-pulmonary resuscitation
CRP	C-reactive protein
CSF	Cerebrospinal fluid
CSM	Carotid sinus massage
CT	Computerised tomography
CTA	CT angiography
CTPA	CT pulmonary angiography
CXR	Chest X-ray
DKA	Diabetic ketoacidosis
DNAR	Do not attempt resuscitation
ECG	Electrocardiogram
ED	Emergency department
EEG	Electroencephalogram
eGFR	Estimated glomerular filtration rate

ERCP	Endoscopic retrograde cholangiopancreatography
ESR	Erythrocyte sedimentation rate
FAST	Focused assessment with sonography for trauma
FAST	Face, arm, speech time test
FBC	Full blood count (US – complete blood count)
GCS	Glasgow coma scale
GEM	Geriatric emergency medicine
GI	Gastrointestinal
GP	General practitioner (US – primary care provider)
HDU	High dependency unit (US – step down unit)
HHS	Hyperglycaemic hyperosmolar syndrome
HR	Heart rate
IA	Intra-arterial
ICP	Intracranial pressure
ICU	Intensive care unit
IM	Intramuscular
INR	International normalised ratio
IV	Intravenous
JVP	Jugular venous pressure
LACS	Lacunar circulation stroke
LFT	Liver function test
LP	Lumbar puncture
LV	Left ventricle
LVF	Left ventricular failure
MDT	Multidisciplinary team
MI	Myocardial infarction
MRI	Magnetic resonance imaging
MRSA	Methicillin resistant staphylococcus aureus
MSU	Mid stream urine
NG	Nasogastric
NHS	National Health Service
NICE	National Institute of Health and Care Excellence
NIHSS	National Institute for Health Stroke Scale
NIV	Non invasive ventilation
NSAIDs	Non steroidal anti inflammatory drugs
NSTEMI	Non ST segment elevation myocardial infarction
$PaCO_2$	Arterial partial pressure of carbon dioxide
PACS	Partial anterior circulation stroke
PaO_2	Arterial partial pressure of oxygen
PE	Pulmonary embolism
POCS	Posterior circulation stroke
PPI	Proton pump inhibitor
PT	Prothrombin time
PUD	Peptic ulcer disease
QALY	Quality adjusted life year
RV	Right ventricle
SC	Subcutaneous
SSRI	Selective serotonin reuptake inhibitor

STEMI	ST segment elevation myocardial infarction
SVT	Supraventricular tachycardia
TACS	Total anterior circulation stroke
TB	Tuberculosis
TCA	Tricyclic antidepressant
TFTs	Thyroid function tests
TIA	Transient ishchaemic attack
U&E	Urea and electrolytes (US – urea nitrogen and chemistries)
UK	United Kingdom
US	United States
USS	Ultrasound scan
UTI	Urinary tract infection
V/Q scan	Ventilation perfusion scan
VBG	Venous blood gas
VF	Ventricular fibrillation
VT	Ventricular tachycardia
WCC	White cell count
WHO	World Health Organisation
X-ray	Radiograph

CHAPTER 1

Introduction to geriatric emergency medicine

Demographics

Population ageing is an international phenomenon, in terms of both the increasing number of people reaching old age and the rise in median age. Between 2000 and 2050, the proportion of the world's population over 60 years of age will double from about 11% to 22%, with the absolute number of people aged over 60 years expected to increase from 605 million to 2 billion over the same period (1). The number of people aged 80 years or older will have almost quadrupled to 395 million between 2000 and 2050 (1) (Figures 1.1 and 1.2). An ageing population brings potential benefits but also imposes particular challenges, particularly a growing demand for health and social care services. Whilst many people are staying healthy and active into old age, the number of older people who are reliant on care or have multiple health problems is increasing.

Over 65% of patients admitted to hospital are over 65 years old in the United Kingdom (UK) and many have complex medical conditions (2). In the United States (US), 19.6 million emergency department visits were made by patients aged over 65 in 2009–2010 (3). Those aged 65 years and older are twice as likely to be admitted than those under 65, rising to over 10 times more likely in those aged 85 and above (4).

Emergency department attendance as an older patient is associated with adverse outcomes, including an increased rate of subsequent (separate) hospitalisation, increased re-attendance to the ED, increased rate of functional decline and reduced capacity for independent living (5).

> **KEY POINT:** The beginning of this potential cascade of adverse events is at the front door of the emergency department, where a rushed or inadequate assessment resulting in hastened discharge or inappropriate disposition places complex older patients in a vulnerable position.

Emergency presentations

Illnesses in the older patient presenting to the ED are more likely to be of a higher acuity compared to younger patients. They are more likely to arrive by ambulance, they are more likely to be acutely unwell even when they appear stable on initial evaluation, and they are more likely to require immediate critical care.

Geriatric Emergencies, First Edition.
Iona Murdoch, Sarah Turpin, Bree Johnston, Alasdair MacLullich and Eve Losman.
© 2015 John Wiley & Sons, Ltd. Published 2015 by John Wiley & Sons, Ltd.

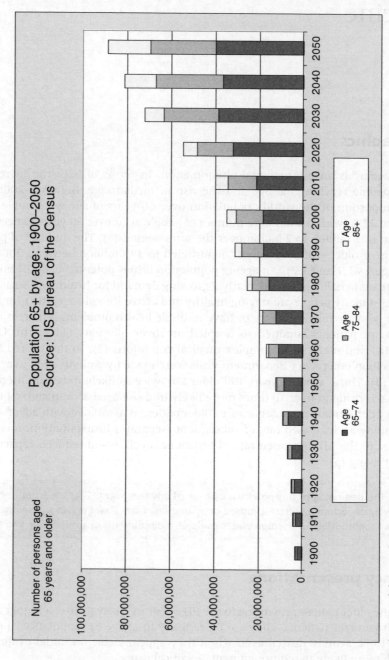

Figure 1.1 Projections of the population by age and sex for the United States: 2010–2050 (NP2008-T12), Population Division, US Census Bureau; Release Date: August 14, 2008.

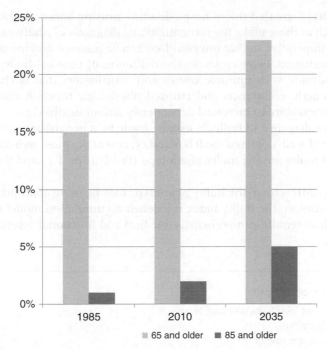

Figure 1.2 Percentage of older people in the United Kingdom 1985, 2010, 2035. Source: Office for National Statistics, National Records of Scotland, Northern Ireland Statistics and Research Agency.

Older patients often present with non-specific problems including the classic 'geriatric giants': falls, delirium, immobility and incontinence. These presenting complaints are often representative of multi-factorial disorders including underlying illness and comorbidity that require consideration of a broad differential; the assessment of these older patients requires skilful history and examination.

> **KEY POINT: Older patients with decreased functional reserve have the potential to deteriorate extremely quickly when placed under physiological stress.**

Frailty at the front door

The presentation of frail patients to the ED and acute medical unit (AMU) is attracting increasing interest. These patients have previously not been a priority and have fallen through gaps in an environment designed to treat condition-specific problems rather than address the more complex issues which can present in a patient who is 'frail'. Mortality rates of frail older patients presenting to EDs and AMUs is high and as such, this condition must be addressed by emergency physicians and acute physicians.

A large study on frail adults who were discharged from the ED showed they have a poorer 30-day outcome that non-frail patients, with between 10% and 45% (depending on level of frailty) increased risk of hospitalisation, nursing home admission and death (6). Studies such as these make the recognition and diagnosis of frailty early in an acute illness episode imperative so that interventions can be planned and initiated.

A recent international consensus on the definition of physical frailty defines it as, 'a medical syndrome with multiple causes and contributors that is characterised by diminished strength, endurance, and reduced physiologic function that increases an individual's vulnerability to increased dependency and/or death' (7).

The definitive diagnosis of frailty is usually made by a geriatrician and can be based on any number of well-validated models of frailty; two of the most well-known theoretical concepts of frailty are the frailty phenotype (Fried) (Box 1.1) and the frailty index (Rockwood).

In the ED or AMU setting, the frailty phenotype may be more appropriate as it can be applied at first contact; the frailty index is a deficit accumulation model that has many strengths but does require comprehensive medical and functional assessment before it can be applied.

Box 1.1 The frailty phenotype (8)

Unintentional weight loss (10 lbs over past year)
Self-reported exhaustion
Weakness (reduced grip strength)
Slow walking speed
Low physical activity

No criteria = Robust
1–2 criteria = Pre-frail
3 or more criteria = Frail.

There are several rapid screening tests that are aimed at helping acute care physicians to objectively identify frail patients early in their admission and target early interventions to help prevent deterioration in health or increased dependency (Table 1.1).

Another way of identifying frail patients in the emergency or acute care setting is if they present with a classic frailty syndrome. These syndromes are falls, delirium and dementia, polypharmacy (Chapter 2), incontinence, immobility and the receipt of end of life care (10).

If a patient is identified as frail or pre-frail using a screening test on admission, then plans should be made for early comprehensive geriatric assessment (CGA) with an aim

Table 1.1 The FRAIL scale, a rapid screening tool for older patients presenting to medical services (9).

3 or greater = Frailty; 1 or 2 = Pre-frail

Fatigue: 'Are you fatigued?'
Resistance: 'Cannot walk up one flight of stairs?'
Aerobic: 'Cannot walk one block?'
Illnesses: 'Do you have more than five illnesses?'
Loss of weight: 'Have you lost more than 5% of your body weight in the past 6 months?'

Source: From Van Kan GA, Rolland YM, Morley JE, Vellas B. Frailty: toward a clinical definition. *J Am Med Dir Assoc.* 2008 Feb;9(2):71–72. Reproduced with permission of Springer.

of facilitating appropriate discharge and preventing progression from pre-frail to frail. Where the service is available, such patients should also strongly be considered for referral or transfer to specialist geriatric care. Patients in earlier states of frailty may benefit more from CGA than patients who are approaching end-stage frailty (10).

KEY POINT: Omitting a frailty assessment in an older patient in the ED in the interests of time pressure is a false economy.

Comprehensive geriatric assessment (CGA)

CGA is defined as 'a multidimensional, interdisciplinary diagnostic process to determine the medical, psychological, and functional capabilities of a frail older person in order to develop a coordinated and integrated plan for treatment and long-term follow-up' (11). CGA is carried out by a multi-disciplinary team and often utilises standardised assessment tools. CGA is a highly effective process: it leads to improved discharge rates, reduced readmissions, reduced long-term care, greater patient satisfaction and lower costs (12).

Owing to time constraints, it is not usually possible to undertake CGA in the ED. However, research has shown that it is possible to embed aspects of the CGA into the ED, thus creating an 'Emergency Frailty Unit' with associated improvements in patient and operational outcomes. Work in the United Kingdom has shown that embedding CGA into the ED was associated with a reduction in readmission rates from 26% to 19.9% at 90 days (13). Frailty assessment units and AMUs are increasingly utilising versions of CGA in the emergency setting (Table 1.2).

Table 1.2 Components of comprehensive geriatric assessment (14).

Medical	Active medical problems
	Comorbid conditions and disease severity
	Medication review
	Nutritional status
Mental health	Cognitive assessment
	Mood and anxiety
Functional capacity	Activities of daily living and instrumental activities of daily living
	Activity levels and exercise tolerance
	Gait and balance
Social circumstances	Social support from family, neighbours or friends
	Daytime activities and social network
	Eligibility for care resources
Environment	Home situation, facilities and safety
	Use of local resources and community services
	Transport facilities

KEY POINT: CGA can be delivered in the ED and the limited research available has shown it is associated with reduced readmission rates.

Pathways in geriatric emergency care

Services available for older patients presenting in an emergency vary depending on geographical location. Most patients are admitted to hospital via the ED. As a zone of transition between primary and secondary care, the ED offers an ideal opportunity to identify and direct the care needs of the older adult with the support of inpatient and multidisciplinary care teams.

Unfortunately, many EDs tend to be loud, fast-paced, focused on crises and impersonal, and are thus particularly challenging environments for older patients. At least three approaches are necessary to address these challenges:

1 Creating care systems that minimize ED visits for the frailest, sickest elders.
2 Creating EDs that are 'elder-friendly' – more quiet, calm, and comfortable, with enhanced social services.
3 Improving the competence of all emergency personnel to deal with the special needs of older people. It is to the last approach that this book is primarily focused, but the other two approaches are at least as important.

Geriatric Emergency Medicine (GEM) is an established subspecialty of Emergency Medicine in the United States, and similar programmes are emerging in the United Kingdom. A number of hospitals have established a Geriatric ED; a clinical area alongside the main ED dedicated to providing acute care for the older person (15) (Table 1.3).

An awareness of the particular needs of the older population, and the oldest old, has resulted in the increasing development of services tailored to dealing with geriatric syndromes. These may be accessed directly by the primary care physician or via the ED. Available facilities in a growing number of centres may include:

• *Multidisciplinary teams* which may contain a physiotherapist, occupational therapy, social worker and/or community nurse. They are able to assess mobility in the ED or AMU and provide mobility aids, review social circumstances and arrange for personal care to be delivered in the patient's home on a temporary basis if required. They can be essential in enabling safe discharge of older patients.
• *Frailty assessment units* are specific short-stay or day wards where stable patients with geriatric syndromes can undergo prompt CGA. If admission is required they can be referred on to an inpatient bed.
• *Ambulatory care pathways*: For the patient who is able to be discharged home, these offer a means of prompt follow-up and expert review. These may include rapid access falls clinics, syncope service or outpatient antibiotic therapy clinics for conditions such as cellulitis.
• *Geriatric liaison teams* may assess patients in the ED or AMUs.

The transition between care facilities (hospital to home; hospital to enhanced care facility/skilled nursing facility) is one of the most vulnerable points in a patient's journey and is wrought with the risk of communication errors and resulting poor outcomes. A careful approach when transferring older, complex patients may mitigate this risk. Optimising transitions of care is discussed in Chapter 2.

Table 1.3 Components of an elder-friendly emergency department (16–18).

Environmental adaptations	Non-glare lighting
	Access to visual and hearing aids (e.g. portable amplifiers), large print information, clear signage
	Non-skid flooring and hand rails
	Less 'sensory chaos': fewer beeping machines, reduced background noise
	Pressure-relieving mattresses and more pillows and padding
	Calmer environment with embedded culture of respectful approach to older people
Screening and referral	Specialist nurse involvement with the use of screening tools for geriatric syndromes such as delirium, falls, immobility and polypharmacy
	Access to rapid referral for specialist clinics
	Pharmacist in department for medicines reconciliation
Improved transitions	Links with primary care
	Rapid access to social work
	Multidisciplinary team based in the ED
	Telephone follow-up system
	Geriatric follow-up clinic
Staff education	Specialist training programmes for staff working in the emergency department relating to geriatric patients and their differences in the emergency setting.
	'GEM champions' based in the department to promote gold standard care and lead by example

References

1 World Health Organisation (WHO). *Health Topics: Ageing.* http://www.who.int/topics/ageing/en/ [cited 2014 Apr 17].

2 Royal College of Physicians. *Future Hospital Commission. 2013.* http://www.rcplondon.ac.uk/projects /future-hospital-commission [cited 2014 May 15].

3 Centers for Disease Control and Prevention (CDC). *Products – Data Briefs – Number 130 Emergency Department Visits by Patients Aged 65 and Over – October 2013.* http://www.cdc.gov/nchs/data/databriefs /db130.htm [cited 2014 May 15].

4 Aminzadeh F, Dalziel WB. Older adults in the emergency department: a systematic review of patterns of use, adverse outcomes, and effectiveness of interventions. *Ann Emerg Med.* 2002;39(3): 238–247.

5 Grief CL. Patterns of ED use and perceptions of the elderly regarding their emergency care: a synthesis of recent research. *J Emerg Nurs.* 2003;29(2):122–126.

6 Hastings SN, Purser JL, Johnson KS, Sloane RJ, Whitson HE. Frailty predicts some but not all adverse outcomes in older adults discharged from the emergency department: frailty and adverse outcomes after ED discharge. *J Am Geriatr Soc.* 2008;56(9):1651–1657.

7 Morley JE, Vellas B, van Kan GA, Anker SD, Bauer JM, Bernabei R, et al. Frailty consensus: a call to action. *J Am Med Dir Assoc.* 2013;14(6):392–397.

8 Fried LP, Tangen CM, Walston J, Newman AB, Hirsch C, Gottdiener J, et al. Frailty in older adults evidence for a phenotype. *J Gerontol A Biol Sci Med Sci.* 2001;56(3):M146–M157.

9 Van Kan GA, Rolland YM, Morley JE, Vellas B. Frailty: toward a clinical definition. *J Am Med Dir Assoc.* 2008 Feb;9(2):71–72.

10 Royal College of Physicians (RCP). *Acute Care Toolkit 3: Acute Medical Care for Frail Older People.* http://www.rcplondon.ac.uk/resources/acute-care-toolkit-3-acute-medical-care-frail-older-people [cited 2014 May 15].

11 Rubenstein LZ, Stuck AE, Siu AL, Wieland D. Impacts of geriatric evaluation and management programs on defined outcomes: overview of the evidence. *J Am Geriatr Soc.* 1991;39(9 Pt 2):8S–16S; discussion 17S–18S.

12 Ellis G, Whitehead MA, Robinson D, O'Neill D, Langhorne P. Comprehensive geriatric assessment for older adults admitted to hospital: meta-analysis of randomised controlled trials. *BMJ.* 2011;343(oct27_1):d6553.

13 Conroy SP, Ansari K, Williams M, Laithwaite E, Teasdale B, Dawson J, et al. A controlled evaluation of comprehensive geriatric assessment in the emergency department: the 'Emergency Frailty Unit'. *Age Ageing.* 2014;43(1):109–114.

14 British Geriatric Society. Comprehensive Assessment of the Frail Older Patient. 2010.

15 Hogan TM, Olade TO, Carpenter CR. A profile of acute care in an aging America: snowball sample identification and characterization of United States geriatric emergency departments in 2013. *Acad Emerg Med.* 2014;21(3):337–346.

16 Walsh K, Stiles M, Foo CL. *New Age: Why the World Needs Geriatric Emergency Medicine Emergency Physicians International.* 2013; issue 11. http://www.epijournal.com/articles/100/new-age-why-the-world-needs-geriatric-emergency-medicine [cited 2014 May 15].

17 Meet the needs of aging patients with a senior-friendly ED. *ED Manag.* 2011;23(8):85–88.

18 American College of Emergency Physicians (ACEP). *13 – The Geriatric Emergency Department.* http://www.acep.org/content.aspx?id=87577 [cited 2014 May 15].

CHAPTER 2

Essentials of assessment and management in geriatric emergency medicine

Introduction

Assessment of older adults in the emergency setting is relatively resource-intensive. History taking may be challenging in patients with acute or chronic cognitive impairment, and obtaining the essential collateral history from carers or a long-term care facility can be time-consuming. Two-thirds of people over the age of 65 have multiple chronic health conditions (1), which along with polypharmacy complicates the clinical presentation and makes decision-making on clinical management intellectually complex.

Atypical, multifactorial, and non-specific presentations are par for the course in older adults. A thorough assessment can rarely be done rapidly. This contributes to the pressure on providers in today's crowded emergency departments.

This chapter aims to provide help with the initial triage of acutely ill older people and provide guidance on history taking and examination of older patients with particular focus on making the assessment efficient, taking a brief functional history and considering an overview of initial investigation and management strategies.

Triage and initial assessment

Older patients attending the ED are more likely than younger patients to have severe illness or injury (2). Prompt triage is vital to ensure timely identification of life-threatening presentations, address acute pain and initiate appropriate investigations.

In older patients, the degree of illness severity may be underestimated, leading to delays in medical assessment or inappropriate placement within the ED.

> KEY POINT: Standardised triage tools have been shown to frequently miss critical illness in the older patient (3).

Geriatric Emergencies, First Edition.
Iona Murdoch, Sarah Turpin, Bree Johnston, Alasdair MacLullich and Eve Losman.
© 2015 John Wiley & Sons, Ltd. Published 2015 by John Wiley & Sons, Ltd.

Triage also offers an opportunity to identify frailty, delirium or other specific conditions which may prompt early involvement of specialised services, such as early comprehensive geriatric assessment. Identifying patients likely to be admitted (including use of tools such as the ISAR (identification of seniors at risk) score – see below) may reduce the risk of prolonged boarding in the ED whilst awaiting an inpatient bed.

Box 2.1 Reasons for undertriage (3).

Physiological and pharmacological factors that may mask changes in vital signs with illness or injury

Presentation with non-specific symptoms or geriatric syndromes such as immobility, which may be mistaken for a more trivial complaint

Difficulties with history taking or lack of information about the patient's baseline mental and physical function

Lack of awareness of past medical problems, which may significantly impact on presentation

Failure to appreciate symptoms and signs which may be of higher risk in the older patient, such as abdominal pain.

Patients with a high illness severity score, abnormal vital signs or who appear critically unwell should be transferred to the resuscitation room or a monitored area and a systematic ABCDE approach to primary assessment should be undertaken in line with Advanced Life Support guidelines (4).

Note: The initial assessment of trauma patients is covered in Figure 11.1, Chapter 11.

Box 2.2 An ABCDE approach to the initial assessment of an acutely ill older person.

Airway	Ensure the airway is patent. Factors affecting the airway in an older patient are highlighted in Figure 11.2, Chapter 11
	Provide high-flow oxygen in critical illness or trauma in the first instance
Breathing	Measure respiratory rate, depth and work of breathing. Record oxygen saturations. Auscultate the chest, noting symmetry of chest expansion, air entry and crackles or wheeze. Sit the patient up if their work of breathing is increased
	Tachypnoea may be the first sign of serious undifferentiated illness
	The older patient has a reduced or delayed response to hypoxia and hypercapnia
Circulation	Assess pulse rate, volume and regularity. Measure blood pressure. Assess skin colour, capillary refill and hydration status. Attach cardiac monitoring and obtain an ECG. Obtain intravenous access and take blood samples. Obtain a venous or arterial blood gas and measure lactate level if there are signs of acute illness
	Pre-existing hypertension may result in a blood pressure in the normal range despite severe illness or haemorrhage
	Tachycardia may be absent due to cardiac medication or lack of response to sympathetic stimulation with ageing
	Medications such as beta-blockers, anti-hypertensives or the presence of a pacemaker may mask shock

Disability	Record alertness according to the AVPU (alert, response to voice, response to pain, unresponsive) scale or Glasgow coma scale (GCS). Assess pupillary responses and measure blood sugar *A reduced conscious level may indicate delirium (5) and thus severe acute illness. It is rarely due to chronic causes, such as dementia*
Exposure	Measure temperature and instigate warming measures to prevent or treat hypothermia. Assess the patient for injuries, abdominal tenderness, pressure areas, joint swelling or other signs. Assess pain and administer analgesia *Fever is absent in a third of older patients with sepsis*

 KEY POINT: Critically ill older patients should be discussed early with a senior clinician. Appropriate management plans including decisions regarding suitability for intensive care, resuscitation status and ultimate goals of care need to be considered.

Decisions and discussions regarding goals of care and resuscitation in older patients are covered in Chapter 3.

Communication with older patients

Once acute life-threatening illness and associated physiological disturbance has been identified or excluded and the critically ill patient has been appropriately stabilised, a more thorough assessment can begin. Optimising communication before beginning any further assessment can make the history and examination process more efficient.

Positioning and body language

Sit or crouch down so you are at the patient's level and able to make eye contact and appear non-threatening. Relaxed and open body language is particularly important and appropriate physical contact, for example, hand-holding can provide reassurance for some patients. Do not appear impatient, even if you feel overwhelmed by a large volume of work because many older patients already feel they are a burden. If you appear rushed, patients may react by becoming withdrawn or omitting details from the history in an attempt to save you time.

Vision and hearing

Ensure any visual or hearing aids are in place and working correctly. If a patient is blind, then make sure they know where you are positioned; touch and verbal explanation can be useful. Very deaf patients pose a challenge. Every effort should be made to optimise their hearing: ensure hearing aid batteries are fresh (there is usually a supply on most medical wards) and speak slowly and loudly into their good ear without shouting. If this fails, write things down, this is quicker, more effective and more respectful than needing to repeat questions several times. Many providers find that portable amplifiers (also called 'pocket talkers') can be an invaluable communication tool to have available.

Communicating with the cognitively impaired

Smile, maintain eye contact as much as possible, speak clearly using short clusters of words, and do not rush. Use a friendly and positive tone of voice. Closed questions may be easier for cognitively impaired patients to answer; however, before embarking on a list of medical questions, try to establish a rapport. Be patient and respectful throughout, do not patronise.

Initial cognitive assessment

Before taking any detailed history, a quick assessment of your patient's cognitive state is necessary, as patients who are cognitively impaired may be less able to provide a detailed history of recent events or answer functional assessment questions accurately.

Box 2.3 The 4AT.

		CIRCLE

[1] ALERTNESS
This includes patients who may be markedly drowsy (e.g. difficult to rouse and/or obviously sleepy during assessment) or agitated/hyperactive. Observe the patient. If asleep, attempt to wake with speech or gentle touch on shoulder. Ask the patient to state their name and address to assist rating

Normal (fully alert, but not agitated, throughout assessment)	0
Mild sleepiness for <10 s after waking, then normal	0
Clearly abnormal	4

[2] AMT4
Age, date of birth, place (name of the hospital or building), current year

No mistakes	0
One mistake	1
Two or more mistakes/untestable	2

[3] ATTENTION
Ask the patient: 'Please tell me the months of the year in backwards order, starting at December.' To assist initial understanding, one prompt of 'what is the month before December?' is permitted

Months of the year	Achieves 7 months or more correctly	0
backwards	Starts but scores <7 months/refuses to start	1
	Untestable (cannot start because unwell, drowsy, inattentive)	2

[4] ACUTE CHANGE OR FLUCTUATING COURSE
Evidence of significant change or fluctuation in alertness, cognition, other mental function (e.g. paranoia, hallucinations) arising over the last 2 weeks and still evident in last 24 h

No	0
Yes	4

---

4 or above: possible delirium ± cognitive impairment.
1–3: possible cognitive impairment.
0: delirium or severe cognitive impairment unlikely (but delirium still possible if [4] information incomplete).

Many patients will have cognitive impairment, often with overlying delirium. Despite this, in most centres, over 50% of older people are not screened for signs of cognitive impairment on admission.

Screen for evidence of cognitive impairment after introducing yourself and establishing rapport. A possible way of introducing such an exercise could go as follows:

> So, before we really get started on why you are here, I was hoping to ask you a few quick questions to just check that you are up-to-date with everything, and that your concentration is OK. We ask everyone over 65 these questions, and some of them might seem a bit strange, so try not to worry if you have any trouble with them ...

The 4 'A's Test or 4AT (www.the4AT.com) is a recently validated rapid assessment for delirium. It also incorporates two short cognitive items so as to avoid requiring a separate cognitive testing instrument at the point of initial assessment. The 4AT generally takes only 2 minutes to complete and its brevity makes it suitable for acute situations. There are many other screening tests that can be used in the ED including the Mini-Cog, the Ottawa 3DY (O3DY), the Brief Alzheimer's Screen (BAS), the Short Blessed Test (SBT) and the caregiver-completed AD8 (cAD8) which are not discussed here (6, 7).

History of presenting complaint

The history of presenting complaint in an older person without cognitive impairment is much the same as in a younger person, although there are some additional challenges that need to be considered.

Chronic versus acute symptoms

Try to begin with open questions, but be aware of the fact that many older patients have longstanding symptoms that are attributable to chronic comorbidity and are present most of the time. The key thing here is establishing whether these chronic symptoms have changed in any way recently or are affecting the patient's function in a way they previously had not. Statements such as 'has this changed over the last few days or weeks?' or 'does this feel the same as it always has or is it different to normal?' can help clarify these issues.

Cognitive impairment

Patients with cognitive impairment may find it difficult to recall the events leading up to their admission or to identify any recent changes in their health; however, this does not mean that cognitively impaired patients are unable to provide any meaningful history. Cognitively impaired patients are mostly still able to answer questions about any symptoms they are having at the time of your assessment and express any fears or worries that they have.

Collateral history

The ability to take a collateral or ancillary history is an essential skill in anybody involved with caring for older people. It provides crucial information and also helps place the patient in the context of their wider social circumstances. Finally, a conversation with friends or family also provides an excellent opportunity to identify carer stress.

 KEY POINT: Patient wishes and confidentiality are paramount; be sure to establish the patient's feelings and worries about their home situation, and remember that you are the patient's advocate first.

What to ask
See Table 2.1.

Whom to ask
Family and friends

When?
Immediately following your initial assessment if they are in attendance or as soon as possible following admission.

How?
Ideally in person although telephone calls are acceptable.

Family, friends or neighbours can provide enormous informal support to older people living alone in their homes. Whoever is closest to the patient will probably be able to provide the richest source of information. Remember, family who visit once every 2 or 3 weeks may be less aware of problems than a neighbour who pops in most days to help with tasks such as taking the rubbish out or collecting the weekly shopping.

The primary care physician
When?
During working hours within the first few days of admission.

How?
Usually by telephone.

The primary care physician (PCP) may know the patient very well, possibly over a number of years, and have a good knowledge of any social or interpersonal factors contributing to the admission such as family anxiety or social problems. They are also able to provide an up-to-date list of medications and detailed medical history.

The homecare providers
When?
During the course of an admission or when discharge planning.

How?
Usually by telephone, often made by the nursing staff.

Care staff visiting patients at home can be difficult to track down; however, contacting the care agency manager can sometimes provide useful information on observations carers may have made about issues such as increasing dependency, poor living conditions or generally declining health.

Table 2.1 How to take a collateral history.

What you are checking	How to check it
Cognition and behaviour	Normal cognitive function?
	Are they more confused than normal?
	Any suggestion of decline in cognitive function over months/years?
	Previous episodes of delirium?
	Other changes in behaviour: sleeping, eating, going out unexpectedly
Physical health	Symptoms suggestive of recent illness or new incontinence?
	Recent visits to the primary care physician/recent stays in hospital?
	Recent falls or head injuries?
	Eating and drinking normally?
	Weight loss?
Medications	Who deals with the tablets?
	Any recent changes?
	Over-the-counter use?
	Evidence of non-compliance?
Functional status	What do they get help with?
	ask specifically about bathing/dressing/transferring to
	the toilet/housework/shopping/meal preparation/bedtime
	Who provides the help?
	Family/friends/formal carers?
	How often does the help come?
	Daily (how many times?)/weekly
	Any day centre attendance?
	Is the house in a mess?
Alcohol	Is there evidence of excess alcohol intake?
	Who buys the alcohol and how much, how often?
	Have there been alcohol-related health problems in the past?
Strong feelings (patient and carer)	Any particular fears or worries? E.g. refusal to accept help/recent bereavement
	Carer stress: do they feel overburdened? Are they struggling to provide all the support required?
	Any strong feelings about care homes?

The paramedics
When?
At presentation to the emergency department or acute medical unit.

How?
In person. If you don't catch them now, you never will.

Having literally just come from the patient's place of residence, they can tell you what it is like and whether there are obvious problems that need to be addressed.

The nursing home
When?
During your initial assessment as part of the history taking process.

How?
By telephone, 24 hours a day.

Collateral history from a nursing home is slightly different, and the patient will often come with formal transfer documents detailing medications, functional ability, cognitive ability and observations. Despite this useful information, there is sometimes little detail regarding the actual presenting complaint. For example, 'blacked out in lounge' is not enough information, so most nursing home admissions should be followed-up with a telephone call and a collateral history of presenting complaint taken from the care staff. Care home staff should also be asked about the resident's normal level of cognition and behavioural functioning.

Systematic enquiry

In an older person with many chronic problems, a systematic enquiry can seem a daunting task. However, much important information can be revealed, some of which will be useful in the immediate diagnostic summary and management plan. A more accurate history will save time in the long run as the treatment and management of the patient can often be more targeted than would otherwise be possible.

Box 2.4 Important things not to miss in the systemic enquiry.

Falls
Pain
Incontinence
Memory loss
Depression
Anxiety
Eyesight and hearing change
Weight loss
Change in eating pattern
Sleep disturbance.

Benefits of a thorough systematic enquiry:
1 Identifying specific causes for a relatively non-specific presenting symptom, e.g. recent urinary incontinence and frequency in a patient who has presented with falls.
2 Unearthing incidental serious underlying pathology in patients with relatively mild presenting complaints, e.g. weight loss and altered bowel habit in an older patient presenting with cellulitis.
3 Establishing chronic symptoms which may not be related to the presenting complaint but which may have an impact on rehabilitation goals, for example, chronic dyspnoea and an exercise tolerance of 10 yards secondary to severe COPD (chronic obstructive pulmonary disease) is useful background information for a patient who may require physiotherapy.

4 Many older people erroneously attribute pathological symptoms such as weight loss or exertional chest tightness as simply a sign of 'old age'. A careful systematic enquiry should be performed as a screening tool for identifying early signs of preventable or at least modifiable severe illness.

Social and functional history

> KEY POINT: A questions-based functional screen takes less than 5 minutes and should be done during the initial assessment of any older person who presents acutely.

Relatively minor changes in health can lead to a major decline in functional status and patients presenting with poor functional status as a primary complaint have increased mortality. This aspect of assessment in older patients is one of the key differences between the acute assessment of older versus younger adults.

In an acute environment, a brief assessment of a patient's social and functional status is a key part of the evaluation and constitutes a major component of assessing frailty. Any problems identified on initial screening should prompt referral for more detailed assessment by an appropriate provider.

Brief screens of functional assessment can be done using a questions-based approach and these questions take less than 5 minutes. Questions should address the basic and then instrumental activities of daily living (ADL) (Table 2.2). Scales of functional status are available with different scoring systems, for example, the Barthel Index and the Nottingham ADL Index.

Example questions for quick functional screening:
1 Do you have anyone coming in to help at home?
   (a) Be specific: ask directly about professional carers, district nurses, relatives and neighbours.
   (b) How often do they come? Is it every day? How many times per day?
2 Do you use anything to help you walk? Do you have a wheelchair? How about long distances?
3 Does anyone help you get washed or dressed?
4 Do you need help using the toilet and do you wear pads?
5 Do you get any help with shopping or cooking?
6 Who does the housework?
7 How do you manage your tablets?
8 Who sorts out the bills?
9 Do you get out and about much? How about day centres? Can you drive?

Medications and polypharmacy

It is generally recognised that as patients age, they tend to take more medications. There is no consensus definition of polypharmacy, but it is generally accepted to be the presence of several daily medications, some of which may be inappropriate (8). Indeed, 'inappropriate versus appropriate' prescribing is a simple alternative to a number-based

Table 2.2 Activities of daily living.

Basic activities of daily living	Instrumental activities of daily living
Bathing	Shopping
Dressing	Cooking
Toileting	Housework
Transfers	Telephone use
Continence	Transport
Feeding	Medications
	Finances

definition of polypharmacy. An accurate list of current medications should be obtained on presentation, and medicines reconciliation should occur within the first 24 hours of admission. Patients noted to be on multiple medications should undergo a structured medication review by a pharmacist or a geriatrician later in their admission.

Some medications may be life-saving; however, others may be unnecessary and detrimental to an older person's health and quality of life. Polypharmacy is a risk factor for falls and places older patients at increased risk of adverse drug reaction.

Polypharmacy is particularly prevalent in the United Kingdom and the United States; two-thirds of UK patients aged over 75 are prescribed four or more medications and a large review in the United States showed nearly 30% of older patients were on six or more medications (9, 10).

Tools to assist with structured medication reviews include the updated Beers criteria; the STOPP (screening tool of older person's prescriptions) and START (screening tool to alert doctors to right treatment) criteria exist to help with structured medication reviews in older patients (11, 12).

Examination

Older patients have a higher prevalence of physical signs and these signs are often relevant to the acute presentation and/or chronic health problems. In patients presenting with non-specific syndromes such as falls or delirium, physical examination can help elicit an underlying diagnosis of, for example, lobar pneumonia or subdural haematoma.

When facing a frail, confused or immobile older person, remember that they may be frightened, exhausted, confused or a combination of all of these things. They should be approached with kindness and respect and treated with time, care and consideration.

General examination

Much information can be gained from systematic end-of-the-bed observation. Documentation of pertinent facts regarding general appearance and behaviour can provide very valuable information on overall state, which can used as baseline for judging future deterioration or recovery.

'Sitting up in a chair, alert, lucid and well-kempt, doing Sudoku'.

'Lying sideways in the bed, intermittently obeying commands but not speaking, unkempt, hair matted, strong odour of urine'.

'Agitated, anxious, repeatedly lashing out, trying to get out of bed, shouting for "Mum"'.

The examination of an older person can pose challenges not present when examining a younger person. Yet there are ways to approach the process of examining an older person which may help overcome these challenges.

Box 2.5 Approach to optimising the examination of an older person (PACE).

Positioning: Ensure the patient is positioned comfortably, ideally on a bed or a stretcher, usually sitting slightly upright with their legs straight and their arms by their sides. Ensure they have appropriate support with pillows or blankets to compensate for any kyphoscoliosis or contractures. If possible, avoid examining somebody in their wheelchair or sitting on the edge of their bed. Patients who are unable to lay flat can usually still lie down with the head of the bed raised.

Assistance: Get help manoeuvring the patient. Having the assistance of a nurse, nursing assistant or relative can make a big difference when an immobile patient is required to lean forward, roll over or transfer from chair to bed. It is hard to focus on chest auscultation when you are straining to steady a patient from toppling over as they lean forward!

Communication: It is easier to examine anyone if they understand what you are trying to do. Ensure hearing aids and glasses are worn and in working order, try to reduce background noise and seek out communication aids such as amplifiers or picture charts. If necessary, write instructions down.

Exposure: Older patients often present wearing many layers of clothes and with chronic wounds or ulcers dressed with bandages and dressings. These may cover a multitude of important signs and are a barrier to your examination; they must be removed.

 KEY POINT: You are not able to detect wound infection through three layers of compression bandages nor are you able to comment on pressure areas through underwear, a corset, a vest and a jumper.

Specific areas of focus on examination
Cognition
It is important to assess and document an older person's cognitive state at the time they present to hospital.

Skin
Pressure areas, particularly the heels and sacrum should be checked on admission and any pressure damage documented; this is important for monitoring progress and changes in skin integrity throughout an older person's hospital stay. For advice on how to assess and grade pressure damage, see Chapter 8. There is a high prevalence of incidental skin cancers in older people, so abnormal looking skin blemishes should be referred appropriately.

Genito-urinary
Silent urinary retention is a common cause of non-specific functional decline, recurrent UTI (urinary tract infection) and delirium. It should be considered in every patient and if in doubt, bladder scanners are usually readily available. Genital skin inflammation secondary to chronic incontinence or a strong smell of stale urine can be a useful indicator of continence problems that patients may be too embarrassed to divulge or too confused to be aware of.

Respiratory examination

Basal crepitations are a relatively common finding in chest examination in otherwise healthy older patients. It is important to document the nature and location of the crepitations, and to check to see whether they clear on coughing. This will help in assessing any changes. Chest wall deformity secondary to kyphoscoliosis can have significant effects on ventilatory capacity and should be documented. Chest wall tenderness from rib fractures should be checked for.

Cardiac examination

Many older patients have heart murmurs and these may be an incidental finding (aortic sclerosis) or may be directly relevant to their presenting symptom (critical aortic stenosis and syncope). Examine closely for signs of cardiac failure such as jugulovenous distention and pedal oedema.

Neurological examination

Globally decreased power, loss of ankle jerks or non-specific signs secondary to generalised white matter change can all present as aspects of 'normal' findings in older patients. Acute illness such as delirium (Chapter 18) can exacerbate previous neurological signs such as weakness from a previous stroke. Tremor is common in older patients and the presence and features of tremor should be documented. Patients who present with falls and reduced mobility require a full neurological examination, and signs suggestive of parkinsonism should prompt referral for specialist assessment.

Fluid status

This is more difficult to assess in older patients because skin turgor is frequently decreased due to age-related changes in connective tissue. Lone pedal oedema in the absence of other signs of heart failure does not necessarily suggest fluid overload and may be secondary to chronic vascular changes, gravitational dependency, reduced blood albumin levels or medications such as amlodipine.

Vascular

Examination and documentation of peripheral pulses is an important baseline screen as older patients are at increased risk of acute limb ischaemia during admission. Abdominal aneurysms are potential incidental findings and increased age is a risk factor. Chronic venous skin changes in the legs are a common finding and can be mistaken for cellulitis.

Rectum

Check for faecal impaction as a cause for non-specific decline or delirium.

Breasts

In women, breast examination to check for lumps should be performed at some point during admission, particularly in cases of weight loss or confusion.

Joints

Evidence of arthropathy, inflammation and previous arthroplasty should be documented. Range of movement should be tested and acute pain identified and managed.

Gait and mobility

This is an essential part of assessment, and can be done as a quick screen (less than 5 minutes) in the ED or on a ward.

Document the type and quality of footwear and the use of a walking aid. Ensure that the patient is wearing appropriate and correctly fitting shoes, and there is a relatively uncluttered space available: move tables and drip stands aside.

The timed up and go test

Ask the patient to stand up and walk a short distance (10 feet) turn round, and come back again: 10 seconds or less is a normal score time, 10–20 seconds is intermediate and patients may require further evaluation. Patients who take longer than 20 seconds to complete this test require further evaluation of their mobility and transfers by a physiotherapist.

Observe and document:

1 Ability to go from sitting to standing: independent? Assistance of one or two people?
2 Base of support: narrow, normal or wide?
3 Stride length: small and shuffling? Normal?
4 Arm swing: preserved, reduced or absent?
5 General balance: steady or unsteady?
6 Any particular gait pattern? Antalgic, parkinsonian, ataxic, high stepping?
7 Steadiness on turning
8 Use of walking aid.

Note: if there are concerns that the patient is unsteady or unsafe, ensure there is a bystander present to support the patient and terminate the assessment early if they are clearly at high risk of falling when attempting to walk. Clearly abnormal gait patterns picked up on a general mobility screen can help direct further examination and investigations such as assessment for parkinsonism or need for joint radiographs.

Functional assessment

Brief functional assessment should and can be done as an integral part of general history and examination. Document the patient's ability to dress/undress, do up buttons, put on socks. Detailed functional assessment is the role of an occupational therapist or, in the United States, the primary care provider.

Investigations

For a given presentation, the older patient usually requires a greater number of investigations than their younger counterpart. Even in a minor complaint, basic blood tests may identify gross derangements that require addressing as a cause or consequence of the presenting problem, which if not identified may result in re-admission or poor outcome. A balanced approach is required when selecting investigations in the older patient, considering the need for diagnosis and prognostication whilst not prolonging the patient's stay unnecessarily or exposing them to complications of invasive investigations. The clinician should be aware of the limitations of certain investigations in the older patient (Table 2.3).

Consider undertaking basic investigations in most older patients presenting in an emergency.

Table 2.3 Tests associated with reduced sensitivity or specificity in the older patient.

Reduced sensitivity (increased false negatives) A normal test result may be present in the older patient despite significant pathology	Reduced specificity (increased false positives) A positive test may be due to a number of causes in the older patient and should be interpreted carefully
The older patient may not demonstrate a *leucocytosis or left shifted white blood count* despite pneumonia, cholecystitis or other inflammatory or infective processes (13)	*Troponin* may be a marker of myocardial ischaemia, but is also raised in other conditions such as pulmonary embolus, acute kidney injury and systemic, with uncertain prognostic value. An appropriately timed negative result is useful in ruling out non-ST elevation myocardial infarction
Chest radiograph in pneumonia may appear normal initially. In frail patients, a supine chest radiograph may be necessary, missing pleural effusions or other abnormalities	*D-dimer* specificity reduces to approximately 5% in patients aged over 80. It may be raised in older patients due to pathologies other than pulmonary embolus such as infection or malignancy. A normal D-dimer result, however, may be useful in excluding pulmonary embolus, and a higher cut-off in the older patient has been shown to safely exclude venous thromboembolism (14)
Chest and abdominal radiographs may appear normal in up to 40–50% of confirmed abdominal viscus perforations. Distended bowel loops may not be visible on plain films in bowel obstruction	
A *creatinine* measurement in the normal range may still be compatible acute kidney injury in the frail older patient with reduced muscle mass. Compare with previous results if available	Older patients frequently have *leucocytes* and *nitrites* present in the urine, which often represents asymptomatic bacteriuria. As such UTI may be over diagnosed, without careful thought of other more serious causes of the patient's presentation. Urine dipstick testing should only be considered in patients with unexplained systemic sepsis, which may present as delirium
	C-reactive protein (CRP) or erythrocyte sedimentation rate (ESR): Long-term immobility and malignancy may be associated with high levels and this does not necessarily indicate infection, although a high value should prompt further history and examination to find a cause. The upper limit for a normal ESR is higher in older patients

Choice of investigations will depend on the clinical presentation but a basic set should include:
- Electrocardiogram (ECG)
- Urea and electrolytes
- Chest radiograph.

Liver function tests and bone profile are often omitted in younger patients, but in older patients may be useful to pick up previously undiagnosed liver disease or hypercalcaemia. Thyroid function, vitamin B12 and folate or amylase and lipase may be required in delirium or abdominal pain, respectively. Coagulation studies and blood typing are required in patients who are on anticoagulants, bleeding, anaemic or likely to undergo surgery.

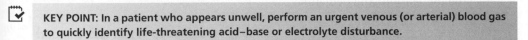

KEY POINT: In a patient who appears unwell, perform an urgent venous (or arterial) blood gas to quickly identify life-threatening acid–base or electrolyte disturbance.

KEY POINT: The clinician should always be wary of prescribing antibiotics based on raised inflammatory markers alone, without evidence of infection from the history and examination.

Computed tomography (CT) scans in older patients

There is a generally lower threshold for older patients to undergo CT scanning in emergency situations and these are discussed in context relating to specific emergency presentations throughout this book. The risks associated with radiation exposure are much less of a consideration in older patients. However, CT investigations involving radiographic contrast agents, such as coronary angiography, are associated with a greater risk of nephropathy, particularly in patients with pre-existing renal disease. If time allows, stop nephrotoxic drugs, and provide intravenous hydration before contrast CT. Evidence for other strategies to prevent contrast nephropathy is lacking at the time of writing (15).

When not to investigate

A pragmatic approach is required when an older patient with multiple morbidities or advanced frailty presents with a new symptom requiring evaluation. Advance directives, knowledge of the patient's wishes or discussion with the proxy decision maker may make it clear that further investigations would not be warranted. If a certain procedure, such as coronary stenting, abdominal or neurosurgery would not be consented to or considered in the patient's best interests, there may be a question as to whether imaging would change the patient's management. However, it is recognised that an understanding of the pathological process underlying deterioration can assist with management of the patient's symptoms, identify other potential palliative treatments and help a patient and family members come to terms with their decline. The benefits and burdens of investigations should be considered at each stage.

Management

Examples of different management strategies in the older patient compared to their younger counterpart include a lower threshold for admission in infection; wider spectrum of antibiotics in nursing home residents to cover for healthcare associated infections; consideration of advanced monitoring and pain management techniques in chest trauma; and earlier surgical management of intra-abdominal infection such as cholecystitis. Specific details are discussed in individual chapters.

Increasingly, quality indicators for older patients admitted to hospital are being utilised (16, 17), with the aim of auditing particular areas of geriatric care. These include:
• Rationalising urinary catheterisation
• Prevention of falls and pressure injuries

- Screening for delirium and dementia
- Undertaking structured medication reviews.

Anticipatory care planning in the ED, including resuscitation status and appropriateness of escalation of therapy to the intensive care unit, should be considered and documented in all unwell older patients; for further information on how to approach these issues, see Chapter 3.

How to make a problem list

A problem list is a key part of geriatric practice. The list helps crystallise the health professional's thoughts at the end of an assessment in a patient with multiple presenting issues or complex comorbidity. Problem lists can be created and updated at any time and they provide a useful overview of current issues pertaining to that individual. Items on the problem list are not restricted to diagnoses or other medical issues, but can include functional and social issues.

Problems lists are usually divided into 'active' and 'inactive' problems.

Active problems
These problems usually relate to the initial presenting symptom or diagnosis and the causes or consequences directly relating to that which are acute issues at the time of presentation. It is often helpful to also document initial management plans relating to each active problem as part of the list so that you do not forget about them later on in the patient's admission.

Inactive problems
These problems relate to stable aspects of the patient's medical or social condition which are not directly relevant to the presenting problem but may benefit from 'tweaking' to ensure they are being optimally managed and are not contributing to issues such as polypharmacy.

Box 2.6 How to make a problem list, a case example.

A 90-year-old lady presents with a fall and subsequent reduced mobility. Assessment reveals she is in pain from a vertebral compression fracture, constipated due to a combination of opioid analgesia and immobility and in acute kidney injury due to use of over-the-counter ibuprofen purchased by her daughter. She has a history of osteoarthritis, type 2 diabetes, stable angina, chronic kidney disease and cataracts.

Active problems:
1 Falls and reduced mobility: multifactorial in nature secondary to arthritis, poor vision and back pain
  (a) Undergoing physiotherapy assessment
  (b) Awaits ophthalmology input? Cataract removal?
  (c) Regular paracetamol and low-dose opiates commenced
  (d) Orthopaedics to consider kyphoplasty
2 Constipation: secondary to analgesia and immobility

(a) On daily/routine laxatives
(b) Opioid dose reduced
(c) Needs PR examination.
3 Acute on chronic kidney injury: secondary to use of ibuprofen.
(a) Ibuprofen stopped
(b) On IV fluids: check urea and electrolytes daily until AKI resolved
(c) Renal USS (ultrasound scan) awaited to check for additional obstructive uropathy.

Inactive problems:
1 Type 2 diabetes
(a) On oral hypoglycaemic agents: monitor blood glucose three times daily.
2 Ischaemic heart disease
(a) Multiple anti-anginal agents. Can these be rationalised? → cardiology opinion awaited
(b) Needs erect and supine blood pressure checks? Postural hypotension.

Discharging a patient from hospital

Unplanned hospital admission in the older patient is associated with increased risk of functional decline, delirium, nosocomial infections and complications of investigations and treatments. Hospital admissions should be avoided where possible. However, discharges from the ED or after a stay in hospital are associated with an increased risk of adverse events (18). Discharge planning, where this is a possibility, should be commenced from the time of initial assessment.

Patients with mild illness, good social support and mobility and no significant comorbidity may be considered for immediate discharge home, provided they are aware of signs and symptoms of worsening illness, have a means of contacting help if required and have follow-up arranged.

Various screening tools are available to assist with identifying patients most at risk of poor outcomes following an emergency presentation, such as the ISAR score (Box 2.7, (19)). Unfortunately, due to the complexity of older people's presentations and healthcare needs, these scoring systems have poor predictability (20). They do have some value as an adjunct to clinical decision-making, and to stimulate further assessment of the patients function and social status (19).

Box 2.7 Identification of seniors at risk (ISAR) score.

1 Before the injury or illness, did you need someone to help you on a regular basis?
2 Since the injury or illness, have you needed more help than usual?
3 Have you been hospitalised for one or more nights in the past 6 months?
4 In general, do you see well?
5 In general, do you have serious problems with your memory?
6 Do you take more than three medications daily?
   >1 positive response is considered high-risk.

If discharging the patient to his or her own home is not possible or considered to be unsafe, there may be alternatives to hospital admission. Options may differ depending on region but include a rehabilitation or community hospital, intermediate care facility or nursing or residential home placement. If it is possible to discharge the patient to his or her own home, temporary provision of carers or a re-enablement team may be an option. Consider referral to ambulatory care services such as a falls clinic or a frailty assessment unit (Table 2.4). If the patient is being admitted to hospital, an estimated discharge date should be established on the first day, to ensure that any care required on discharge is organised in advance.

Re-admission is usually defined as a further admission within 30 days following discharge. Depending on the local healthcare system, this may be associated with a financial or other penalty to the hospital. Risk factors for re-admission include prolonged length of previous hospital stay; a previous admission within the last 6 months; four or more comorbidities; six or more prescribed medications; and moderate to severe functional deficits (21, 22).

Transitions of care

A *transition of care* is defined as a time when a patient moves to a different site or healthcare facility, or when the team responsible for their care changes. Owing to their more complex medical needs, older patients are more likely to be transferred between facilities or specialty teams. For the complex older patient, any transition or handover in care is extremely risk-prone and success depends on careful communication of their medical history and management plan. A simple miscommunication or omission may result in a significant adverse drug event, unnecessarily repeated tests, missed diagnosis or other poor outcome.

KEY POINT: Avoid transferring an older patient between wards at night. This can increase the risk of delirium and adverse events due to poor communication (24).

In terms of location, a transition of care may be from the patient's home to the ED via an ambulance, from the ED to a medical or surgical ward or from the ED back to their long-term care facility.

Even if the patient does not move location, the responsibility for their management may change from the emergency physician to the inpatient geriatrician or surgeon or from the nursing team at a rehabilitation facility to a community nursing team. There may be conflicting understandings of who is responsible for care, particularly in admitted patients boarding in the ED.

KEY POINT: Communication issues are most frequently responsible for failed transition of care (25) and a standardised communication proforma for transitions of care may be helpful in reducing errors related to diagnostic uncertainty and care planning.

The key to reducing risk in transition of care is meticulous attention to detail and clear, direct and robust communication. This may be a significant challenge in a busy, crowded ED but is of vital importance. The advent of effective information technology

Table 2.4 A checklist of items to consider before the disposition of an older adult from hospital.

Mobility	Assess mobility and compare it to the patient's baseline. Arrange for a physiotherapy assessment if necessary. Consider whether further mobility aids or adaptations to the house are necessary
Cognition	Is the patient at baseline cognition or is there ongoing delirium requiring further assessment? If they have dementia, are they still safe to be at home alone?
Safety	Consider the risks to the patient on hospital discharge and whether these have been mitigated as far as possible. Consider whether the patient would benefit from a falls alarm or safety buzzer. If the patient does not have carers, is anyone able to check on them after the first day of discharge home? If they have dementia, does the risk of wandering or gas safety need to be addressed?
Social support	Does the patient live alone? Have they been coping at home? Are relatives or carers managing? Have carers been reinstated on hospital discharge if the patient has been admitted for some time? If possible, arranging carers to be present for when the patient gets home from hospital can smooth the transition of care
Equipment	Check the availability and delivery of medical (e.g. home oxygen) or mobility (e.g. bathroom rails) equipment if required. Have they got food and functional heating at home?
Advanced care planning	If the person has a progressive chronic disease, consider discussion about future admissions, ceilings of care and resuscitation status. Consider whether community palliative care needs to be involved. If appropriate, discuss the possibility of advance directives or power of attorney
Follow-up and continuing care	Ensure the primary care physician is aware of the patient's discharge and is up-to-date with their ongoing medical issues. Ensure that the other community services such as palliative care or heart failure teams are also aware. Arrange a follow-up appointment if required
Timing	The morning, or at least during daylight hours, is usually the best time of day for a planned hospital discharge to ensure that community services are available if there are any initial problems. If discharge is delayed, consider keeping the patient overnight and arranging transport for early the next morning
Medication	Frequent problems include drug interactions, missing drugs, unnecessarily long duration of treatment, incorrect dosage and incorrect drug selection (23). Drug-related problems are associated with an increased risk of hospital re-admissions, morbidity and mortality. Ensure the patient understands their medication regime and the potential drug side effects to be aware of. Is the patient still able to swallow tablets or remove them from their packaging?
Education of patients and their relatives	Ensure that the patients and their relatives understand the reasons for their admission, the investigations and treatment they have undergone. Provide a discharge summary and other written material about their condition if relevant (available in large print if necessary). Explain the ongoing treatment plan and indicators for return. Give patients and their relatives time to ask questions
Discharge summary	Ensure that an adequate summary of events, investigations and treatments during the hospital admission is provided for the patient, primary care physician, community care team and other clinicians or agencies involved in their care (with patient consent). Highlight any outstanding test results, when these are due and who will action them
Final medical review	It is important to examine the patient before discharge. Check for worrying symptoms, change in mental state, vital signs and perform a focused physical examination to make sure that there are no acute infections or other complications that require urgent attention
Transport	Consider whether the patient requires trolley or wheelchair transport home. Will they manage the steps to their front door? Check that they have got keys to get into their house (these issues can be handled by the social worker or discharge planner)

systems may improve transfer of information between teams but in many healthcare systems, this is some way off.

When passing on information to the next healthcare provider, it is useful to provide both verbal and written information.

When discharging an older patient:

- Call the long-term care facility or community nursing team and handover to the nurse in charge. At the end of the conversation, ask them to repeat the information you have given to ensure adequate understanding.
- Send written information back with the patient
- Fax or email a copy of the chart and/or discharge summary to the primary care provider and all other specialties involved in the patient's care (if the patient consents to this).
- Give the patient a copy of the discharge summary and ensure they understand all aspects of it. Ensure the patient and relatives have a chance to ask questions.

KEY POINT: Accurate and detailed written information following discharge is a key aspect in enabling high-quality ongoing care and preventing re-admission.

If the patient is being admitted, ensure a verbal handover to the specialty taking over care, and document clearly in the chart which investigations have been requested and which are still outstanding.

References

1 Centers for Disease Control and Prevention (CDC). *The State of Aging and Health in America 2013*. http://www.cdc.gov/aging/pdf/state-aging-health-in-america-2013.pdf [cited April 25 2014].
2 Aminzadeh F, Dalziel WB. Older adults in the emergency department: a systematic review of patterns of use, adverse outcomes, and effectiveness of interventions. *Ann Emerg Med*. 2002;39(3):238–247.
3 Grossmann FF, Zumbrunn T, Frauchiger A, Delport K, Bingisser R, Nickel CH. At risk of under-triage? Testing the performance and accuracy of the emergency severity index in older emergency department patients. *Ann Emerg Med*. 2012;60(3):317–325.e3.
4 Resuscitation Council (UK). *Systematic Approach to Acutely Ill Patient*. http://www.resus.org.uk/pages /alsABCDE.htm [cited 2014 May 17].
5 Tieges Z, McGrath A, Hall RJ, Maclullich AMJ. Abnormal level of arousal as a predictor of delirium and inattention: an exploratory study. *Am J Geriatr Psychiatry*. 2013;21(12):1244–1253.
6 Carpenter CR, Bassett ER, Fischer GM, Shirshekan J, Galvin JE, Morris JC. Four sensitive screening tools to detect cognitive dysfunction in geriatric emergency department patients: brief Alzheimer's Screen, Short Blessed Test, Ottawa 3DY, and the caregiver-completed AD8. *Acad Emerg Med*. 2011; 18(4):374–384.
7 Lin JS, O'Connor E, Rossom RC, Perdue LA, Burda BU, Thompson M, et al. Screening for Cognitive Impairment in Older Adults: An Evidence Update for the U.S. Preventive Services Task Force. Rockville (MD): Agency for Healthcare Research and Quality (US); 2013 http://www.ncbi.nlm.nih .gov/books/NBK174643/ [cited 2014 May 17].
8 Bushardt RL, Massey EB, Simpson TW, Ariail JC, Simpson KN. Polypharmacy: misleading, but manageable. *Clin Interv Aging*. 2008;3(2):383–389.
9 Fitzgerald R, Pirmohamed M. Polypharmacy and the elderly. *GM*. 2007;37:41–45 http://www.gm journal.co.uk/polypharmacy_and_the_elderly_30711.aspx [cited 2014 July 25].

10 Maher RL, Hanlon JT, Hajjar ER. Clinical consequences of polypharmacy in elderly. *Expert Opin Drug Saf*. 2014;13(1):57–65.

11 Beers MH. Explicit criteria for determining potentially inappropriate medication use by the elderly: an update. *Arch Intern Med*. 1997;157(14):1531–1536.

12 Gallagher P, Ryan C, Byrne S, Kennedy J, O'Mahony D. STOPP (screening tool of older person's prescriptions) and START (screening tool to alert doctors to right treatment). Consensus validation. *Int J Clin Pharmacol Ther*. 2008;46(2):72–83.

13 Potts F, Vukov L. Utility of fever and leukocytosis in acute surgical abdomens in octogenarians. *J Gerontol Biol Sci Med Sci*. 1999;54:M55–M58.

14 Douma RA, le Gal G, Söhne M, Righini M, Kamphuisen PW, Perrier A, et al. Potential of an age adjusted D-dimer cut-off value to improve the exclusion of pulmonary embolism in older patients: a retrospective analysis of three large cohorts. *BMJ* 2010;340:c1475.

15 Solomon R. Preventing contrast-induced nephropathy: problems, challenges and future directions. *BMC Med*. 2009;7(1):24.

16 Geriatric Emergency Department Guidelines – Joint Statement by the American College of Emergency Physicians, American Geriatrics Society, Emergency Nurses Association, and Society for Academic Emergency Medicine. 2013.

17 Banarjee J, Conroy S, O'Leary V, Al E. Quality Care for Older people with Urgent & Emergency Care needs '*The Silver Book*'. 2011.

18 Forster AJ, Murff HJ, Peterson JF, Gandhi TK, Bates DW. The incidence and severity of adverse events affecting patients after discharge from the hospital. *Ann Intern Med*. 2003;138(3):161–167.

19 McCusker J, Bellavance F, Cardin S, Trépanier S, Verdon J, Ardman O. Detection of older people at increased risk of adverse health outcomes after an emergency visit: the ISAR screening tool. *J Am Geriatr Soc*. 1999;47(10):1229–1237.

20 Edmans J, Bradshaw L, Gladman JRF, Franklin M, Berdunov V, Elliott R, et al. The identification of seniors at risk (ISAR) score to predict clinical outcomes and health service costs in older people discharged from UK acute medical units. *Age Ageing*. 2013;42(6):747–753.

21 García-Pérez L, Linertová R, Lorenzo-Riera A, Vázquez-Díaz JR, Duque-González B, Sarría-Santamera A. Risk factors for hospital readmissions in elderly patients: a systematic review. *QJM Mon J Assoc Physicians*. 2011;104(8):639–651.

22 Franchi C, Nobili A, Mari D, Tettamanti M, Djade CD, Pasina L, et al. Risk factors for hospital readmission of elderly patients. *Eur J Intern Med*. 2013;24(1):45–51.

23 Ahmad A, Mast MR, Nijpels G, Elders PJ, Dekker JM, Hugtenburg JG. Identification of drug-related problems of elderly patients discharged from hospital. *Patient Prefer Adher* 2014;8:155–165.

24 Royal College of Physicians (RCP). *Acute Care Toolkit 3: Acute Medical Care for Frail Older People*. http://www.rcplondon.ac.uk/resources/acute-care-toolkit-3-acute-medical-care-frail-older-people [cited 2014 May 15].

25 Kessler C, Williams MC, Moustoukas JN, Pappas C. Transitions of care for the geriatric patient in the emergency department. *Clin Geriatr Med*. 2013;29(1):49–69.

CHAPTER 3

Special skills in geriatric emergency medicine

Geriatric Emergency Medicine presents multiple clinical and ethical challenges. These challenges require the clinician to have distinct areas of skills and knowledge including assessment and treatment of pain, assessment of decision-making capacity, palliative and end-of-life care in the emergency department and discussion of resuscitation, escalation and intensive care treatment.

Owing to the differences in healthcare systems globally, local and national guidance should be sought when confronted with ethical and legal issues in acute geriatric care.

Pain in the older patient

Older patients commonly present with acute or chronic pain to the ED. Despite this, pain in older patients is often under-recognised and undertreated. Older adults are 20% less likely to receive treatment for pain than younger patients (1). There is often a delay to administration of analgesia (2). Regardless of the underlying cause, effective treatment of acute pain is important for relieving suffering, enabling early mobilisation and preventing delirium and chronic pain. Pain should be considered a fundamental part of the initial assessment.

Box 3.1 Potential reasons for inadequate treatment of pain in the older patient.

Reduced reporting of pain
Communication difficulties, e.g. dysphasia
Cognitive impairment, leading to difficulty using standard pain assessment scales
Cultural factors, stoicism, reluctance to 'be a burden'
Fear of hospital admission or loss of independence
Fear of dependence or addiction to analgesia
Pain is considered an 'inevitable' part of ageing

Reduced recognition of pain
Lack of awareness of atypical presentations of pain in the older patient
Lack of appreciation of painful conditions or injuries

Reluctance to administer analgesia
Fear of drug side effects, interactions and comorbidities
Concerns over polypharmacy

Geriatric Emergencies, First Edition.
Iona Murdoch, Sarah Turpin, Bree Johnston, Alasdair MacLullich and Eve Losman.
© 2015 John Wiley & Sons, Ltd. Published 2015 by John Wiley & Sons, Ltd.

Table 3.1 Atypical observations in older patients with pain (3).

Type	Description
Autonomic features	Pallor, sweating, tachypnoea, tachycardia, altered breathing, hypertension
Facial expressions	Grimacing, wincing, frowning, brow raising, brow lowering, nose wrinkling, lip puckering
Body movements	Hand wringing, repetitive movements, rocking, increased tone, guarding, bracing
Vocalisation	Sighing, grunting, groaning, moaning, screaming, calling out, aggressive/offensive speech
Interpersonal interactions	Aggression, withdrawal, resisting, refusal of care
Mental status changes	Confusion, crying, distress, irritability, agitation

Optimal pain management is made more complex by reduced drug metabolism and clearance with ageing, potential drug–drug interactions, adverse drug events and comorbidities. Many painkillers, such as NSAIDS, are considered high risk in the older patient, reducing the number of potential analgesics.

Pain assessment

Identifying pain may be challenging in the older patient due to the points in Box 3.1. Alternative expressions such as 'is it sore?', 'does it hurt?' and 'are you uncomfortable?' may be useful. In the patient with dementia or communication difficulties, agitation or a change in behaviour (Table 3.1) may indicate poorly controlled pain, and carers or family members may detect this better than clinicians unfamiliar with the patient.

The location and cause of the pain may be obvious or further history, examination and investigation may be required. A pain map or diagram which the patient can annotate may be useful. A patient may have more than one type of pain simultaneously. Pain has physical, psychological, spiritual and social contributions, as well as a variable impact on functional ability, and to provide adequate treatment, all these factors should be assessed.

Patients who are fully alert and orientated will be able to report pain severity according to a verbal rating scale (Figure 3.1). Observational pain tools, of which there are

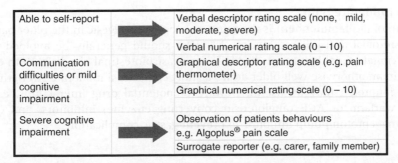

Figure 3.1 Methods of assessing pain intensity in the older population (3).

	YES/NO	
1−Facial expressions: frowning, grimacing, wincing, clenched teeth, inexpressive	☐	☐
2−Look: inattentive, blank stare, distant or imploring, teary-eyed, closed eyes	☐	☐
3−Complaints: 'ow-ouch', 'that hurts', groaning, screaming	☐	☐
4−Body position: withdrawn, guarded, refuses to move, frozen posture	☐	☐
5−A typical behaviours: agitation, aggressiveness, grabbing onto something or someone	☐	☐
Total YES	/5	

Figure 3.2 Algoplus® pain scale: acute pain-behaviour scale for older persons with inability to communicate verbally. Source: From Rat P, Jouve E, Pickering G, et al. Validation of an acute pain-behavior scale for older persons with inability to communicate verbally. *Eur J Pain* 2011;15(2):198.e191–10; with permission from Wiley & Sons.

a number available, may be required for patients with cognitive impairment. A simple validated tool for the older patient, which takes less than 1 minute to perform and incorporates some of the features in Table 3.1, is the Algoplus® pain scale (Figure 3.2).

Management of acute pain
Treat the underlying cause
Acute onset of pain may represent a life-threatening emergency, such as ST elevation MI, or bowel perforation, and resuscitation and other management should take place simultaneously. Sometimes providing definitive treatment, e.g. reducing a fracture, may reduce the need for further analgesia.

Non-pharmacological pain management strategies
Reassurance and an explanation of symptoms should be provided. In traumatic injuries, positioning, elevation, splinting, a cold compress or wound dressings may be effective.

Regional anaesthesia such as fascia iliaca block or femoral nerve block in hip fractures can be very effective and is opioid-sparing (Chapter 12).

Pharmacological pain management
Analgesia should be given promptly after identifying pain. Older patients may have concerns about the over-use of analgesia for fear of developing tolerance, dependence or addiction (4), and this should be addressed if necessary.

Mild to moderate pain
Paracetamol (acetaminophen) is the safest non-opioid analgesic in the older patient.

Non-steroidal anti-inflammatories (NSAIDs) should generally be avoided as they may precipitate renal failure, cardiac failure or gastrointestinal bleeding. With extreme caution in an otherwise well older adult, a short course of a moderate strength NSAID such as ibuprofen may be useful. Beware of potential drug interactions, e.g. with aspirin, warfarin or ACE (angiotensin converting enzyme) inhibitors, and consider prescribing a proton pump inhibitor to prevent gastric complications.

Moderate acute pain

Moderate to acute pain is likely to require the addition of opioid analgesia. Starting doses should be 25–50% lower than with younger adults, especially in the presence of renal failure. Side effects such as constipation, nausea and vomiting, delirium, drowsiness and increased falls risk are more common in the older patient. There is no ideal opioid; all have slightly different side effect frequencies and clinician preference varies. Many hospitals have formularies which may limit the choice of drugs available.

Consider a mild opioid such as codeine or hydrocodone, or prescribe regular small doses of oxycodone or morphine. Morphine and codeine have metabolites that accumulate in impaired renal function. Oxycodone has a shorter half-life and little to no toxic metabolites. Regular opioids should be co-prescribed with a stool softener and/or stimulant laxative (5).

Severe acute pain

This will usually require parenteral opioids. 'Start low and go slow' is a useful maxim (4). A small initial bolus should be given, e.g. 1–2 mg of morphine. Peak effects may be delayed: allow time to assess effectiveness before repeat dosing. It may take several doses over the course of 1 hour to achieve pain control. Careful monitoring for hypotension or respiratory depression is required in the older patient.

Reassessment of pain severity should occur after any intervention; this is as important as assessing pain initially.

Chronic pain management

The management of chronic pain is discussed below under 'Palliative Care'.

Palliative care in the acute setting

Advanced terminal illness is a relatively common presentation to the ED, and all physicians should be aware of the key management interventions necessary to provide comfort care at the end of life. This section discusses patients presenting with a terminal illness who are not necessarily at the end of life, and those who are actively dying.

> KEY POINT: Palliative care includes end-of-life care, but not all palliative care patients are at the end of life.

Introduction

The focus of medicine is traditionally on preserving life and preventing death. Palliative care may be somewhat counterintuitive in the emergency environment; however, for the patient with advanced disease, such as malignancy or dementia, interventions to prolong life may not be appropriate or wanted by the patient.

Presentation to hospital may represent a palliative care emergency, rapid or unexpected deterioration, unrelated medical or surgical problem, poorly controlled symptoms or inconsistent community palliative care services. Patients may present with a requirement for end-of-life care, with family being unable to cope in their usual place of residence.

Definition

Palliative care aims to improve the quality of life of patients and their families facing life-threatening illness, through the prevention and integrated treatment of pain, and other symptoms, whether physical, psychosocial or spiritual (6). It also incorporates care given during the last few hours or days of a patient's illness, termed 'end-of-life care'.

Background

Diagnosis of terminal illness is often easier in cases of advanced malignancy, where decline frequently occurs in a linear manner, affording some degree of predictability. However, other life-limiting diagnoses, such as dementia, cardiac or respiratory failure also have substantial palliative care needs (7). In these cases, deterioration may occur

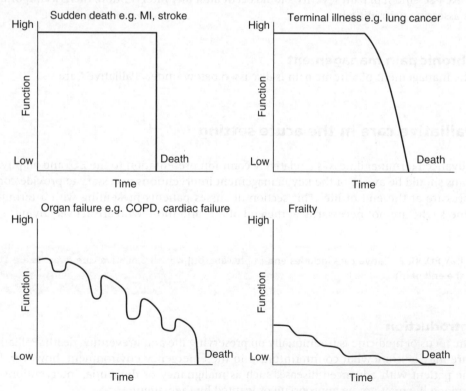

Figure 3.3 Trajectories of dying. Source: Reproduced from Lunney JR, Lynn J, Hogan C. Profiles of Older Medicare Decedents. *J Am Geriatr Soc.* 2002 Jun;50(6):1108–12 with permission from Wiley & Sons.

more slowly and gradually, interspersed with exacerbations of illness followed by recovery (Figure 3.3).

Identifying patients requiring palliative care

Palliative care services can assist in identifying patients who, whilst not imminently dying, require improved control of difficult symptoms such as pain, dyspnoea or nausea; help avoid burdensome or futile treatments; and facilitate further support in the community or hospice care. 70–75% of people older than 65 years known to have a life-limiting condition visit an ED within the last few months of their life (8, 9). Box 3.2 highlights factors that may assist in identifying patients in the ED who would benefit from palliative care services.

Box 3.2 Factors indicating potential need for palliative care referral in the ED (10).

The patient has a life-limiting diagnosis such as dementia, malignancy, chronic cardiac, respiratory, renal or liver failure in addition to one or more of the following factors:

1 Surprise: You would not be surprised if the patient died within 12 months
2 Bounce backs: more than one ED or hospital visit in the last few months for the same condition
3 Difficult to control symptoms: ED visit prompted by increased intensity of physiological or psychological symptoms
4 Complex care requirements: dependent on carers, home oxygen, feeding or ventilatory support.
5 Functional decline: decline in weight, reduced mobility or impaired cognition, carers struggling to cope.

General approach to the patient with palliative care needs

As mentioned above, patients with advanced illness may present with a range of problems related to or unrelated to their principle diagnosis. Box 3.3 outlines the approach to initial assessment.

Box 3.3 Initial assessment of the patient with a life-limiting illness presenting to acute care facilities.

- History (including collateral history from informant), examination and investigations to identify acute medical or surgical problems or a palliative care emergency (Table 3.2).
- Assess the patient's symptoms and how well they are controlled
  - Pain, dyspnoea, nausea and vomiting, constipation, low mood, anxiety, sleep disturbance and poor appetite
  - Psychological, spiritual and social care needs.
- Seek advice from inpatient and community palliative care services.
- Assess the patient and family's current understanding and need for further information.
- Establish goals of care after discussion with the patient, their family or carers.
- Consider advance care planning and review resuscitation status as well as an appropriate ceiling of care.
- Identify the best location for further care: patient's usual place of residence, hospice care, care home or hospital admission.

Table 3.2 Management of palliative care emergencies (11).

	Causes	Symptoms and signs	Management
Bowel obstruction	Compression or intraluminal obstruction by tumour	Abdominal pain, vomiting, constipation	Conservative, e.g. NG decompression, anti-spasmodic medication, antisecretory agents (e.g. octreotide) or surgical management (Chapter 15)
Hypercalcaemia	Bone invasion or secretion of PTHrP*	Thirst, nausea, delirium, constipation, renal stones	IV fluid resuscitation, bisphosphonates (Chapter 17)
Spinal cord compression or cauda equina syndrome	Vertebral metastasis or oedema following radiation	Worsening back pain, loss of pain and temperature sensation, leg weakness and reduced mobility, bowel or bladder sphincter disturbance	Steroids, urgent neurosurgical or radiotherapy referral (Chapter 12)
Dyspnoea or respiratory failure	Pleural effusion, fluid overload, pulmonary embolus, pneumonia, anaemia	Reduced exercise tolerance, wheeze, cough, orthopnoea	Small doses of opioids or benzodiazepines. Drainage of pleural effusions may be useful. Consider diuretics if appropriate. Oxygen may help (Chapter 6)
Superior vena cava obstruction	Tumour invasion or compression Intraluminal thrombosis	Periorbital oedema, facial swelling, dyspnoea, cough, engorged neck veins, headache	Steroids ± diuretics Intravascular stenting, thrombolysis or radiotherapy
Delirium	Medications such as opioids and steroids, sepsis, raised ICP or brain metastases	Fluctuating mental state. Altered concentration, attention and disordered thinking	Exclude easily treated causes such as hypoglycaemia and hypercalcaemia. Small doses of antipsychotics may be required (Chapter 18)
Severe haemorrhage	Tumour invasion of a major blood vessel	Haemoptysis, haematemesis, rectal or vaginal bleeding	May require urgent intervention or palliation with subcutaneous midazolam if thought to be an end-of-life event

NG, nasogastric; ICP, intracranial pressure.
*PTHrP, parathyroid hormone related peptide.

Palliative care emergencies

A palliative care emergency is an unexpected change in a patient's condition in the context of an underlying life-limiting illness. When embarking on investigation and treatment, consider the likely outcome and reversibility, current functional status, life expectancy, risks and benefits of treatment and the wishes of the patient and their family.

Emergencies in palliative care usually result from advancing malignancy and include the conditions featured in Table 3.2.

Addressing symptom management

Pain is the commonest symptom in palliative care, experienced in 70% of patients with both malignant and non-malignant terminal illnesses. As mentioned above, pain management includes consideration of physical, psychological, spiritual and social factors. The choice of regime for analgesia depends on multiple factors including setting, available routes and the presence of any renal impairment. Regular reassessment of pain is required.

Regular analgesia should be prescribed along with 'breakthrough' doses if needed. Ensure laxatives are also administered if opioid analgesia is used. Once stable pain control is achieved, an equivalent dose of modified-release opioid may be given. Certain types of pain may require adjuvant analgesics such as antidepressants, anticonvulsants and corticosteroids. Bone pain may respond to bisphosphonates or radiotherapy. Local topical treatment with gels or patches may be valuable. Neuropathic pain may improve with pregabalin, gabapentin or (with appropriate supervision), non-steroidal anti-inflammatory drugs.

Nausea and vomiting are common in terminal illness, often significantly impacting on quality of life. Causes may be the underlying disease process or secondary to opioid analgesia, chemotherapy agents, brain metastases, constipation or bowel obstruction. Consider both pharmacological and non-pharmacological treatments: good mouth care may make a significant difference. Choice of antiemetic will depend on the underlying cause; consult local palliative care guidelines.

Other symptoms such as constipation, low mood, anxiety and sleep problems should be assessed and treated by the palliative care team.

Communication with patient, carers and family

Patients have concerns and unanswered questions on presentation to the ED. Identifying and addressing these is a crucial. Although the busy and crowded environment of the ED often makes discussion difficult, a few simple questions as suggested in Box 3.4 may help clarify the patient's wishes and help form the management plan.

Box 3.4 Useful discussion points in the palliative care patient.

- How has your illness affected your daily activities?
- What symptoms affect you the most?
- Have you been feeling worried or sad about your illness? What are your biggest fears?
- Knowing that time is short, what is most important to you at this point?

- How much would you be willing to go through for the possibility of gaining more time?
- Are there abilities so critical to your life that you can't imagine living without them (such as being able to communicate with loved ones)?
- What are your goals for this last phase of your life?
- Have you thought about how and where you would like to be cared for at the time of death?

Managing the dying patient in the emergency department

Most patients with life-limiting illness will prefer to die in their home environment, although currently 58% of deaths occur in hospital (12). Some patients with terminal illnesses may present to acute services in the last few hours or days of their life. Despite community support, patients and their family are often frightened as their condition worsens and may seek the relative security of the hospital environment.

Commencing end-of-life care in the ED, where the sole focus is on controlling symptoms, may be appropriate in certain circumstances (Box 3.5). This decision should be made after careful discussion with the patient and/or their relatives or proxy decision maker.

Box 3.5 Circumstances where end-of-life care may be appropriate.

- An advanced illness has progressed or is associated with a new complication for which treatment is not wanted or would be futile.
- A valid advance directive (AD) refuses further treatment or resuscitation.
- The patient has an acute condition which is deemed non-survivable, e.g. massive intracerebral haemorrhage.

In the emergency situation, it may be difficult to predict whether the presenting symptoms represent end-of-life or not. In patients with advanced malignancy, signs of dying include (13):
- Profound weakness: bedbound, needing assistance with all care
- Diminished intake of food and fluid, difficulty swallowing tablets
- Reduced conscious level.

In non-malignant disease, the downward trajectory may be interrupted with acute exacerbations, from which there may be a good recovery (Figure 3.1), even if the patient initially appears to be dying. Severe hypoactive delirium may mimic end of life, and may be potentially reversible with treatment of the underlying cause. In such cases, palliative symptom control can be delivered alongside life-prolonging treatments such as antibiotics or intravenous fluids. Infection is often the terminal event in end-stage disease and treatment of this may assist with palliation of symptoms (14).

A good death is the one that is 'free from avoidable distress and suffering for patients, families and caregivers; in general accord with patients' and families' wishes; and reasonably consistent with clinical, cultural and ethical standards' (15). If the patient is recognised to be dying, integrated pathways utilised in some hospitals may facilitate the treatment of troublesome symptoms (Table 3.3). A quiet side room, where relatives may spend time with the patient in their last hours, should be identified.

Table 3.3 Palliating symptoms associated with end of life.

Pain and breathlessness	A subcutaneous opioid by SC injection or syringe driver eases pain and palliates dyspnoea. Consult guidelines on opioid conversion and dose calculation
Noisy breathing (death rattle)	This is often more upsetting for family members than the patient. Reassure the family that the patient is not choking. Increased bronchial and salivary secretions are best treated prophylactically with anti-muscarinics (e.g. hyoscine, glycopyrroneum). Position the patient on their side to facilitate postural drainage of secretions. Occasional suctioning may be beneficial but may cause more distress to the patient
Agitation, twitching, myoclonic jerks	Subcutaneous administration of a benzodiazepine (e.g. midazolam) or a phenothiazine (e.g. levomepromazine). A subcutaneous infusion via a syringe driver may be required
Reduced oral intake	Reduced interest in food and fluid is a normal part of the dying process. Artificial hydration in the dying patient will not affect survival and may lead to increased respiratory secretions and dyspnoea due to fluid overload. Good mouth care is important in improving any symptoms associated with dehydration
Anxiety and distress of patient and relatives	Good communication, explanation of symptoms and signs of dying and uncertainties regarding time course

Decision-making capacity

Decision-making capacity refers to the patient's ability to understand and communicate choices related to medical treatment and other aspects of care. Autonomy is a key principle of medical ethics and a decision must be intentional, made with an understanding of the potential outcomes and without undue external influence. Capacity to make autonomous decisions should always be assumed until proven to be lacking.

Various legislation such as the Mental Capacity Act 2005 (England) and Adults with Incapacity Act 2000 (Scotland) provide guidance on assessment of capacity and on making best-interest decisions in patients who lack capacity. Local and up-to-date legislation should be consulted.

A capacity assessment should be carried out if the patient is considered to have an impairment in cognitive or psychological functioning and there is concern regarding their ability to make decisions. Impairments may include delirium, dementia, depression, acquired brain injury, alcohol intoxication or acute medical conditions that cause cognitive impairment, drowsiness or loss of consciousness. Quantitative measures of cognitive function such as the mini-mental status examination may not reliably predict a patient's capacity to make medical decisions (16). Assessment of capacity relates to a particular decision, e.g. consenting to abdominal surgery or self-discharging from hospital and should be undertaken by the physician responsible for the patient's care.

The key questions in assessing capacity are highlighted below in Box 3.6.

Ensure that any reversible or partially reversible barriers to communication, such as hearing or visual impairment, language barrier, dysarthria or dysphasia, are addressed.

Dysphasia may require the assistance of a speech and language therapist or specialist communication tools. It is important to note that a patient does not lack decision-making capacity just because they make an odd decision, as long as they fully understand the consequences and can explain their choice.

Box 3.6 Two-stage decision-making capacity assessment (17, 18).

STAGE 1: Does this person have an impairment of, or a disturbance in the functioning of, their mind or brain?
STAGE 2: Does the impairment or disturbance mean that the person is unable to make a specific decision when they need to?

1 Can the patient *understand* the information necessary to make a decision?
   The patient should be able to explain the diagnosis and treatment in their own words or recognise prompts.
2 Can the patient *retain* the information for long enough to make an effective decision?
3 Can the patient *weigh up* the benefits and risks of their decision? Can they justify their choice and their processes of rationalisation?
4 Can the patient *communicate* their decision? Are they consistent in their decision?

How to assess decision-making capacity
Box 3.7 summarises the key practical aspects of assessment of decision-making capacity.

Box 3.7 Practical assessment of decision-making capacity.

1 Explain the treatment or procedure, the risks, potential side effects in simple language. Outline the alternatives and the likely consequences of not undertaking treatment. Answer any questions.
2 Explore the patient's understanding and retention of information by asking a series of questions.
   • 'In your own words, please tell me about what we've just discussed, regarding your current illness and the decisions we need to make.'
   • 'What medical problem do you have at the current time?'
   • 'What are the treatment options?'
   • 'What is your understanding of what will happen if nothing is done?'
   • 'What could happen if you have surgery or don't have surgery?'
   More directed questions may be required depending on the patient's ability to communicate:
   • 'Do you have a problem with your leg?'
   • 'Is surgery an option'?'
   • 'Could you get more unwell or die if you don't have surgery?'
   At this stage, provide further information if necessary followed by reassessment.
3 Assess the patient's ability to weigh up the facts to make a decision and their ability to communicate their decision.
   • 'Can you help me understand how you have reached your decision?'
   • 'What factors are most important to you in deciding about your treatment?'
   • 'What are the reasons you do not want to go ahead with the surgery?'

Carefully document the discussion and the outcome of the assessment. In cases of uncertainty, the decision-making capacity assessment should be repeated and a second opinion, possibly by a psychiatrist, may be required. Instruments to aid decision-making capacity assessments such as the aid to capacity evaluation (19) provide a structured approach to assessment in more difficult cases and also a means to documenting the process (20).

If a patient makes an unexpected decision, it is important to explore this in greater depth by assessing whether the patient fully understands the treatment options and their consequences. In some cases, the patient's decision may be influenced by depression or a delusional state which may be more difficult to detect. Further questions may bring this to light and a psychiatric review will be required.

Some patients feel that they are a burden to their family or healthcare facilities and will decline treatment based on this sentiment. It is important to be aware of this and try to address the underlying issues to allow them to choose the treatment that is right for them.

When the patient lacks decision-making capacity

If the patient is found to lack decision-making capacity, consider if this may be temporary and whether the decision can wait until their condition improves. In many cases, the situation is urgent and a decision will need to be made on their behalf. Consider firstly if the patient has an advance directive (AD) or has appointed a proxy decision maker (e.g. power of attorney).

In an emergency, physicians may treat patients in their best interests without consent where the condition is life- or limb-threatening, time-critical and it is considered that a reasonable person would consent under the same circumstances (21). This should consider the least restrictive option for the patient and if there is any doubt, life-sustaining treatment should always be pursued (22). Where possible, the decision should be the consensus of a clinical team rather than an individual.

Once the patient has been stabilised or more information is available, who makes decisions about a patient's care will depend on statutory law in the United States, and in the United Kingdom is guided by the Mental Capacity Act 2005 (England) and Adults with Incapacity Act 2000 (Scotland). This may be a proxy decision maker as appointed by a Lasting Power of Attorney (UK), surrogate decision maker as per a hierarchy of next of kin (US) or the clinician responsible for the patient's care. In the latter case, decisions should be made in the patient's best interests after seeking knowledge of the patient's past and present wishes, beliefs and values. If disagreement occurs, seek urgent advice from colleagues, seniors or the hospital ethics and legal team.

Advance directives

Advance care planning includes both *advance directives* and *proxy directives*. An *AD* or 'living will' is a formal statement of a patient's wishes with regard to their future care, in the event of them not having decision-making capacity at a future time. A *proxy directive* involves the appointment of a surrogate decision maker or power of attorney to make decisions in the event of the patient being unable to do so.

The legislation concerning ADs, power of attorney and surrogate decision makers varies internationally. The following is intended as a guide to the principles, but local legal advice should be consulted in all circumstances. Official paperwork should be examined at the earliest possible opportunity to verify the patient's wishes.

The 'living will' is a stipulation of interventions to be provided or withheld, usually in terminal illness or persistent vegetative state, but increasingly covering a wider variety of potential circumstances. These allow patients to state their values with regard to medical interventions such as artificial nutrition and hydration, ventilation and resuscitation. The AD may specifically refuse a particular treatment (e.g. blood transfusion in Jehovah's Witnesses); provide a particular directive such as 'do not resuscitate, do not hospitalise; do not intubate' or provide more general guidance about ongoing care priorities.

Documents may vary widely, from being very specific and clear to vague and difficult to interpret. Advance directives are popular with patients and professional organisations but implementation may be inconsistent and problematic. Patients may not have a physical copy of their AD with them or may forget to inform the physician of the AD. When presented with an AD, a physician must first assess its validity and applicability (Box 3.8). In some states, the AD may need to be activated by another physician to confirm lack of decision-making capacity (21). If the AD cannot be produced at the time of presentation to hospital, clinical decisions should be made with respect towards the patient's previously stated views, whilst being wary of potential conflicts of interest. In an emergency, immediate medical care should be provided until the first opportunity the AD can be consulted.

Advance directives must be respected as a key tool of patient autonomy. The Mental Capacity Act 2005 (England) code of practice states that healthcare professionals must follow an advance decision if they are satisfied that it exists, is valid and is applicable to their circumstances (18). However, a number of problems may arise. Language in living wills is often ambiguous, leading to difficulty applying instructions to urgent ED-specific decisions (23). The general intent of the patient's wishes should be carefully considered in such cases.

Box 3.8 Assessing the validity and applicability of an advance directive.

1 Does the patient have decision-making capacity? If they do, decisions should be made after discussion with the patient in the usual way. If they do not, proceed to step 2.
2 Ask to see the advance directive and check it is signed, dated and witnessed by an independent signatory. Check that it has been reviewed if a review time frame is given in the document. When potentially life-sustaining treatment is to be refused, this should be stated explicitly.
3 Validity: Make a judgment on the validity of the advance directive. Was the patient likely to have had decision-making capacity at the time the AD was made; did they understand and evaluate the pros and cons of refusing or consenting to medical treatment? Discuss with any proxy decision maker, family or carers as to whether the advance directive reflects the patients last known wishes. Ensure that the AD has not been withdrawn. Establish that the person has not recently behaved in a way that is inconsistent with the AD (e.g. actively seeking life-sustaining treatment if the AD emphasises palliation).
4 Applicability: Consider if the advance directive applies to the current circumstances. Is the proposed treatment the same as specified in the AD? Are the circumstances different to those referred to in the AD? Ambiguous or unclear wording with too few or too many specific details may make this process more difficult.

Patient's relatives or a proxy decision maker may disagree with an AD and request active treatment where the patient has expressly refused this. The patient's preferences, life-circumstances or indeed available medical treatment may have changed since the AD was written. The patient's presentation to the hospital may appear to be a contraindication to their previously stated wishes. The patient's autonomy should always be respected but in the cases of such concerns, and in an emergency situation, withholding life-sustaining treatment may not be appropriate and active treatment should be provided until further discussion and clarification is possible (24). Urgent hospital legal advice may be necessary.

Cardiopulmonary resuscitation (CPR)

The chances of survival to hospital discharge following cardiorespiratory arrest are 15–20% in hospital inpatients, dropping to 5–10% in out-of-hospital cardiac arrest patients, with some populations experiencing much worse outcomes (25). Resuscitation is more likely to be successful with prompt initiation of CPR (cardiopulmonary resuscitation); in shockable cardiac rhythms (ventricular fibrillation and ventricular tachycardia) with early defibrillation; with a short duration of CPR and in a patient with few pre-arrest comorbidities. Patients with cardiac pathology who are closely monitored in hospital before arresting are more likely to survive. Age has not been demonstrated to be a significant independent variable contributing to survival (24, 26). However, older people with chronic, progressive illnesses or with multiple comorbidities are less likely to survive following a cardiac arrest and if they do survive are more likely to have neurological damage.

> **KEY POINT: Age is not a reliable predictor of poor outcome in cardiac arrest, and decisions not to pursue resuscitation should not be based on age alone.**

CPR usually encompasses chest compressions, defibrillation, advanced airway management and intravenous medication. Reversible causes resulting in return of spontaneous circulation include thrombosis (myocardial infarction or pulmonary embolus) and electrolyte disturbances such as hyperkalaemia, airway obstruction or hypovolaemia, amongst others. In the event of return of spontaneous circulation, aftercare will usually be required on an intensive care unit (ICU), involving treatment of the underlying cause, ventilation, organ support or targeted temperature management whilst assessing neurological improvement.

Many patients and their relatives have a limited understanding of what CPR involves, and its potential complications and limitations. They may have unrealistic expectations about the chances of successful resuscitation. When discussing resuscitation in the older patient, it is important to establish their understanding and explain the process sensitively and clearly. Written information or further discussion with staff may be helpful in providing detailed explanation and answering the patient's questions.

Resuscitation decisions

Whether to perform CPR in the event of cardiorespiratory arrest is an important, but often difficult, decision to be made. Cardiac arrest requires immediate intervention

Table 3.4 Potential risks and benefits of CPR in the older patient.

Risks	Benefits
• Potential for traumatic, undignified death • Hypoxic brain injury and resulting disability, leading to a requirement for long-term care • Prolonged admission to the intensive care unit, requirement for multi-organ support and artificial ventilation. • Rib, sternal and thoracolumbar fractures (24) • Injuries to the heart, lungs and great vessels • Hepatic or splenic injuries	• Prolonging life • The patient will not survive without CPR • Small potential for hospital discharge with good function if immediate CPR with reversible causes

without the possibility to ask the patient about their wishes at that time. CPR is an emotive topic of discussion in a patient who has just been admitted to hospital and is acutely unwell.

> **KEY POINT: Approaches differ significantly between the United States and the United Kingdom. Clarify local policy.**

In the United Kingdom, guidance suggests that decisions regarding CPR should be made in patients admitted to hospital with a 'foreseeable risk of cardiopulmonary arrest' (25, 27). Currently some decisions are not discussed with families or patients, such as when the patient has advanced dementia and multiple other comorbidities. In the United States, 'code status' should be discussed with every older patient on admission to the hospital.

A decision not to undertake CPR in the event of a cardiac arrest may be recorded as a do not attempt resuscitation (DNAR), not for resuscitation (NFR) or allow a natural death (AND) order. Some will be part of more detailed statements regarding goals of care and limits of treatment. All assessments should be clearly documented and discussed with the team caring for the patient. As with any life-prolonging treatment, resuscitation can be considered in terms of a balance of benefits and harms (Table 3.4).

Difficulties may arise if the patient requests resuscitation when the clinician feels that the chances of a positive outcome are minimal. This is a controversial, topical area with very different approaches internationally. It is important to consult local hospital policy and if required, seek a second opinion or hospital legal or ethics advice.

How to discuss resuscitation decisions

Box 3.9 highlights some useful phrases that may assist the physician in discussing advance care planning, resuscitation status and escalation of care with patients and their relatives. Each approach should be tailored to individual circumstances and not all of the examples will be appropriate. These discussions take time but are a valid investment in improving understanding and satisfaction of patients and their relatives. Generally, there should be involvement of senior clinicians in such conversations and decisions.

Box 3.9 Possible phrases that can be used whilst discussing resuscitation, escalation and advance care planning.

Establishing understanding

'What have you been told about the status of your illness and what to expect in the near future?'

'Are there any plans for new treatments that will help you extend your life?'

'Has anyone talked to you about your prognosis and how much time you likely have?'

Opening the topic

'At the moment, we are concerned that you are quite unwell. We are hoping for the best, but I think we also need to prepare for the worst. If your condition were to get worse, have you given any thought to what kinds of treatment you would want (and not want), if you became unable to speak for yourself?'

'I understand that discussing the worse case scenario is very difficult. Have you given any thought as to what you would like to happen towards the end of your life?'

Discussing CPR

'If your heart were to stop, we could try and restart it by doing chest compressions. Occasionally, this is successful, but you would most likely need to spend some time on a ventilator (breathing machine) in an intensive care unit. In addition, it may result in a situation which some people may find unacceptable, such as living with brain injury or in a care home. Are you the type of person that would prefer to err on the side of life-sustaining treatments or on the side of focusing on comfort, even if it might mean a shorter life?'

If you feel that the patient is extremely unlikely to benefit from CPR, you might say

'As a medical team, we want to do everything that we can to help you, but we also don't want to provide you with treatments that are likely to make you suffer without providing benefit. With your conditions, we believe that chest compressions and other advanced procedures would be very unlikely to help you. If that were to happen, we believe that the best care for you would be to focus on comfort and allowing a peaceful and dignified death. How do you feel about that recommendation?'

Ceilings of care

Resuscitation status is just one aspect of advance care planning. As ADs gain in popularity amongst patients, decisions such as whether to provide intravenous fluids, artificial nutrition or intubation and ventilation may have already been discussed before hospital presentation. However, in many cases, these interventions will not have been explored previously. There is sometimes a concern that a DNAR order, although only referring to the decision to carry out CPR in the event of a cardiac arrest, tends to influence other aspects of treatment. Physicians and nursing staff may interpret a DNAR order as indicating a preference for end-of-life care, and may not offer other interventions or take as aggressive action to prevent deterioration (23, 28, 29). When a DNAR order is made, it is useful if a statement about other active care is also documented (30), following discussion with the patient or their relatives. In some centres, a specific document may be in use for this purpose. This may include a statement as to whether the patient would be for interventions such as non-invasive ventilation, intubation and ventilation or renal dialysis. Such decisions may involve collaboration with other clinical teams (such as intensive care, see below), to establish whether it might be beneficial to offer these interventions to the patient.

 KEY POINT: A DNR order does not mean 'do not treat'. A DNR decision refers specifically to CPR and not to other treatment.

Critical care referral

The number of ICU admissions amongst older patients, and the oldest old, is increasing, and is likely to continue to increase given demographic changes, increased undertaking of high-risk surgeries in the older patient, medical advances and increasing expectations of patients and their relatives (31–33). Indications for intensive care admission include mechanical ventilation, haemodialysis, inotropic or vasopressor therapy or advanced monitoring. Early recognition and prompt treatment of the seriously unwell or deteriorating older patient with the aim of avoiding ICU admission are vital.

The provision of ICU facilities and case mix therein varies globally. Some centres may have a high ratio of ICU beds to hospital beds and/or a 'no refusal' policy, resulting in a higher proportion of older patients admitted to the ICU. Half of all hospital deaths involve intensive care in the United States, compared with only 1 in 10 in England (34). Higher capacity of intensive care beds in some areas may result in less unwell patients being admitted, leading to difficulty comparing mortality data between ICUs.

Although comparing mortality rates between older people and younger people admitted to intensive care is fraught with confounding factors, older patients have worse outcomes following ICU admission (31, 33). Older patients have higher ICU mortality, in-hospital mortality and 1 year mortality in those who are discharged from hospital (35). The risk of death is concentrated in the first 6 months following hospital discharge and highest amongst those who required mechanical ventilation (31). One

Table 3.5 Risks and benefits of ICU admission in the older adult.

Risks	Benefits
• Barotrauma and ventilator-associated pneumonia, delayed respiratory weaning and chronic respiratory failure	• Prolonging life
	• Prolonging time available for decision-making and discussion with relatives and physicians
• Nosocomial infections	• Potential for hospital discharge with good function
• Iatrogenic complications from invasive procedures or monitoring (e.g. pneumothorax)	
• ICU delirium	
• Prolonged ICU or hospital length of stay	
• Increased morbidity, cognitive impairment and functional disability	

study reported mortality rates of up to 89% at one year in those aged 80 years and older with unplanned medical or surgical admission, although those that survived appeared to have a reasonable longer-term outcome (36). The oldest ICU patients often have treatment limitations, and may not be offered mechanical ventilation, dialysis, inotropes or vasopressors (37), potentially skewing mortality data. Intubation and mechanical ventilation are often withheld in the older patient due to concerns regarding weaning the patient from the ventilator, due to factors such as reduced respiratory muscle mass, poor pre-morbid nutritional state or underlying chronic lung disease. Non-invasive ventilation may be considered in order to avoid intubation, and may be an appropriate ceiling of care.

Physiological changes with ageing as highlighted elsewhere in this book, along with medications and comorbidities, all impact the ability to compensate in the presence of severe illness. It seems that age alone should not be a barrier to ICU admission; however, functional ability and the severity of the acute illness are more useful measures of likely outcome (38). Box 3.10 summarises some of the factors that should be considered.

Box 3.10 Factors to consider when considering referring an older patient for intensive care treatment.

- Preferences of the patient or surrogate decision makers or contents of an advance directive
- Nature and severity of the acute illness
- Likely treatment or organ support required
- Comorbidities, including other life-limiting conditions
- Pre-hospital functional status, mobility, exercise tolerance and level of independence
- Frailty score.

If time allows, discussion with the patient, their proxy or relatives should take place before intensive care referral. Consideration must be given to the possibility of an increased length of stay, increased risk of complications in an older patient (Table 3.5) and a longer recovery time with the potential of failure to return to baseline function. Decisions are often difficult and based on intuition rather than any evidence-based criteria. Occasionally, a time-limited trial of intensive care treatment may be most appropriate choice. If the patient fails to improve with supportive treatment on ICU, withdrawal of care and palliation of symptoms may be considered.

Take home messages

- Pain is underappreciated and undertreated in the older patient and observational assessment tools may be useful in patients with cognitive impairment or communication difficulties
- Palliation of symptoms associated with terminal illnesses and end-of-life care is a core skill of any clinician working in an acute speciality
- Assessment of decision-making capacity requires careful assessment and should not be based on age, cognitive impairment or previous assessments. Each assessment is

decision-specific and the patient should be assumed to have decision-making capacity until proven otherwise. Everything should be done to facilitate the patient exercising their right to autonomy

- Advance directives are a useful tool in facilitating patient choice towards the end of life. However, their interpretation may be problematic in the emergency environment
- Clinicians may find discussing CPR with their patients difficult. Clear and continual communication with the patient and their relatives is essential to making sensitive and realistic decisions with regard to resuscitation status. Discussing the balance of benefit and burdens and being transparent about the chances of success are important
- Assessing when aggressive life-saving treatment is indicated, and where palliation of symptoms is required is often a difficult judgment even in the most experienced hands. There may be difficult ethical decisions to make regarding ceilings of treatment
- The benefit of intensive care treatment in the older person may be difficult to quantify. Difficult decisions often need to be made. For selected older patients with a treatable reversible cause, ICU care is worthwhile. In the emergency situation, it may be appropriate to start a trial of intensive care treatment with the possibility of treatment withdrawal if there is no response. Further time is often required to fully assess illness severity and establish the patient's values and wishes.

References

1 Platts-Mills TF, Esserman DA, Brown DL, Bortsov A V, Sloane PD, McLean SA. Older US emergency department patients are less likely to receive pain medication than younger patients: results from a national survey. *Ann Emerg Med*. 2012;60(2):199–206.

2 Jones JS, Johnson K, McNinch M. Age as a risk factor for inadequate emergency department analgesia. *Am J Emerg Med*. 1996;14(2):157–160.

3 The assessment of pain in older people: a series of evidence-based guidelines for clinical management. British Pain Society; British Geriatric Society; Royal College of Physicians. 2007.

4 Hwang U, Platts-Mills TF. Acute pain management in older adults in the emergency department. *Clin Geriatr Med US* 2013;29(1):151–164.

5 Abdulla A, Adams N, Bone M, Elliott AM, Gaffin J, Jones D, et al. Guidance on the management of pain in older people. *Age Ageing*. 2013;42 Suppl 1(suppl_1):i1–i57.

6 World Health Organisation. *Definition of Palliative Care*. http://www.who.int/cancer/palliative /definition/en/ [cited 2014 Mar 23].

7 Grudzen CR, Richardson LD, Morrison M, Cho E, Morrison RS. Palliative care needs of seriously ill, older adults presenting to the emergency department. *Acad Emerg Med*. 2010;17(11):1253–1257.

8 Rosenwax LK, McNamara BA, Murray K, McCabe RJ, Aoun SM, Currow DC. Hospital and emergency department use in the last year of life: a baseline for future modifications to end-of-life care. *Med J Aust*. 2011;194(11):570–573.

9 Smith AK, McCarthy E, Weber E, Cenzer IS, Boscardin J, Fisher J, et al. Half of older Americans seen in emergency department in last month of life; most admitted to hospital, and many die there. *Health Aff (Millwood)*. 2012;31(6):1277–1285.

10 Weissman DE, Meier DE. Identifying patients in need of a palliative care assessment in the hospital setting: a consensus report from the Center to Advance Palliative Care. *J Palliat Med*. 2011;14(1):17–23.

11 Rosenberg M, Lamba S, Misra S. Palliative medicine and geriatric emergency care: challenges, opportunities, and basic principles. *Clin Geriatr Med*. 2013;29(1):1–29.

12 End of life care strategy 4th annual report. Department of Health. 2012.

13 Ellershaw J, Ward C. Care of the dying patient: the last hours or days of life. *BMJ.* 2003;326(7379): 30–34.

14 Gibbins J, McCoubrie R, Alexander N, Kinzel C, Forbes K. Diagnosing dying in the acute hospital setting – are we too late? *Clin Med.* 2009;9(2):116–119.

15 Field M, Cassell C. Institute of Medicine Report – approaching death: improving care at the end of life. Washington DC; 1997.

16 Blais CM. Bioethics in practice: a quarterly column about medical ethics – assessment of patients' capacity to make medical decisions. *Ochsner J.* 2012;12(2):92–93.

17 Appelbaum PS. Clinical practice: assessment of patients' competence to consent to treatment. *N Engl J Med* 2007;357:1834–1840.

18 Mental Capacity Act 2005: Code of Practice. United Kingdom: Office of the Public Guardian; 2007.

19 Community Tools: Aid to Capacity Evaluation (ACE), University of Toronto, Joint Centre for Bioethics. http://www.jointcentreforbioethics.ca/tools/ace.shtml [cited 2014 Apr 11].

20 Dunn LB, Nowrangi MA, Palmer BW, Jeste D V, Saks ER. Assessing decisional capacity for clinical research or treatment: a review of instruments. *Am J Psychiatry.* 2006;163(8):1323–1334.

21 Limehouse WE, Feeser VR, Bookman KJ, Derse A. A model for emergency department end-of-life communications after acute devastating events – part I: decision-making capacity, surrogates, and advance directives. *Acad Emerg Med.* 2012;19(9):E1068–E1072.

22 Church M, Watts S. Assessment of mental capacity: a flow chart guide. *Psychiatr Bull.* 2007;31(8): 304–307.

23 Mirarchi FL, Costello E, Puller J, Cooney T, Kottkamp N. TRIAD III: nationwide assessment of living-wills and do not resuscitate orders. *J Emerg Med.* 2012;42(5):511–520.

24 Narang AT, Sikka R. Resuscitation of the elderly. *Emerg Med Clin North Am.* 2006;24(2):261–272, v.

25 Decisions relating to cardiopulmonary resuscitation. A joint statement from the British Medical Association, the Resuscitation Council (UK) and the Royal College of Nursing. 2007.

26 Van de Glind EMM, van Munster BC, van de Wetering FT, van Delden JJM, Scholten RJPM, Hooft L. Pre-arrest predictors of survival after resuscitation from out-of-hospital cardiac arrest in the elderly a systematic review. *BMC Geriatr* 2013;13:68.

27 Baskett PJF, Steen PA, Bossaert L. European Resuscitation Council guidelines for resuscitation 2005. Section 8. The ethics of resuscitation and end-of-life decisions. *Resuscitation.* 2005;67(Suppl 1): S171–S180.

28 Chen JLT, Sosnov J, Lessard D, Goldberg RJ. Impact of do-not-resuscitation orders on quality of care performance measures in patients hospitalized with acute heart failure. *Am Heart J.* 2008;156(1): 78–84.

29 Scarborough JE, Pappas TN, Bennett KM, Lagoo-Deenadayalan S. Failure-to-pursue rescue: explaining excess mortality in elderly emergency general surgical patients with preexisting "do-not-resuscitate" orders. *Ann Surg.* 2012;256(3):453–461.

30 End of life care for adults in the Emergency Department: Best Practice Guidance. London, UK. 2012.

31 Fuchs L, Chronaki CE, Park S, Novack V, Baumfeld Y, Scott D, et al. ICU admission characteristics and mortality rates among elderly and very elderly patients. *Intensive Care Med.* 2012;38(10): 1654–1661.

32 Bagshaw SM, Webb SAR, Delaney A, George C, Pilcher D, Hart GK, et al. Very old patients admitted to intensive care in Australia and New Zealand: a multi-centre cohort analysis. *Crit Care.* 2009;13(2):R45.

33 Nielsson MS, Christiansen CF, Johansen MB, Rasmussen BS, Tønnesen E, Nørgaard M. Mortality in elderly ICU patients: a cohort study. *Acta Anaesthesiol Scand.* 2014;58(1):19–26.

34 Wunsch H, Linde-Zwirble WT, Harrison DA, Barnato AE, Rowan KM, Angus DC. Use of intensive care services during terminal hospitalizations in England and the United States. *Am J Respir Crit Care Med.* 2009;180(9):875–880.

35 Nguyen Y-L, Angus DC, Boumendil A, Guidet B. The challenge of admitting the very elderly to intensive care. *Ann Intensive Care*. 2011;1(1):29.

36 De Rooij SEJA, Govers AC, Korevaar JC, Giesbers AW, Levi M, de Jonge E. Cognitive, functional, and quality-of-life outcomes of patients aged 80 and older who survived at least 1 year after planned or unplanned surgery or medical intensive care treatment. *J Am Geriatr Soc*. 2008;56(5):816–822.

37 Boumendil A, Aegerter P, Guidet B. Treatment intensity and outcome of patients aged 80 and older in intensive care units: a multicenter matched-cohort study. *J Am Geriatr Soc*. 2005;53(1):88–93.

38 Ryan D, Conlon N, Phelan D, Marsh B. The very elderly in intensive care: admission characteristics and mortality. *Crit Care Resusc*. 2008;10(2):106–110.

CHAPTER 4
Vulnerable adults and elder abuse

Introduction

Elder abuse is common, serious, and under-reported. Abused older adults have a three-fold increased risk of dying when compared to their non-abused counterparts. Despite this, many professionals working with older adults lack awareness of reporting guidelines and referral pathways (1).

This chapter will suggest a practical and structured approach to elder abuse, identify the different types of elder abuse, describe common presenting features to aid identification and provide structured guidance on the most direct way to report concerns about abuse.

Definition

The WHO defines elder abuse as *'a single or repeated act, or lack of appropriate action, occurring within any relationship where there is an expectation of trust which causes harm or distress to an older person'* (2). Although self-neglect is not uniformly considered a type of elder abuse, it is the most commonly reported form of elder mistreatment in the United States.

Background

Elder abuse is considered under the umbrella term 'family violence' and can either be 'domestic violence grown old' or a phenomenon developing in later life due to changing circumstances of the abused or the abuser (3).

Who does it?

Ninety percent of abusers are known to their victims, the most common perpetrators being an adult child or a spouse (4).

Anybody can abuse an older adult.

What constitutes a 'vulnerable adult'?

In England and Wales a vulnerable adult is defined as, 'a person who is or may be in need of community care services by reason of mental or other disability, age or illness and who is or may be unable to take care of himself or herself, or unable to protect him or herself against significant harm or exploitation' (5).

Geriatric Emergencies, First Edition.
Iona Murdoch, Sarah Turpin, Bree Johnston, Alasdair MacLullich and Eve Losman.
© 2015 John Wiley & Sons, Ltd. Published 2015 by John Wiley & Sons, Ltd.

In Scotland, the 2007 Adult Support and Protection (Scotland) Act defines an adult at risk as

1 Unable to safeguard their own well-being, property, rights or other interests,
2 At risk of harm, and
3 Due to being affected by disability, mental disorder, illness or physical or mental infirmity, they are more vulnerable to being harmed than adults who are not so affected.

In the United States, a vulnerable adult is defined as a person who is being mistreated or is in danger of mistreatment and who, due to age and/or disability, is unable to protect himself or herself (6).

Prevalence

The prevalence of elder abuse is hard to determine because the nature of the problem means it often occurs behind closed doors. It is also under-reported by both victims and health professionals. Adding to the challenge, studies that have attempted to estimate prevalence rates have been of variable quality, and have used different definitions and sampling methods. The National Elder Mistreatment study in the United States suggested that up to 11% of older people in the US had experienced some type of abuse in the previous year (7) and a large systematic review in 2008 reported a prevalence of 6% in general population, which is nearly double the reported prevalence rates 10 years previously (8). The prevalence of abuse in particularly vulnerable subgroups, such as people with dementia, is even more difficult to measure, but is suspected to be as high as 1 in 4 (8). All experts in the field agree that the documented prevalence of elder abuse underestimates the true magnitude of the problem.

Types of elder abuse

The United Kingdom recognises five main types of elder abuse; the United States also recognises these and has included a further two types of abuse, which are highlighted below (9, 10).

Physical

Inflicting, or threatening to inflict, physical pain or injury on a vulnerable elder, or depriving them of a basic need.

Psychological/emotional

Inflicting mental pain, anguish or distress on an elder person through verbal or non-verbal acts.

Financial/material

Illegal theft, misuse or concealment of funds, property or assets of a vulnerable elder.

Sexual

Non-consensual sexual contact of any kind, including coercing an elder to witness sexual behaviours.

Neglect

Refusal or failure by those responsible to provide food, shelter, healthcare or protection for a vulnerable elder. Neglect is not always intentional, many family members or carers are doing their best and have the best of intentions, but neglect in the context is still a form of abuse.

Self-neglect

A person's refusal or failure to provide himself or herself with adequate food, water, clothing, shelter, personal hygiene, medication and safety precautions.

Abandonment

The desertion of a vulnerable elder by anyone who has assumed the responsibility for care or custody of that person.

History

Think about it

A key factor in identifying elder abuse is a high index of suspicion; clinicians will not see it if they have never been taught to consider it in the first place.

Box 4.1 Risk factors for elder abuse (3).

- Decreased physical health (e.g. requiring more assistance with activities of daily living)
- Dementia or other cognitive impairment
- Female
- History of violence
- Increased age
- Shared living arrangements
- Social isolation
- Victim or caregiver with mental health or substance abuse issues.

  Source: From Bond MC, Butler KH. Elder abuse and neglect: definitions, epidemiology, and approaches to emergency department screening. *Clin Geriatr Med*. 2013;29(1):257–273. Reproduced with permission of Elsevier.

Ask about it

Patients are often reluctant to report abuse, and in the hospital setting, doctors may be less likely than nurses or other therapy staff to identify abuse, often because their interaction with patients is limited to briefer clinical encounters. Despite the difficulties identifying elder abuse, an initial encounter with an older patient still provides an important window of opportunity in which to consider and potentially identify signs of abuse. It is critical that clinicians create an opportunity to interview a vulnerable adult alone without family members or other potential perpetrators present.

The elder abuse suspicion index (EASI) takes approximately 2 minutes and is appropriate for use in the emergency department. It can be used in patients at high risk or if there are particular reasons to suspect elder abuse. It has been validated in primary and ambulatory care settings.

KEY POINT: Initial contact with the patient is a critical opportunity to identify and act on suspected elder abuse; often, analysis of prior cases shows that during encounters with healthcare providers, although signs of elder abuse were evident and documented, no concerted action was taken.

Box 4.2 The elder abuse suspicion index (EASI) (11).

Questions should be answered Yes or No or Unsure and ideally asked in an environment where the patient is alone with the interviewer.
Questions 1–5 are answered by the patient; question 6 is answered by the interviewer.
An answer of 'yes' to one or more of questions 2–6 should prompt concern for abuse or neglect:

Questions to the patient:

1 Have you relied on people for any of the following: bathing, dressing, shopping, banking or meals?
2 Has anyone prevented you from getting food, clothes, medication, glasses, hearing aids or medical care, or from being with people you wanted to be with?
3 Have you been upset because someone talked to you in a way that made you feel shamed or threatened?
4 Has anyone tried to force you to sign papers or to use your money against your will?
5 Has anyone made you afraid, touched you in ways that you did not want or hurt you physically?

To the interviewer:

6 (a) Elder abuse *may* be associated with findings such as poor eye contact, withdrawn nature, malnourishment, hygiene issues, cuts, bruises, inappropriate clothing or medication-compliance issues. Did you notice any of these today or *within the last 12 months*?
   (b) Aside from you and the patient, is anyone else in this room during this questioning?
   Source: From Mark J. Yaffe MD MCISc, Christina Wolfson PhD, Maxine Lithwick MSW & Deborah Weiss MSc (2008): Development and Validation of a Tool to Improve Physician Identification of Elder Abuse: The Elder Abuse Suspicion Index (EASI)©, *J Elder Abuse & Neglect*, 20:3, 276–300. Reproduced with permission of Taylor & Francis.

Examination

Physical examination

All patients should undergo a thorough examination, although there are often no distinct abnormalities in patients experiencing elder abuse. Particular attention should be paid to the patient's overall state, in particular, the level of grooming, cleanliness, clothing and nutritional status. In addition, a patient presenting with an advanced, untreated condition (e.g. pressure ulcer, infection or heart failure) may suggest that the person is being neglected. Examination of intimate areas such as genitals, rectum and breasts should be performed with a chaperone present.

Specific areas of focus
In the case of suspected sexual or physical abuse

Forensic evidence should not be removed until the patient has been examined by a professional trained in forensic medical examination, usually in conjunction with a police investigation.

Mental state examination

Patients with cognitive impairment are still able to report abuse and are at increased risk of suffering it. The patient should be examined for evidence of cognitive impairment and observed for signs of depression or anxiety. It is critical to determine whether the patient has decision-making capacity; patients who lack decision-making capacity are particularly vulnerable and may need intervention to ensure their safety (see Chapter 3 for further discussion on assessing decision-making capacity). Patients with decision-making capacity have the right to remain in an environment that is suboptimal.

The patient–carer dynamic

This may be relevant and should be observed and documented. Many informal carers can unknowingly abuse their loved ones due to lack of access to help, mental health issues or ignorance of what is considered appropriate levels of care. If possible, the provider should look at the carers' interaction with the patient. Is the caregiver caring, or callous disinterested, or dismissive? Is there visible hostility or aggression present? Does the caregiver seem exhausted, emotionally unstable or intoxicated with drugs or alcohol? Documenting observations carefully can be extremely helpful for future investigations (Table 4.1).

Investigation

Initial investigations

Serum levels of certain drugs such as epileptic medications can be measured to identify whether medications are being administered correctly at home.

Physical examination findings raising the concern of fractures or contusions should be followed up with appropriate imaging. At present, unlike suspected child abuse, there is no standard imaging set for injuries associated with elder abuse (13).

> **KEY POINT:** It is not your job to investigate abuse, but it is your responsibility, and sometimes your legal obligation, to refer it.

Management

Documentation

Meticulous documentation is essential during any encounter where abuse is suspected.
1 Document who has raised concerns about abuse.
2 Use direct quotes from both the patient and the caregiver; this is particularly important if the abuse is later formally investigated or prosecuted.
3 Time and date your entry in the notes.
4 Use a body chart diagram to record any physical examination findings such as bruises or abrasions.
5 Document who else was present in the room during the interview, include other doctors, nurses, therapists and relatives or friends of the patient.
6 Document clearly your planned actions and why you feel these actions are necessary or appropriate.
7 Document whom you have referred to/liaised with and any follow-up plans that have been made.
8 Use specific names and dates and specify a timescale if possible.

Table 4.1 Elder abuse typologies, possible manifestations and potential indicators (12).

Type of abuse	Manifestations	Potential indicators
Physical abuse	Hitting, slapping, pushing, kicking, spitting, medication misuse, restraint, force-feeding or inappropriate sanctions	Bruising, cuts lacerations, scratches, sprains, hair loss, missing teeth, fractures, slap or kick marks, eye injuries, burns
Sexual abuse	Rape, sexual assault or acts the older person has not consented to or has not got the ability to consent to or was compelled to consent	Trauma around the genitals, breasts, rectum or mouth
Psychological abuse	Humiliation, intimidation, threats of abandonment, ridicule, causing fear/anxiety, bullying, blaming, controlling, coercion, harassment, verbal abuse, lack of acknowledgement, isolation/withholding social contact, denial of basic rights, overprotective	Demoralisation, depression, withdrawal, apathy, feeling hopeless, insomnia, appetite change, unexplained paranoia, agitation, tearfulness, excessive fears, confusion, ambivalence towards perpetrator
Neglect	Ignoring physical/medical needs, failing to provide access to appropriate services (health/social/educational) of life and/or aids for activities of daily living (such as medication, heating)	Dehydration, malnutrition, inappropriate clothing, poor hygiene, unkempt appearance, over/under-medication, unattended medical needs, exposure to risk/danger, absence of aids (zimmer/hearing aid), pressure sores
Financial abuse	Sudden reduction in financial funds, removal of material property, coerced signing over of property/funds/material goods or change of will	Sudden/unexplained inability to pay bills or buy necessities, uncharacteristic withdrawal of funds, diverted funds for another's use, damage to property, disappearance of property, absence of required aids or medication, refusal to spend money, disparity of assets and living conditions, extraordinary interest by others in older persons assets, dramatic financial decisions
Ageism	Towards older people (individual/group)	Stereotypically, discriminatory and demeaning ways of viewing older people. Manifests in the way older people are spoken of, treated and cared for by individuals, groups and society. For example, paternalism, infantilisation or actions which imbue inequality with other age groups

Source: From Phelan A Elder Abuse in the Emergency Department in Int Emerg Nurs. 2012 Oct;20(4):214–20. Reproduced with permission of Elsevier.

Referral

Referral guidance and investigative procedure vary depending on the local area of practice; this section contains general guidance about when to refer to social care or adult protection agencies with links to area-specific protocols based on country or state.

When to refer

Referral should take place if there are any concerns arising from the history and examination that abuse is a possibility. The patient may directly divulge information about abuse, or more subtle clues may be evident.

What if the patient does not want the abuse to be reported?

The decision of an adult with capacity to remain in a potentially harmful situation is a complex one, and consideration of the most appropriate course of action in these cases is beyond the scope of this text.

In Scotland (but not the rest of the United Kingdom) and in many US states, healthcare workers are required to report suspicions of abuse even if a patient with decision-making capacity has asked them not to.

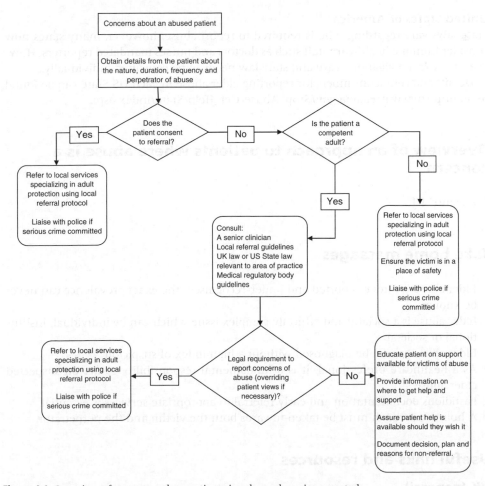

Figure 4.1 Overview of an approach to patients in whom abuse is suspected.

In this situation, consult a senior clinician and state or UK law regarding specific legal position and duties. The relevant medical regulatory body will also provide guidance on these situations.

 KEY POINT: A patient can be suffering abuse without being aware of it.

How to refer
United Kingdom

In hours: Call the local social care department and ask to speak to the adult protection officer on duty for the day.
Out of hours: Ensure the patient is in a place of safety and not at risk of immediate further harm. Call the social care department urgently the following morning.

United States of America
State laws vary regarding who is required to report abuse; however, many states now consider frontline healthcare staff such as doctors and nurses mandated reporters. However, the exact obligations vary and state law needs to be consulted individually.

Details and contact numbers for reporting elder abuse in each US State can be found here: http://www.ncea.aoa.gov/Stop_Abuse/Get_Help/State/index.aspx

Overview of an approach to patients where abuse is a concern

See Figure 4.1.

Take home messages

- Elder abuse is under-reported and under-recognised; the exact prevalence can never be known
- Elder abuse is a socially and ethically complex issue which can be individual, institutional or societal
- Elder abuse cannot be diagnosed without a high index of suspicion
- As a healthcare professional, it is a fundamental responsibility to act on suspected elder abuse
- Fastidious documentation and early referral to appropriate services is essential
- A holistic approach must be taken towards both the victim and the perpetrator.

Useful links and resources

UK (general)

http://www.elderabuse.org.uk/index.html

http://www.gmc-uk.org/guidance/good_medical_practice.asp
http://www.cqc.org.uk/

England

http://www.elderabuse.org.uk/Documents/Other%20Orgs/No%20Secrets.pdf

Northern Ireland

http://www.dhsspsni.gov.uk/index/hss/safeguarding_vulnerable_adults/safeguarding
_vulnerable_adults-resourcelibrary.htm

Scotland

http://www.legislation.gov.uk/asp/2007/10/part/1
http://www.actagainstharm.org/

Wales

http://wales.gov.uk/topics/health/publications/socialcare/reports/ishnov09/?lang=en

USA

Details and contact numbers for reporting elder abuse in each US State can be found
here:
http://www.ncea.aoa.gov/Stop_Abuse/Get_Help/State/index.aspx
http://www.ncea.aoa.gov/index.aspx
http://www.americanbar.org/groups/law_aging/resources/elder_abuse.htm

Case Studies

Case study 1: Newly admitted older patient to the acute medical unit

You are working in the acute medical unit and are clerking a newly admitted patient.

Joan is 84 years old and lives with her husband, John, who is 80. Joan has macular
degeneration, severe rheumatoid arthritis and osteoporosis. She is unable to walk and
relies on John for help with personal care, toileting and meal preparation.

Joan is admitted to hospital with severe back pain and L1/2 vertebral crush fractures
sustained when she fell whilst transferring from her wheelchair to the toilet.

On examination, Joan is mentally alert but extremely frail with multiple bruises on
her shins and wrists. She has a small sacral pressure sore and her mouth is ulcerated due
to poorly fitting false teeth, which do not appear to have been cleaned for several days.

Whilst taking a history from Joan, you ascertain that Joan and John have no support
at home and no equipment in the house to assist with transfers. John is adamant that
he will not allow carers into the house and that he has looked after Joan for years and
does not need help from 'interfering women and busybodies'.

Joan is able to communicate and there are no signs of dementia or delirium, and she wishes to come into hospital to get the pain under control, but ultimately wishes to return home to live with John once her pain killers are adjusted.

How would you proceed?

Case study 2: Emergency department admission

You are on duty in the emergency department.

Maria is 79 years old and is brought to the ED by paramedics following a fall at home. On arrival, the paramedics report to you that Maria lives with her daughter who has not attended, but who appeared intoxicated and was verbally abusive to the paramedics when they arrived at the home.

Maria's daughter is well-known to the ED as an intravenous drug abuser whose children are in care. Until now, it was not known that Maria was living in the house.

Maria has mild dementia and is unable to provide details on what happened or why the ambulance was called. On examination, she appears withdrawn and confused; her clothes are soiled with faeces and she smells strongly of urine. She has no physical injury but appears dehydrated and malnourished.

How would you proceed?

Case study 3: Inpatient

You are working on the orthopaedic ward.

Simon is 84 years old and is an inpatient undergoing a lengthy rehabilitation following a complicated elective total hip replacement. Before admission, he managed independently at home and was well aside from osteoarthritis. He is a retired bank manager who has no family but an active social life.

Whilst on the ward, nursing staff have noticed that his most regular visitor is a woman who Simon refers to as 'his guardian angel'. It transpires that Simon regularly gives this woman his bank cards and PIN number so she can pay his bills and maintain any household upkeep whilst he is in hospital. She has joked with the staff about 'helping herself' as an extra for all the work she has been doing for Simon, and he has mentioned that he paid for her car insurance this year 'as a thank you' for all the help she has given him over the last few weeks. The nursing staff are concerned about the possibility of financial abuse.

How would you proceed?

Case study 4: Nursing home resident

Nancy, a nursing home resident who is bedbound and unable to communicate due to advanced dementia has been admitted to the gynaecological assessment unit due to concerns from her carers and GP about offensive smelling vaginal discharge. The GP is concerned about the possibility of an advanced cervical tumour and has referred her urgently for further assessment.

On examination, there is no evidence of cervical pathology and she is discharged back to her nursing home pending an ultrasound scan and high vaginal swab results.

Two days later, swabs taken on admission have returned positive for *Neisseria gonorrhoeae*.

How would you proceed?

References

1 Cooper C, Selwood A, Livingston G. Knowledge, detection, and reporting of abuse by health and social care professionals: a systematic review. *Am J Geriatr Psychiatry*. 2009;17(10):826–838.

2 WHO *Elder Maltreatment*. WHO. http://www.who.int/mediacentre/factsheets/fs357/en/index.html [cited 2013 Mar 23].

3 Bond MC, Butler KH. Elder abuse and neglect: definitions, epidemiology, and approaches to emergency department screening. *Clin Geriatr Med*. 2013;29(1):257–273.

4 The National Center on Elder Abuse. The National Elder Abuse Incidence Study: Final Report. The Administration for Children and Families and the Administration on Aging in the US Department of Health and Human Services; 1998, p. 108.

5 The National Archives. *Who Decides?: Making Decisions on Behalf of Mentally Incapacitated Adult*. http://webarchive.nationalarchives.gov.uk/; http://www.dca.gov.uk/menincap/meninfr.htm [cited 2013 Apr 3].

6 Department of Health and Human Services, NCEA. *Adult Protective Services*. http://www.ncea.aoa.gov /Stop_Abuse/Partners/APS/index.aspx [cited 2013 Apr 14].

7 National Institute of Justice. *Extent of Elder Abuse Victimization*. http://www.nij.gov/nij/topics/crime /elder-abuse/extent.htm [cited 2013 Apr 3].

8 Cooper C, Selwood A, Livingston G. The prevalence of elder abuse and neglect: a systematic review. *Age Ageing*. 2008;37(2):151–160.

9 Department of Health and Human Services, NCEA. *Frequently Asked Questions*. http://www.ncea.aoa .gov/faq/index.aspx. [cited 2013 Apr 14].

10 Mosqueda L and Dong X. Elder abuse and self-neglect. "I don't care anything about going to the doctor, to be honest". *JAMA* 2011; 306: 532–540.

11 Yaffe MJ, Wolfson C, Lithwick M, Weiss D. Development and validation of a tool to improve physician identification of elder abuse: the elder abuse suspicion index (EASI)©. *J Elder Abuse Negl*. 2008;20(3):276–300.

12 Phelan A. Elder abuse in the emergency department. *Int Emerg Nurs*. 2012; 20(4):214–220.

13 Murphy K, Waa S, Jaffer H, Sauter A, Chan A. A literature review of findings in physical elder abuse. *Can Assoc Radiol J*. 2013;64(1):10–14.

CHAPTER 5

Chest pain and atrial fibrillation

Part 1: Chest pain

Introduction

Chest pain in an older person can signify a wide range of conditions from the benign and self-limiting to the life-threatening and rapidly fatal. The spectrum of causes of chest pain in older people is similar to that in younger people, but a higher index of suspicion is required because of reduced severity of symptoms in relation to the seriousness of the cause in some older people.

Many of the management principles for a patient with chest pain are the same in young and older patients; this chapter will provide guidance on how to efficiently assess an older person presenting with chest pain. Basic general management principles of the three most common life-threatening causes of chest pain will be suggested under the subheading 'therapies to consider', but this chapter will focus on particular anomalies or challenges relating to the presentation and management of these conditions in older people. For detailed advice on disease-specific management, supplementary use of general medical texts and local protocols is recommended.

Background

Chest pain is a common symptom, accounting for 5% of ED visits in the United Kingdom and 25% of emergency hospital admissions. In the United States, over 6 million patients present with chest pain to the ED each year. Despite the common nature of chest pain as a presenting complaint, it is a complex clinical phenomenon with a wide range of causes.

Chest pain in older adults is more likely to be associated with a serious underlying cause; however, older adults are more likely to present with vague or atypical symptoms and a delay in seeking medical care (1, 2). Older patients presenting with chest pain have a higher overall mortality (2, 3) and healthcare professionals responsible for assessing older adults with chest pain need to be systematic and thorough in their initial evaluation in order to safely rule out life-threatening causes (Table 5.1).

History

A focused history of the nature of the chest pain is necessary to obtain potentially useful information when formulating a differential diagnosis.

Geriatric Emergencies, First Edition.
Iona Murdoch, Sarah Turpin, Bree Johnston, Alasdair MacLullich and Eve Losman.
© 2015 John Wiley & Sons, Ltd. Published 2015 by John Wiley & Sons, Ltd.

Table 5.1 Common causes of chest pain in older patients.

Life-threatening causes	Non-life-threatening causes
Acute coronary syndrome	Gastro-oesophageal reflux
Pulmonary embolism	Pleurisy
Aortic dissection	Costochondritis
Myocarditis	Herpes zoster
Pneumonia	Musculoskeletal pain
Tension pneumothorax	Anxiety disorders
Sickle cell crisis	Mitral valve prolapse
Oesophageal rupture	Pericarditis
Peptic ulcer disease	
Acute pancreatitis	
Acute cholecystitis	
Renal colic	

Source: Adapted from Kelly BS. Evaluation of the elderly patient with acute chest pain. *Clin Geriatr Med.* 2007 May;23(2):327–349, vi. Reproduced with permission of Elsevier.

Patients with cognitive impairment may have difficulty providing this information, and obtaining a collateral history is important in these circumstances. For more information on collateral history-taking, see Chapter 2.

Particular challenges in taking a history from patients with:
Acute coronary syndrome (ACS)
In a large review (4), a third of older patients with acute myocardial infarction did not present with chest pain but instead had 'atypical' presenting features. These included:
- Dyspnoea (49.3%)
- Diaphoresis (26.2%)
- Nausea and vomiting (24.3%)
- Syncope (19.1%).

Other 'atypical' symptoms experienced by older patients include worsening cardiac failure, fatigue and delirium.

Pulmonary embolism (PE)
This is common and underdiagnosed; chest pain is the second most common presenting symptom, occurring in 40–60% of patients as a presenting feature (5, 6). The PIOPED (prospective investigation of pulmonary embolism diagnosis) study found no significant difference in the frequency of chest pain as a presenting feature between young and old patients, although it did note that other common features such as dyspnoea and tachycardia were present in fewer older patients than younger patients (5). Some smaller studies have found that older patients are less likely to present with chest pain and more likely to present with non-specific symptoms such as syncope (7, 8).

Co-existing chest pathology such as cardiac failure or COPD (chronic obstructive pulmonary disease) can complicate the diagnosis of PE placing it further down on the list of differentials. Dyspnoea and chest pain can be erroneously attributed to 'old age' and significantly delay patients seeking medical help. A high index of suspicion is required when assessing an older patient with any chest symptoms, as morbidity and mortality associated with PE increases with age (1, 9).

Pre-test probability of D-dimer is less helpful in older patients, as many patients will have a raised D-dimer. This means that the clinician should have a lower threshold for requesting CTPA (computed tomography of pulmonary angiogram) to exclude PE in older patients.

Aortic dissection

This is an uncommon but often fatal condition, and peak incidence is in adults aged between 60 and 80 years. Timely diagnosis and early treatment have a significant impact on survival. Abrupt onset, severe central chest pain remains the commonest presenting symptom in older patients, although it occurs in only 76% of cases compared to 85–95% of younger patients (10).

Other symptoms that occur more commonly in older patients are:
• *Syncope*: this is the primary presenting symptom in 12–13% of cases and the only presenting symptom in 3% (1).
• *Symptoms suggestive of branch vessel involvement*: differing blood pressure in upper limbs, acute neurological symptoms or ischaemic limbs presenting in combination with chest pain should be considered as diagnostic of aortic dissection until proven otherwise.

A useful mnemonic (SOCRATES) to assist in taking a focused chest pain history can be found in Table 5.2.

Table 5.2 'Typical' associated features of the three most common life-threatening causes of chest pain.

History	Acute coronary syndrome (likelihood ratio of acute MI)	Pulmonary embolism	Aortic dissection
Site	Central and left arm pain (2.7)	Lateralising	Anterior chest wall or intrascapular
Onset	Gradual and worsening. Time of worst pain and time of onset is important for checking cardiac biomarkers	Sudden onset	Sudden onset and maximal severity at onset
Character	'crushing' 'dull' 'heavy'	'sharp' pleuritic	Abrupt onset, sharp or 'tearing' 'stabbing'
Radiation	Into right shoulder (2.9) Left arm (2.8) Both arms (7.1)	–	Into back and then abdomen
Associated symptoms	Sweating (2.0) Nausea and vomiting (1.9)	Shortness of breath/ haemoptysis/syncope	Neurological symptoms/syncope
Timing	Worsens over 5–15 min	Abrupt onset maximally severe	Abrupt onset maximally severe
Exacerbating and relieving factors	Worsened by exertion, cold weather, emotional stress, relieved by rest or GTN	Worsened by deep breathing or position	–
Severity	Severity is a subjective feature useful for comparison after treatment	Severity is a subjective feature useful for comparison after treatment	Severity is a subjective feature useful for comparison after treatment

Likelihood ratios from Panju AA, Hemmelgarn BR, Guyatte GH, et al. Is this patient having a myocardial infarction? *JAMA* 1998;280(14):1256.

Examination

Physical examination: general

Older patients presenting with chest pain are potentially very unwell and require an ABCDE (airway, breathing, circulation, disability, exposure) approach to initial assessment; physiological abnormalities should also be identified and treated at the same time.

General observation is also very important in patients with chest pain. Do they look well or unwell? Do they appear distressed or frightened? In particular, observe for signs of pallor, sweating or elevated respiratory rate.

Box 5.1 How to perform a systematic examination on a patient with chest pain? (11)

Airway	Check for airway patency: if the patient is giving you a history, there is unlikely to be an airway problem
Breathing	Listen to the chest for breath sounds and added sounds. Percuss to ensure equal resonance. Feel for symmetrical chest expansion. Give oxygen to correct hypoxia; do not routinely give oxygen unless there is evidence of hypoxia on saturation monitoring or arterial blood gas. Offer supplemental oxygen to:
	• People with oxygen saturation (SpO_2) of <94% for those who are not at risk of hypercapnic respiratory failure, aiming for SpO_2 of 94–98%
	• People with chronic obstructive pulmonary disease who are at risk of hypercapnic respiratory failure, to achieve a target SpO_2 of 88–92% until blood gas analysis is available
Circulation	*Perform a 12 lead ECG as soon as possible*, ideally ask an assistant to obtain the 12 lead before or during your examination. Listen to the heart for murmurs or added heart sounds, feel the pulse and check the blood pressure. Check the capillary refill time. If there are signs of shock including a low BP, give a small fluid challenge and re-assess
Disability	Check capillary blood glucose and examine for any evolving focal neurology which could suggest acute aortic dissection involving the carotid artery
Exposure	Examine the abdomen for pulsatile masses, feel peripheral pulses and check for signs of peripheral oedema, cyanosis or shock. Enquire about the possibility of a gastrointestinal bleed e.g. recent melaena or haematemesis. Palpate the chest wall to elicit focal areas of tenderness, and if present, ask the patient if this is the same pain as they are reporting. Note, however, that an area of tenderness does not rule out a serious disorder such as PE. Look at the skin for any rash in a dermatomal distribution to suggest Herpes Zoster

---

Specific areas of focus on examination
Acute coronary syndrome

Examine the chest closely for heart murmurs or signs of associated cardiac failure. Check the pulse and promptly obtain an ECG to identify any underlying contributory or resultant arrhythmias.

Consider any underlying factors that may be contributing to the ACS such as sepsis, hypovolaemia, hypoxia or arrhythmia.

Aortic dissection

Hypertension is common in patients with aortic dissection but up to 20% of older patients can present with hypotension.

When considering aortic dissection as a diagnosis, measurement of blood pressure in both arms to identify discrepant pulse pressure of >20 mmHg is an insensitive sign of aortic dissection.

Peripheral pulse examination and neurological examination can be helpful in identifying branch vessel involvement. The presence of new, peripheral neurological signs is insensitive but highly specific in patients with chest pain.

> **KEY POINT: Discrepant pulse pressure or asymmetrical pulses depend on the location of the aortic dissection; a significant number of patients with aortic dissection have symmetrical pulses and blood pressures, and many have a normal chest radiograph. There must be a low threshold for clinical imaging.**

> **KEY POINT: In a patient presenting with chest pain and acute neurologic deficit, aortic dissection is the diagnosis until proven otherwise**

Pulmonary embolus

Examine the legs for signs of deep vein thrombosis (DVT) and consider any other underlying prothrombotic factors such as malignancy, recent surgery or prolonged immobility.

Look for signs of right ventricular failure, haemoptysis and cyanosis.

Investigations

Initial investigations

All patients presenting with chest pain should have:

Blood tests

FBC (full blood count), U&Es (urea and electrolytes), LFTs (liver function tests), appropriately timed cardiac biomarkers, amylase, lactate and consideration of D-dimer.

ECG

Serial ECGs every 5–15 minutes may reveal evolving ischaemic changes in a symptomatic patient. Right side ECG or extended, 15 lead, ECG can be helpful in identifying a posterior or right ventricular infarct. See Figures 5.1 and 5.3.

Chest radiograph

Chest radiograph is an essential investigation in all patients with chest pain. It may be normal; however, it may show relevant abnormalities, for example, pulmonary oedema in patients with cardiac failure, or a widened mediastinum in patients with aortic dissection (Figures 5.4 and 5.5).

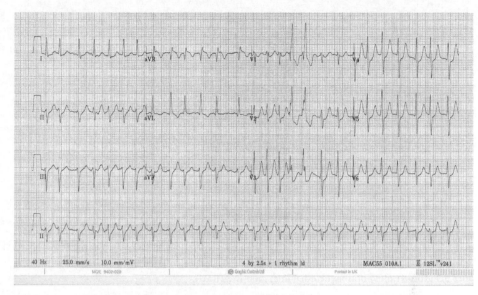

Figure 5.1 Uncontrolled atrial fibrillation with lateral ischaemia.

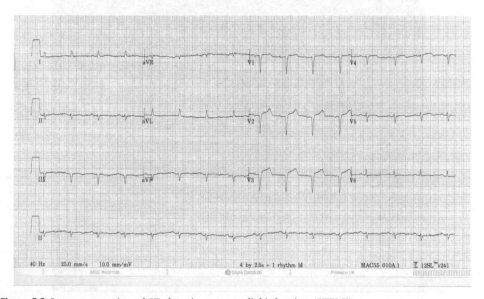

Figure 5.2 Late presentation of ST elevation myocardial infarction (STEMI).

Bedside ultrasound

In an ED or AMU with access to ultrasound, a quick bedside echocardiogram or thoracic ultrasound performed by an emergency physician or cardiology consultant can assess for wall motion abnormalities, pericardial effusion, pleural effusion or pneumothorax.

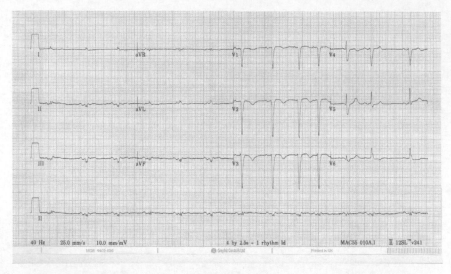

Figure 5.3 Non-ST elevation myocardial infarction (NSTEMI).

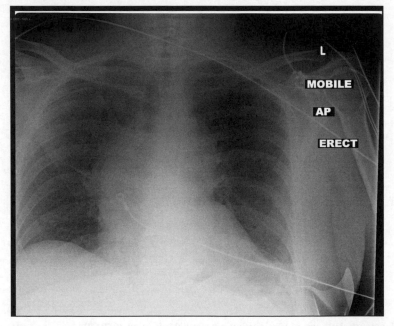

Figure 5.4 Widened mediastinum in aortic dissection. Look also for an indistinct aortic knuckle, apical cap, and pleural effusions.

Further investigation
In suspected acute coronary syndrome
Patients with possible ACS should be connected to continuous cardiac monitoring in an environment with resuscitation equipment nearby. Serial troponin measurement

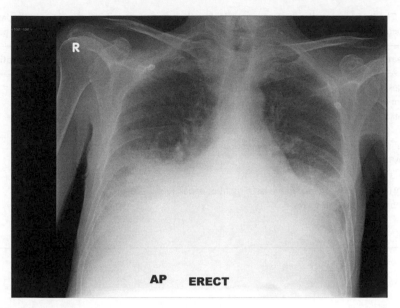

Figure 5.5 Pulmonary oedema.

can be helpful in identifying an evolving ACS. Consider serial ECGs to detect dynamic ST segment changes and repeat the ECG if the patient experiences further episodes of pain.

A historical ECG should be obtained for comparison if possible as many older patients have longstanding ECG abnormalities such as bundle branch blocks which can make assessing for new ischaemic changes challenging.

> **KEY POINT: If a patient has an abnormal, ischaemic looking ECG and there is suspicion of ACS, do not delay giving appropriate treatment whilst locating an old ECG; if in doubt, treat and also refer to a specialist.**

In suspected pulmonary embolism
Arterial blood gas (ABG)
This will typically show type 1 respiratory failure or an increased A-a gradient, and may show a respiratory alkalosis if patients are tachypnoeic. A normal ABG does not exclude a PE.

D-Dimer
PE is usually diagnosed by calculating a pre-test probability using a validated scoring system such as the Well's score (Table 5.3), checking D-dimer and progressing to clinical imaging if necessary. In many older patients, the D-dimer will be raised at baseline and this makes excluding pulmonary embolus using this method more difficult.

> **KEY POINT: The specificity of D-dimer in patients with suspected PE decreases steadily with age.**

Table 5.3 The two-level wells score used to calculate the pre-test probability of a hospital inpatient with suspected pulmonary embolism. Note: This test has not been validated for use in older patients.

Clinical feature	Points	Patient score
Clinical signs and symptoms of DVT (minimum of leg swelling and pain with palpation of the deep veins)	3	
An alternative diagnosis is less likely than PE	3	
Heart rate >100 bpm	1.5	
Immobilisation for >3 days or surgery in the previous 4 weeks	1.5	
Previous DVT/PE	1.5	
Haemoptysis	1	
Malignancy (on treatment, treated in the last 6 months, or palliative)	1	
Clinical probability simplified scores		
PE *likely*	>4 points	
PE *unlikely*	4 points or less	

Clinical imaging

CT pulmonary angiography is the gold standard but is less sensitive at identifying sub-segmental pulmonary emboli. V-Q perfusion scanning is also common and available in most centres, but in older patients, results are commonly affected by co-existing chest pathology (12). Doppler ultrasound of the legs to identify DVT is also useful.

Echocardiography

Acutely unwell patients who are too unstable for CT or VQ scanning can undergo a bed-side echocardiogram to look for acute right heart dysfunction or intra-cardiac thrombus. In older patients, the relevance of right heart dysfunction on echocardiogram should be interpreted with caution as this might reflect pre-existing cardiac or lung disease (12). Current guidance advises that right ventricular dysfunction in the absence of haemodynamic instability is not a criterion for thrombolysis (13).

In suspected aortic dissection
Clinical imaging

National guidelines on imaging in suspected aortic dissection accept that emergency situations will depend on staff experience and availability. The primary aim is to confirm the diagnosis, classify the subtype of aortic dissection and assess for complications and branch vessel involvement (3, 14).

Local guidelines will exist in EDs for recommended emergency imaging in cases of suspected aortic dissection; options include:
- Trans-thoracic or trans-oesophageal echocardiography
- Computed tomography angiography (CTA) or magnetic resonance angiography (MRA).
- Conventional angiography.

Whilst the sensitivity of echocardiography and CTA are similar, echocardiograms require experienced cardiologists on site 24 hours a day whereas CT scanning is more readily available out of hours and less dependent on staff expertise.

Management

General management

> KEY POINT: An older person experiencing chest pain with associated hypotension is a medical emergency requiring urgent review regardless of the underlying cause.

Immediate initial management should focus on the identification and correction of physiological abnormalities and the relief of pain and distress.

Analgesia
If severe, chest pain should be treated with carefully titrated intravenous opioids.

Oxygen
Oxygen should be given if saturations are low (use controlled oxygen in patients with COPD).

IV Fluids
Fluids should be given if there are signs of shock or hypotension, but with caution in patients with pulmonary oedema or known LV systolic dysfunction.

Acute coronary syndrome
Therapies to consider

Reduce clot burden
Anti-platelets, anticoagulants, glycoprotein IIb/IIIa inhibitors.

Reduce myocardial oxygen demand
Beta-blockers.

Enhance coronary artery blood flow
Nitrates, re-perfusion therapy.

> KEY POINT: Older patients with acute coronary syndrome should be treated aggressively. Evidence suggests that older patients with ACS are frequently undertreated and suffer significantly higher mortality from ACS than younger patients (15).

The general management of STEMI (ST elevation myocardial infarction) and NSTEMI (non-ST elevation myocardial infarction) in older patients is the same as in younger patients. This text suggests consulting local protocol.

There are, however, some complicating factors that occur more frequently in older patients, and these are addressed below.

Myocardial infarction induced by systemic illness

This is categorised as a type 2 myocardial infarction and is defined as 'Myocardial infarction secondary to ischaemia due to either increased oxygen demand or decreased supply, e.g. anaemia, arrhythmias, hypertension, or hypotension, coronary artery spasm, coronary embolism' (16).

Older patients frequently have underlying coronary artery disease which, when they are physiologically stable does not cause symptoms, but when unwell, patients may develop chest pain, non-specific ischaemic ECG changes and raised troponin. The management of the underlying condition is the priority in these situations, and a marginally raised troponin in the context of obvious physiological stress should not be treated with anti-platelets and anticoagulant agents unless specialist advice has been sought.

Acute coronary syndrome occurring in warfarinised patients

Older patients who are on long-term oral anticoagulation can present with ACS. Expert opinion advises withholding parenteral anticoagulation (fondaparinux/heparin, etc.) until INR < 2.0 (international normalised ratio) and commencing dual anti-platelet therapy, particularly if there is a plan for percutaneous intervention. There is a lack of robust evidence surrounding the optimal management of these patients, and therefore, contemporary treatment patterns can diverge from formal guidelines on this matter (17).

The WOEST study reported that treating anticoagulated patients presenting with ACS using clopidogrel alone in addition to continuing the patient's warfarin rather than dual anti-platelet therapy appeared to significantly reduce the rate of bleeding complications without increasing the risk of thrombotic events, and this practice has been adopted in some centres (18).

Bleeding complications in patients recently treated for acute coronary syndrome

Older patients are at increased risk of bleeding when treated with dual anti-platelet therapy after ACS. The management of each individual patient will depend on factors such as the type and nature bleeding, how recently their ACS was, and the treatment they received. When faced with a patient on dual anti-platelet therapy, recent ACS and gastro-intestinal bleeding, seek expert help early (19) (Figure 5.6).

Refractory angina

Refractory angina is a chronic condition characterised by coronary insufficiency due to coronary artery disease, which cannot be controlled by a combination of medical therapy, angioplasty and coronary bypass surgery. The presence of reversible myocardial ischaemia should be clinically established to be the cause of the symptoms. Chronicity is defined as a duration of >3 months (20).

Prognosis in these patients is not as poor as previously thought and is comparable to patients with chronic stable angina on maximal medical therapy (21). There is an increasing evidence base and growing interest in the optimal management of such patients.

Managing refractory angina can be challenging and treatment aims to reduce angina symptoms and improve quality of life. Patients presenting with refractory angina should be referred to a specialist to ensure that management options such optimising cardiac medications and providing patient education are fully explored.

If patients are presenting recurrently out of hours, there may be benefit gained from creating a jointly agreed treatment plan involving their own cardiologist, the

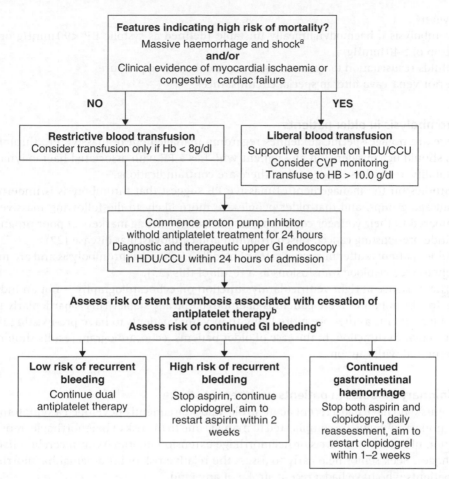

Figure 5.6 An algorithm for assessing and treating patients on dual anti-platelet therapy presenting with non-variceal upper gastrointestinal haemorrhage. From Henriksen PA, Palmer K, Boon NA. Management of upper gastrointestinal haemorrhage complicating dual anti-platelet therapy. *QJM*. 2008 Apr;101(4):261–7. Source: Reproduced with permission of Oxford University Press.

ED clinicians and any other key support services or individuals involved with the patient.

Pulmonary embolus

If the diagnosis of pulmonary embolus is confirmed, or clinical suspicion is very high, treatment should be initiated without delay. Older people are at increased risk of pulmonary embolus and suffer increased mortality and morbidity when compared to their younger counterparts and delayed or missed diagnoses in hospital inpatients are a significant cause of death each year.

Therapies to consider

Therapeutic dose, low-molecular weight heparin (subject to usual cautions, e.g. reduced eGFR)

Oxygen

Thrombolysis if haemodynamically unstable (defined as systolic BP <90 mmHg or BP drop of >40 mmHg)

IV fluids resuscitation to optimise right ventricular filling pressure

Inferior vena-cava filter in special circumstances.

Thrombolysis in older patients

There are no age-specific guidelines regarding management of massive PE; thrombolysis should be considered in any patient who has a PE with associated haemodynamic instability, regardless of age, unless there are contraindications.

Studies on the management of massive PE suggest that thrombolysis is underused in all age groups, and that older people are more likely to die following massive PE compared to their younger counterparts. Particularly strong markers of poor prognosis include pre-existing cancer, raised troponin and cardiovascular disease (22).

Older patients suffer increased rates of bleeding following thrombolysis and are more likely to receive blood transfusions as a result of this (23).

The presence of right ventricular dysfunction on echocardiography is not an indication for thrombolysis if the patient is haemodynamically stable. This is particularly true of older patients as they are more likely than young patients to have pre-existing right ventricular dysfunction. In the case of older patients, echocardiogram results should be interpreted with caution.

Pulmonary embolus in patients with recent stroke

Patients who have had a recent acute stroke and subsequently developed a symptomatic pulmonary embolus are complicated to manage due to the risk of haemorrhagic transformation of ischaemic infarcts or haemorrhage extension in primary intracerebral haemorrhages. Seek senior help early to assess the relative risk of intracranial haemorrhage in patients who have had a recent stroke of any kind.

Treatment options include low-molecular-weight heparin, unfractionated heparin or mechanical intervention (inferior vena cava filter) to prevent further emboli. In general, patients will require treatment but this should be guided by a senior doctor with careful assessment of all risks based on the size and timescale of the stroke and the patient's clinical state.

Formal guidance suggests that (24):

• Patients with ischaemic stroke and symptomatic proximal DVT or PE should receive anticoagulation treatment in preference to treatment with aspirin unless there are other contraindications to anticoagulation.

• Patients with haemorrhagic stroke and symptomatic DVT or PE should have treatment to prevent the development of further pulmonary emboli using either anticoagulation or an inferior vena cava filter.

Aortic dissection

In any patient with suspected aortic dissection, surgical advice and radiological advice should be sought immediately, as diagnosis depends on clinical imaging and management decisions are highly specialised.

Therapies to consider

Oxygen

Intravenous analgesia

Arterial line insertion to facilitate blood pressure monitoring

Aggressive blood pressure (100–120 mmHg systolic) and heart rate (60 bpm) control

Use of IV therapies (e.g. propranolol, labetalol, esmolol, fenoldopam) ± additional intravenous vasodilators

Careful titration of intravenous fluids or blood products in hypotensive patients, with
avoidance of inotropes if possible

Immediate liaison with cardiothoracic surgery, radiology and intensive care

Surgery for aortic dissection in older patients

Historically, older patients are less likely than their younger counterparts to undergo
surgery for aortic dissection due to concerns about operative risk (10).

Increasing numbers of older patients are presenting with aortic dissection and there
are studies emerging which suggest that in selected older patients, surgical management
of aortic dissection carries acceptable risk and confers significant survival benefit over
conservative treatment (25). At present, there are no age-specific guidelines and the
decision to operate on any patient, regardless of age, depends on a complex assessment
of multiple factors including patient characteristics and type of dissection (14, 26).

Overview of an approach to a patient presenting with chest pain

See Figure 5.7.

Part 2: Atrial fibrillation

Atrial fibrillation

Atrial fibrillation (AF) is the commonest arrhythmia, with a prevalence of 10% at the
age of 80, rising to 18% in those aged over 85 (27). New onset or poorly controlled AF is
frequently encountered in the ED or acute medical unit, and often poses clinical dilem-
mas as to the most appropriate management. It may be the primary clinical problem,
a complication of another acute pathology (e.g. sepsis, ACS) or an incidental finding
detected in the work-up of another presentation. Therapeutic decisions are guided by
AF duration and onset; classification (Table 5.4); predisposing and precipitating factors
(Box 5.2 and 5.3); symptoms; and any signs of haemodynamic instability. This section
provides a brief overview of different management strategies, but readers should be
advised to follow local guidance and seek cardiology advice in complex or urgent cases.

Definition

AF is a supraventricular tachycardia resulting from the presence of uncoordinated
re-entrant circuits within the atria, with an associated deterioration in atrial mechanical
function. Lack of atrial systole decreases cardiac output by 10–20%, and predisposes to
atrial thrombi formation leading to embolic phenomena such as stroke. The ventricular
response to chaotic atrial activity depends on the degree of conduction through the
AV node, influenced by factors such as drugs and vagal tone. Fast ventricular response

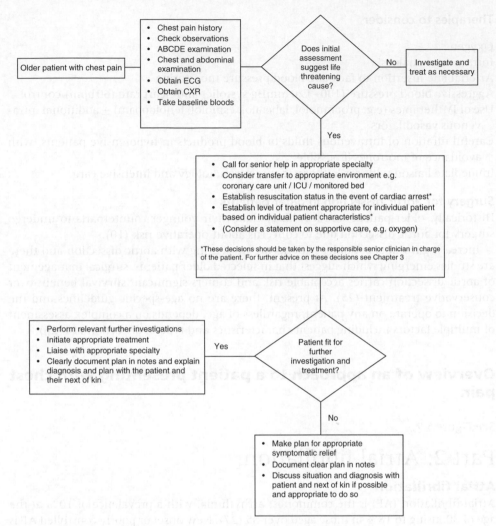

Older patient with chest pain

- Chest pain history
- Check observations
- ABCDE examination
- Chest and abdominal examination
- Obtain ECG
- Obtain CXR
- Take baseline bloods

Does initial assessment suggest life threatening cause?

No → Investigate and treat as necessary

Yes

- Call for senior help in appropriate specialty
- Consider transfer to appropriate environment e.g. coronary care unit / ICU / monitored bed
- Establish resuscitation status in the event of cardiac arrest*
- Establish level of treatment appropriate for individual patient based on individual patient characteristics*
- (Consider a statement on supportive care, e.g. oxygen)

*These decisions should be taken by the responsible senior clinician in charge of the patient. For further advice on these decisions see Chapter 3

- Perform relevant further investigations
- Initiate appropriate treatment
- Liaise with appropriate specialty
- Clearly document plan in notes and explain diagnosis and plan with the patient and their next of kin

Yes ← Patient fit for further investigation and treatment?

No

- Make plan for appropriate symptomatic relief
- Document clear plan in notes
- Discuss situation and diagnosis with patient and next of kin if possible and appropriate to do so

Figure 5.7 An overview of an approach to a patient presenting with chest pain.

reduces cardiac output and increases myocardial oxygen demand, risking ischaemia. Prolonged tachycardia can result in cardiomyopathy.

AF is classified according to its duration as in Table 5.3. Whilst the focus of this section is on the management of new onset AF or AF with a poorly controlled ventricular rate, knowledge of these terminologies is useful when planning further management and follow-up.

AF in an older patient differs from AF in younger patients in a number of ways (27):

- AF may present with atypical symptoms other than palpitations, and is often undiagnosed. Time of onset in new AF may not be clear.
- AF is more likely to be permanent or persistent (Table 5.3) due to other comorbidities or age-related changes to the heart (Chapter 6, Box 6.2). Rate control and anticoagulation is often the most appropriate long-term management in the older adult (28).
- Older patients have a higher risk of both thromboembolism and bleeding. Age is a major risk factor for stroke in patients with AF.

Table 5.4 Classification of atrial fibrillation (27).

Terminology	Clinical features	Pattern
Initial event (first detected episode)	Symptomatic or asymptomatic Time of onset may not be known	May or may not reoccur
Paroxysmal	Spontaneous termination <7 days and usually <48 h	Recurrent
Persistent	Not self-terminating Lasting >7 days or recurring after cardioversion	Recurrent
Permanent	Unsuccessful cardioversion or no cardioversion attempt	Established

- Older patients are more sensitive to pro-arrhythmic effects of drugs, drug interactions and drug toxicity due to decreased renal and hepatic function.
- Tachycardia is less well-tolerated and can lead to acute cardiac failure, myocardial ischaemia and syncope in acute or poorly controlled AF.

Background

Predisposing factors to AF are highlighted in Box 5.2. These factors may prevent restoration of sinus rhythm and lead to persistent or permanent AF.

Box 5.2 Predisposing factors to atrial fibrillation.

- Age-related changes to the myocardium and conduction pathways
- Left atrial enlargement, e.g. secondary to mitral valve disease or LV diastolic dysfunction
- Chronic lung disease
- Hyperthyroidism
- Alcohol excess
- Hypertension.

New onset AF may occur spontaneously, or in the presence of precipitating factors shown in Box 5.3.

Box 5.3 Possible AF precipitating factors.

- Sepsis
- Electrolyte abnormalities, e.g. hypokalaemia, hypocalcaemia, hypomagnesaemia
- Pulmonary embolus
- Acute cardiac failure
- Myocardial ischaemia
- Alcohol intoxification or withdrawal
- Thyrotoxicosis
- Anti-arrythmic toxicity, e.g. digoxin toxicity
- Recent surgery, especially cardiac surgery.

Initial assessment

In the patient presenting with AF with a ventricular rate over 110 bpm, conduct a rapid ABC assessment (29). Signs of haemodynamic instability (Box 5.4) should prompt urgent help from a senior clinician. Apply high flow oxygen, obtain intravenous access and attach cardiac monitoring.

Box 5.4 Features of haemodynamic compromise in AF.

- Symptoms of myocardial ischaemia, e.g. chest pain or tightness, ischaemia on ECG
- Hypotension, BP < 90 mmHg
- Acute cardiac failure
- A ventricular rate greater than 150 bpm
- Signs of end-organ failure or poor tissue perfusion, e.g. syncope or altered mental status, raised lactate, reduced urine output.

History and examination

AF has a wide spectrum of clinical presentations, and may be asymptomatic. Older patients with new onset, or poorly controlled AF, may present with dyspnoea, palpitations, chest pain, dizziness or syncope. Vague symptoms such as fatigue, delirium and reduced mobility may predominate. The patient may present with stroke or overt heart failure.

If there is a clear time of onset of *any* symptom, this should be noted.

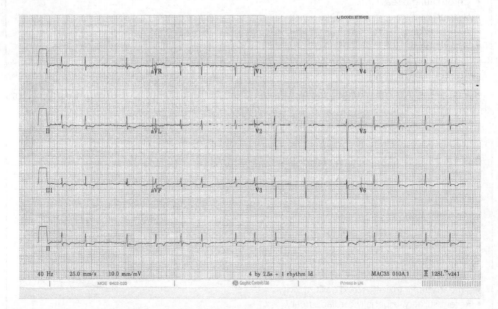

Figure 5.8 Rhythm strip demonstrating atrial fibrillation.

Examine for a precipitating cause of AF, as in Box 5.3, such as sepsis or myocardial infarction. Recent diarrhoea or vomiting or diuretic use may indicate electrolyte disturbance. Look for signs and symptoms of thyroid disease.

When considering anticoagulation, enquire about bleeding risk factors such as coagulopathy, liver failure, alcohol use, previous gastrointestinal bleeding or intracerebral haemorrhage. Consider factors in the past medical history affecting stroke risk such as previous stroke or TIA (transient ischemia attack), hypertension, diabetes or congestive cardiac failure.

Ask about drug allergies and any contraindications to beta-blockers such as asthma, COPD or peripheral vascular disease.

When examining peripheral pulses, be aware that the heart rate may be higher than the pulse rate due to reduced diastolic filling time in high ventricular rates, resulting in low stroke volumes that do not transmit a pulsation to the peripheries.

Investigations

ECG will reveal fibrillatory waves that vary in size and shape and are associated with an irregular ventricular response (Figure 5.8). There is an absence of consistent P waves. Ischaemic changes may be present.

Blood tests should include potassium, calcium, magnesium and thyroid function tests, along with a routine blood screen. In the ED, a venous blood gas may allow rapid identification of major abnormalities and lactate serves as a marker of tissue perfusion. Coagulation studies should be performed as anticoagulation may be required, and if the patient is already on anticoagulants, knowledge of the INR will be important. Cardiac enzymes including troponin may not be useful in distinguishing myocardial ischaemia as the cause rather than a consequence of the AF and should be interpreted with caution.

A *chest radiograph* may identify contributing pulmonary disease or signs of cardiac failure.

Echocardiography can be useful to evaluate for structural changes, such as a dilated left atrium or mitral valve disease, which may influence decisions regarding rate or rhythm control. Echo images will be of better quality if performed once the ventricular rate is controlled.

Transoesophageal echocardiogram may be considered in patients with an unknown onset of AF for whom cardioversion is being planned, in order to exclude atrial thrombi.

Management

The priorities in the management of new onset or poorly controlled AF are as follows:
1 Urgent assessment and treatment of haemodynamic compromise
2 Identify and treat any precipitating cause of the AF
3 Improve cardiac function by control of ventricular rate or restoration of sinus rhythm
4 Protect against thromboembolic events.

1. Haemodynamic compromise
Seek experienced help
A small number of patients will be significantly compromised by new onset or poorly controlled AF. If any of the features in Box 5.4 are present, inform a senior clinician and consult with cardiology. The patient should be managed in a high dependency environment such as the resuscitation room, or other high dependency area where resuscitation facilities are available.

Emergency treatment options for AF with haemodynamically instability include urgent DC cardioversion, pharmacological cardioversion or rate control (28). All these treatments are associated with potential complications.

In many cases, especially in the older patient, it can be difficult to distinguish between circulatory compromise due to the underlying cause of the AF (Box 5.4) and compromise due to the tachycardia. If the underlying cause, such as sepsis or cardiac failure, is responsible, then AF is much more likely to be recurrent even if cardioversion is briefly successful. In these cases, treatment of the underlying cause with careful monitoring of the ventricular rate may be an appropriate initial course of action.

KEY POINT: In cases of severe sepsis or cardiac failure, sedation for electrical cardioversion or negatively inotropic anti-arrhythmics may make the situation much worse. Seek experienced advice.

2. Identify and treat precipitating causes
Treating an underlying condition such as sepsis, hypovolaemia or electrolyte disturbance (Box 5.3) will often result in spontaneous cardioversion or reduced ventricular rate with no need for any further specific management.

3. Improve cardiac function by rhythm or rate control
The choice between acute restoration of sinus rhythm and control of the ventricular rate in a stable patient (i.e. with none of the features in Box 5.4) will depend on the likely duration of AF and the precipitating cause.

KEY POINT: Rate control of AF is often the most appropriate initial therapy in older patients.

Rate control
In patients with permanent AF, where the time of onset is not clear, or for whom sinus rhythm is unlikely to be achieved or maintained due to the presence of predisposing or precipitating factors, the aim should be to control the ventricular rate. Beta-blockers or non-dihydropyridine calcium channel blockers are recommended as first-line agents. They can be given intravenously or orally, depending on the desired speed of action. Digoxin is still considered useful, particularly in older patients with contraindications to beta-blocker therapy, and in patients with cardiac failure, although effective rate control may take 12 hours or longer (27).

KEY POINT: In the acute setting, the target ventricular rate should be 110 bpm (28).

Intravenous amiodarone (see below) may also be used for rate control, particularly in patients with severely depressed LV function. Drug combinations should be used cautiously in the older patient due to the risk of causing conduction blockade.

Rhythm control

Restoration of sinus rhythm may be attempted in older patients with a clear history of AF of <48 hours duration and in whom precipitating causes have been excluded or adequately treated. This may be performed using electrical or pharmacological cardioversion, or a combination of both.

DC cardioversion

Synchronised electrical cardioversion is an effective method of converting AF to sinus rhythm, with a success rate of 90% in the absence of untreated precipitating causes (30). The procedure should be undertaken under sedation unless life-threatening circulatory collapse is present. This will typically be performed in the resuscitation room of the ED, coronary care or intensive care unit, with appropriately experienced personnel present (See Chapter 12 for a discussion on procedural sedation in the older patient). In the older patient, however, DC cardioversion is less commonly used, due to the risks of sedation or anaesthesia combined with a higher probability of AF recurrence. There is a 1–2% risk of thromboembolism without prior anticoagulation when performed within 48 hours of suspected AF onset (31). In patients with structural heart disease, prolonged sinus arrest without an adequate escape rhythm may occur due to sinus node dysfunction (30).

Pharmacological cardioversion

A number of different anti-arrhythmics may facilitate cardioversion. Extreme caution is necessary in the older patient, however, due to increased risk of drug side effects and interactions. Drugs such as propafenone, ibutilide and flecainide should be avoided in patients with abnormal LV function and ischaemic heart disease. Amiodarone may be the safest option in the older patient but can cause hypotension and severe thrombophlebitis. The initial dose may be given via a large bore cannula but a subsequent infusion should be given via a midline or central line.

4. Preventing thromboembolism

In the presence of life-threatening haemodynamic instability, initiation of anticoagulation should not delay emergency DC cardioversion.

Patients presenting with acute AF who are not already on oral anticoagulation, in the absence of contraindications, should receive a therapeutic dose low-molecular-weight heparin or an intravenous infusion of unfractionated heparin. Patients who have sub-therapeutic levels of oral anticoagulants should also receive additional thromboprophylaxis. Local guidelines should be consulted.

Further management

After initial stabilisation, the decision should be made whether to pursue a long-term strategy of rate or rhythm control and whether to start oral anticoagulation. These decisions will depend on the patient's wishes, individual circumstances and past medical history, and should involve a cardiologist, geriatrician or the patient's primary care provider who can provide appropriate follow-up. Risk stratification rules such as the CHA2DS2Vasc score can be invaluable decision aids for making these decisions (see Chapter 19).

Rate control and rhythm control strategies are associated with equivalent mortality and quality of life outcomes and the same rate of thromboembolic events (32). Patients assigned to rhythm control have more hospitalisations from cardiovascular events, and more serious adverse effects from medications (32). Older adults are more likely to develop persistent or permanent AF due to the predisposing factors mentioned in Box 5.2, and therefore, rate control is usually the most appropriate strategy. The target ventricular rate should be 110 bpm in new onset AF (28, 30). Consider stricter rate control, e.g. <90 bpm, if symptoms persist or tachycardiomyopathy occurs. In other cases, lenient rate control (<110 bpm) has been shown to be as effective as strict rate control (28, 33). Oral anticoagulation is recommended for all patients with AF in the presence of significant valvular heart disease or prosthetic heart valves. Generally speaking, in the older patients with non-valvular AF, the overall net clinical benefit favours anticoagulation. The advent of alterative oral anticoagulants such as direct thrombin inhibitors and factor Xa inhibitors may improve the safety of anticoagulation in the older patient with AF. See Chapter 19 for further discussion.

Take home messages

- Older patients presenting with chest pain require a thorough and systematic history and examination to avoid overlooking life-threatening causes
- Diagnosis of life-threatening causes of chest pain in the older patient is more likely to be delayed due to staff and patient factors, so a high level of suspicion is necessary to avoid missing serious underlying conditions
- The incidence and mortality of ACS, PE and aortic dissection increase with age
- Older patients with life-threatening causes of chest pain require expert assessment by the appropriate specialists as soon as possible
- Therapies exist which confer significant survival benefit in older patients, and invasive investigation and aggressive management should be decided on the basis of individual benefit and not chronological age
- Assessment, investigation and management of older patients with multiple comorbidity presenting with chest pain is complex and senior involvement should be sought early
- Atrial fibrillation is common in the older patient and management decisions can be difficult. The key aspects of treatment include recognising haemodynamic compromise, identifying and treating underlying causes, deciding on rhythm or rate control strategies and preventing thromboembolism.

References

1 Kelly BS. Evaluation of the elderly patient with acute chest pain. *Clin Geriatr Med*. 2007;23(2): 327–349, vi.

2 Tresch DD, Brady WJ, Aufderheide TP, Lawrence SW, Williams KJ. Comparison of elderly and younger patients with out-of-hospital chest pain. Clinical characteristics, acute myocardial infarction, therapy, and outcomes. *Arch Intern Med*. 1996;156(10):1089–1093.

3 Corsini F, Scaglione A, Iacomino M, Mascia G, Melorio S, Riccio C, et al. Acute myocardial infarction in the elderly. A case–control study with a younger population and review of literature. (abstract only). *Monaldi Arch Chest Dis*. 2006;66(1):13–19.

4 Brieger D, Eagle KA, Goodman SG, Steg PG, Budaj A, White K, et al. Acute coronary syndromes without chest pain, an underdiagnosed and undertreated high-risk group: insights from the Global Registry of Acute Coronary Events. *Chest*. 2004;126(2):461–469.

5 Stein PD, Beemath A, Matta F, Weg JG, Yusen RD, Hales CA, et al. Clinical characteristics of patients with acute pulmonary embolism. *Am J Med*. 2007;120(10):871–879.

6 Miniati M, Cenci C, Monti S, Poli D. Clinical presentation of acute pulmonary embolism: survey of 800 cases. PLoS ONE. 2012;7(2). http://www.ncbi.nlm.nih.gov/pmc/articles/PMC3288010/ [cited 2013 Sep 14].

7 Berman AR. Pulmonary embolism in the elderly. *Clin Geriatr Med*. 2001;17(1):107–130.

8 Timmons S, Kingston M, Hussain M, Kelly H, Liston R. Pulmonary embolism: differences in presentation between older and younger patients. *Age Ageing*. 2003;32(6):601–605.

9 Masotti L, Ray P, Righini M, Le Gal G, Antonelli F, Landini G, et al. Pulmonary embolism in the elderly: a review on clinical, instrumental and laboratory presentation. *Vasc Health Risk Manag*. 2008; 4(3):629–636.

10 Mehta RH, O'Gara PT, Bossone E, Nienaber CA, Myrmel T, Cooper JV, et al. Acute type A aortic dissection in the elderly: clinical characteristics, management, and outcomes in the current era. *J Am Coll Cardiol*. 2002;40(4):685–692.

11 National Institute for Health and Care Excellence (NICE). *CG95 Chest Pain of Recent Onset: NICE Guideline*. http://www.nice.org.uk/ [cited 2014 May 18].

12 Imperato J, Sanchez LD. Pulmonary emergencies in the elderly. *Emerg Med Clin North Am*. 2006;24(2):317–338, vi.

13 National Institute for Health and Care Excellence (NICE). *Diagnosis and Management of Venous Thromboembolic Diseases*. http://www.nice.org.uk/ [cited 2013 Jul 10].

14 Erbel R, Alfonso F, Boileau C, Dirsch O, Eber B, Haverich A, et al. Diagnosis and management of aortic dissection. *Eur Heart J*. 2001;22(18):1642–1681.

15 Alexander KP, Newby LK, Cannon CP, Armstrong PW, Gibler WB, Rich MW, et al. Acute coronary care in the elderly, part I non-ST-segment–elevation acute coronary syndromes: a scientific statement for healthcare professionals from the American heart association council on clinical cardiology: in collaboration with the society of geriatric cardiology. *Circulation*. 2007;115(19):2549–2569.

16 Thygesen K, Alpert JS, White HD. Universal definition of myocardial infarction. *J Am Coll Cardiol*. 2007;50(22):2173–2195.

17 Subherwal S, Peterson ED, Chen AY, Roe MT, Washam JB, Gage BF, et al. Admission international normalized ratio levels, early treatment strategies, and major bleeding risk among non-ST-segment-elevation myocardial infarction patients on home warfarin therapy: insights from the National Cardiovascular Data Registry.*Circulation*. 2012;125(11):1414–1423.

18 Dewilde WJ, Oirbans T, Verheugt FW, Kelder JC, De Smet BJ, Herrman J-P, et al. Use of clopidogrel with or without aspirin in patients taking oral anticoagulant therapy and undergoing percutaneous coronary intervention: an open-label, randomised, controlled trial. *The Lancet*. 2013;381(9872):1107–1115.

19 Henriksen PA, Palmer K, Boon NA. Management of upper gastrointestinal haemorrhage complicating dual anti-platelet therapy. *QJM*. 2008;101(4):261–267.

20 Mukherjee D. Management of refractory angina in the contemporary era. *Eur Heart J*. 2013;34(34): 2655–2657.

21 Henry TD, Satran D, Hodges JS, Johnson RK, Poulose AK, Campbell AR, et al. Long-term survival in patients with refractory angina. *Eur Heart J*. 2013;34(34):2683-2688.

22 De Bonis S, Rendina D, Vargas G, Minno DD, Piedimonte V, Gallotta G, et al. Predictors of in-hospital and long-term clinical outcome in elderly patients with massive pulmonary embolism receiving thrombolytic therapy. *J Am Geriatr Soc*. 2008;56(12):2273–2277.

23 Spirk D, Husmann M, Hayoz D, Baldi T, Frauchiger B, Engelberger R, et al. Predictors of in-hospital mortality in elderly patients with acute venous thrombo-embolism: the SWIss Venous Thrombo Embolism Registry (SWIVTER). *Eur Heart J*. 2012;33(7):921–926.

24 National Institute for Health and Care Excellence (NICE). *CG68 Stroke: Quick Reference Guide*. http://www.nice.org.uk/ [cited 2014 Feb 11].

25 Yanagisawa S, Yuasa T, Suzuki N, Hirai T, Yasuda N, Miki K, et al. Comparison of medically versus surgically treated acute type A aortic dissection in patients <80 years old versus patients ≥80 years old. *Am J Cardiol*. 2011;108(3):453–459.

26 Santini F, Mazzucco A. Aortic dissection in the elderly: still an unsolved issue requiring rigorous methodology. *J Card Surg*. 2009;24(1):99–100.

27 Camm AJ, Kirchhof P, Lip GYH, Schotten U, Savelieva I, Ernst S, et al. Guidelines for the management of atrial fibrillation: the task force for the management of atrial fibrillation of the European Society of Cardiology (ESC). *Europace*. 2010;12(10):1360–1420.

28 Atrial Fibrillation: National clinical guideline for management in primary and secondary care. National Institute for Health and Clinical Excellence. National Collaborating Centre for Chronic Conditions (UK). London; 2006.

29 Beck H, See VY. Acute management of atrial fibrillation: from emergency department to cardiac care unit. *Cardiol Clin*. 2012;30(4):567–589.

30 Camm AJ, Kirchhof P, Lip GYH, Schotten U, Savelieva I, Ernst S, et al. Guidelines for the management of atrial fibrillation: the task force for the management of atrial fibrillation of the European Society of Cardiology (ESC). *Eur Heart J*. 2010;31(19):2369–2429.

31 Weigner MJ, Caulfield TA, Danias PG, Silverman DI, Manning WJ. Risk for clinical thromboembolism associated with conversion to sinus rhythm in patients with atrial fibrillation lasting less than 48 hours. *Ann Intern Med*. 1997;126(8):615–620.

32 Chen J. Atrial fibrillation and atrial flutter: medical management. *Clin Geriatr Med*. 2012;28(4): 635–647.

33 Van Gelder IC, Groenveld HF, Crijns HJGM, Tuininga YS, Tijssen JGP, Alings AM, et al. Lenient versus strict rate control in patients with atrial fibrillation. *N Engl J Med*. 2010;362(15):1363–1373.

CHAPTER 6
Dyspnoea

Introduction

Acute dyspnoea is a common presenting symptom in older adults and, in contrast to the younger patient, is usually multifactorial in aetiology. Dyspnoea in older patients can be mistakenly attributed to normal ageing, which may result in a delay in presentation and diagnosis (1).

This chapter will provide guidance on the challenges that older age can pose for clinicians managing emergency presentations of obstructive airways disease, end-stage lung disease and cardiac failure. Management of pulmonary embolism and pneumonia are covered in Chapters 5 and 7 respectively.

Definition

Dyspnoea is defined by the American Thoracic Society as a 'subjective experience of breathing discomfort, often derived from the interplay between physiological, psychological, social and environmental factors' (2). Pathological dyspnoea occurs when increased effort in the act of breathing is experienced at rest, or with physical activity that is usually well-tolerated (3). Dyspnoea can be a frightening and distressing symptom.

Background

The sensation of dyspnoea is mediated by detection of hypoxaemia, hypercapnia, irritation and inflammation in the bronchi by chemoreceptors, mechanoreceptors and lung receptors. Age-related changes in the respiratory system (Box 6.1) lead to a functional deterioration, even in the absence of respiratory disease. The consequences of these changes include an increased susceptibility to infection, less capacity of the respiratory system to compensate for increased tissue oxygen demands and a higher likelihood of developing respiratory failure.

Geriatric Emergencies, First Edition.
Iona Murdoch, Sarah Turpin, Bree Johnston, Alasdair MacLullich and Eve Losman.
© 2015 John Wiley & Sons, Ltd. Published 2015 by John Wiley & Sons, Ltd.

> **Box 6.1** Changes in pulmonary structure and function with older age (3).
>
> | | | |
> |---|---|---|
> | *Reduced respiratory muscle mass* more susceptible to fatigue. Increased reliance on diaphragm and abdominal muscles for breathing | *Decreased elastic recoil and size of small airways* resulting in increased airflow resistance, small airways collapse and gas trapping | *Reduced response to hypoxic or hypercapnic stimuli* due to impaired chemoreceptor function |
> | *Reduced chest wall compliance* due to kyphoscoliosis and degeneration of intercostal and costovertebral joints | *Rise in alveolar-arterial (A-a) oxygen gradient* due to impaired gas exchange and increased ventilation-perfusion mismatch | *Reduced cough effectiveness and compromised mucociliary clearance* |

Despite these changes, the age-related changes in the cardiovascular system generally contribute a greater amount to reduced physiological reserve than do changes in the pulmonary system.

> **Box 6.2** Changes in cardiac structure and function with older age.
>
> | | | |
> |---|---|---|
> | *Decline in maximum heart rate and impaired myocardial contractility in response to β-adrenergic stimulation* | *Fibrosis of sinoatrial node, AV node and conducting system* AV block and bundle branch blocks are more common | *Hypertension* causes LV hypertrophy and increased cardiac filling pressures leading to *diastolic dysfunction* |
> | Reduced ability to increase cardiac output. Tachycardia may be absent in acute illness | | |
> | *Increase in left atrial size* due to an increased LV end-diastolic pressure. Predisposition to atrial fibrillation | *Proximal arteries become* thickened and stiffer resulting in *increasing systolic blood pressure* with age | *Impairments in LV diastolic relaxation and compliance* also occur due to increased interstitial collagen content and myocyte hypertrophy |

Initial assessment

The patient may present in extremis, requiring urgent intervention. Here, conduct a rapid primary survey to assess severity and call for senior or critical care help early.

KEY POINT: Acute dyspnoea can be a terrifying experience, and symptoms are compounded by adrenergic drive. Reassurance is essential. Consider titrating small doses of intravenous opioid to relieve distress, with caution (Box 6.9).

Box 6.3 Differential diagnosis of dyspnoea in the older patient.

Pulmonary	*Cardiovascular*	*Neurological*
Pneumonia	Acute myocardial infarction	Neuromuscular disease
Aspiration	Acute cardiac failure	Myasthenia gravis
Pulmonary embolus	Arrhythmia	Guillain–Barre syndrome
Pleural effusion	Pericardial effusion	
Chronic obstructive pulmonary disease		
Asthma		
Non-cardiogenic pulmonary oedema	*Haematological*	*Metabolic*
	Anaemia	Acidosis
Pulmonary malignancy		Sepsis
Pneumothorax	*Upper airway obstruction*	*Psychological*
Tuberculosis	Angiooedema	Anxiety
Chest trauma	Foreign body	Hyperventilation

History

Given the extensive differential diagnosis for dyspnoea in the older adult (Box 6.3), a detailed patient history is vital to exploring and excluding different contributory factors. However, many patients with dyspnoea are unable to provide a comprehensive history until their symptoms are urgently addressed. Bear in mind that older adults often have multiple pathologies contributing to dyspnoea and it is less common for symptoms to fit into one single diagnosis.

 KEY POINT: Dyspnoea is the commonest presenting symptom of acute myocardial infarction in patients aged 75 years and over.

Onset

Timing of symptom onset may help towards diagnosing the cause of dyspnoea. Table 6.1 illustrates some causes of acute dyspnoea and typical associated timings. Note though that atypical presentations are common in the older patient. Dyspnoea of rapid onset, within seconds to minutes, is more likely to be potentially life-threatening.

Comparison with baseline symptoms

The severity of any baseline dyspnoea, including usual maximum exercise tolerance (e.g. the distance the patient can walk on flat ground) should be established. The patient should be asked specifically about the timescale and severity of change in exercise tolerance and impaired ability to perform activities of daily living.

Table 6.1 Causes of acute dyspnoea according to typical timing of symptom onset.

Rapid onset (seconds to minutes)	More gradual deterioration (hours to days)
Acute pulmonary embolism	Pneumonia
Acute coronary syndrome (ACS)	Acute cardiac failure
ACS with interventricular septum rupture,	Exacerbation of COPD or asthma
mitral valve chordae rupture or right	Anaemia
ventricular infarction	Acute kidney injury or worsening chronic
Tachyarrhythmia or severe bradycardia	renal failure
Cardiac tamponade	Poor concordance with drug therapy or
Aortic dissection	fluid restriction
Aspiration	Drug interaction or intolerance, e.g.
Pneumothorax	NSAIDs
Hypertensive crisis	Poorly controlled arrhythmia, e.g. atrial
Fluid overload (usually due to intravenous	fibrillation
fluids)	Uncontrolled hypertension
	Worsening valvular heart disease, e.g.
	aortic stenosis

NSAID, non-steroidal anti-inflammatory drug.

Associated symptoms

Cough, sputum, haemoptysis or fever may indicate pneumonia. Chest pain, palpitations and diaphoresis may indicate acute myocardial infarction, pulmonary embolus or cardiac arrhythmia. Peripheral oedema, paroxysmal nocturnal dyspnoea or orthopnoea suggests cardiac failure.

Previous episodes

Many patients with chronic lung or heart disease will have recurrent presentations with acute exacerbations. Information should be gathered about previous admissions, such as investigations undertaken, treatments provided and requirements for non-invasive ventilation (NIV) or critical care admission. Historical patient records detailing previous arterial blood gas results and ECGs or the results of a recent echocardiogram, high-resolution CT chest or coronary angiogram may prove useful in deciding appropriate treatment.

Past medical history

Comorbidities such as depression and anxiety, chronic kidney disease, osteoporosis and diabetes are common and complicate treatment and increase mortality.

Drug history

A recent change in medication may have precipitated the current presentation, for example, oral or topical β-blocker therapy may trigger an exacerbation of asthma or COPD (chronic obstructive pulmonary disease). Patients on long-term home oxygen or home nebulisers should be identified, as a much lower threshold for admission in these patients is appropriate. Assess concordance with medication, home oxygen therapy, or fluid or salt restriction.

Social history
Many older patients may have a significant passive smoking history despite being 'non-smokers' due to their home or previous working environment. A history of occupational dust, chemical or asbestos exposure, pets, living environment and foreign travel may be relevant.

Systemic enquiry
Weakness, fatigue, weight loss, poor sleep or functional decline may predominate, instead of specific respiratory or cardiovascular symptoms.

Asthma in older patients

Older age onset asthma more closely resembles COPD. It is rarely IgE-mediated, is less likely to have atopic triggers and demonstrates less reversibility with bronchodilators. It tends to be associated with gradually progressive irreversible airways obstruction (4).

> KEY POINT: Asthma is underdiagnosed in older persons, with a prevalence of 7–9% in patients over the age of 70 years (5). It carries a high mortality: two-thirds of deaths attributed to asthma occur in people aged 65 years or older (6).

COPD in older patients

Older adults with an acute exacerbation of chronic obstructive pulmonary disease (AECOPD) may present with a disturbance in daily function and mental status rather than the classical triad of increased dyspnoea and sputum volume and a change in sputum purulence seen in younger patients. Weight loss in COPD may be primarily due to the metabolic demands of an increased respiratory effort, combined with poor nutrition. Patients with COPD, however, are at increased risk of lung malignancy, and symptoms such as chest pain or haemoptysis may necessitate further investigation. Malignancy is the most common cause of death in patients with mild COPD.

Cardiac failure

Symptoms found to correlate most frequently with acute heart failure include paroxysmal nocturnal dyspnoea, orthopnoea and exertional dyspnoea. Other non-specific symptoms may include ankle swelling, bloating, syncope, nocturnal cough, weight gain, fatigue and low mood.

Examination

General examination

If the patient appears critically unwell, a rapid ABCDE assessment should take place with senior help requested early. Provide reassurance and sit the patient upright in a comfortable position.

Box 6.4 ABCDE examination of an acutely breathless patient.

Airway	Ensure the airway is patent. Provide high-flow oxygen in the first instance
Breathing	Assess respiratory rate, depth and use of accessory muscles. Assess the ability of the patient to talk. Record oxygen saturations. Listen for stridor and look for signs of upper airway swelling or obstruction. Expose the chest and assess degree and symmetry of chest expansion. Auscultate the chest for air entry and crackles or wheeze
Circulation	Measure heart rate and blood pressure and connect an ECG monitor. Note whether the pulse is regular or irregular. Secure venous access. If there is evidence of sepsis, take blood cultures before administering intravenous antibiotics. Look for peripheral and sacral oedema.
Disability	Perform an AVPU (alert, voice, pain, unresponsive) assessment. Assess for altered mental state. Note pupil size and check blood glucose
Exposure	Once points A to D have been assessed and any urgent treatment instigated, record temperature and examine the patient fully. Tachypnoea may be due to respiratory compensation for a metabolic acidosis, for example due to peritonitis or limb ischaemia, which may not have been revealed in the history. Severe anaemia may cause tachypnoea, and a cause of this such as an abdominal mass may be evident. Examine the legs for signs of deep vein thrombosis

---

Specific areas of focus on examination

In chronic obstructive airways disease

Observe for evidence of a prolonged expiratory phase, pursed-lip breathing and use of accessory muscles or subcostal recession; the chest is commonly hyperinflated and 'barrel-shaped'. A tracheal tug with reduced cricosternal distance may be visible. On examination, there may be a hyperresonant percussion note and reduced air entry bilaterally.

In severe COPD, pulmonary artery hypertension may develop, leading to right ventricular enlargement and right heart failure – 'cor pulmonale'. Signs of cor pulmonale include jugular venous distension, tender hepatomegaly and peripheral oedema.

In cardiac failure

An elevated jugular venous pressure, third heart sound, cardiac murmur and signs of cardiomegaly such as displacement of the apical impulse are more specific signs suggestive of cardiac failure.

Left-sided heart failure is characterised by pulmonary congestion and systemic hypoperfusion and results in lung crepitations or wheeze. Right-sided heart failure causes systemic congestion leading to findings of raised jugular venous pressure, peripheral and sacral oedema, ascites and hepatomegaly. Older patients most commonly have biventricular failure and therefore display a mixture of signs of left and right heart failure. Examine for potential precipitating factors.

Investigations

Initial investigations
Blood tests
FBC (full blood count), U&E (urea and electrolytes), inflammatory markers, liver function tests and calcium.

Arterial blood gases (ABG)
An ABG should be taken if hypercapnoea or hypoxia is suspected, or if oxygen saturations are less than 94%, according to British Thoracic Society guidelines (7).

Chest radiograph
A chest radiograph may provide vital diagnostic information in cases such as acute pulmonary oedema or lobar consolidation, but can have reduced sensitivity and specificity in older patients. Comparison with previous films to assess whether abnormalities are longstanding is useful. Figures 6.1 and 6.2 illustrate hyperinflation and pulmonary oedema, respectively.

12 lead ECG
The ECG may reveal signs of acute ischaemia, such as ST elevation or new bundle branch block; an arrhythmia such as atrial fibrillation; or right heart strain in the case of pulmonary embolus or chronic pulmonary disease. A previous ECG, if available, may help determine whether any abnormalities are new. A completely normal ECG makes the diagnosis of heart failure unlikely.

Further investigations
If cardiac failure is suspected
Additional blood tests
An appropriately timed troponin, B-type natriuretic peptide (BNP) level and thyroid function tests may be required.

Echocardiography
Echocardiography will help establish the degree and type of ventricular dysfunction, estimate ejection fraction and identify valve disease. It may demonstrate other causes of acute cardiac failure (as in Table 6.1).

Other investigations will depend on the likely cause of cardiac failure and any interventions that are being considered. These may include coronary angiography, myocardial perfusion imaging or cardiac magnetic resonance imaging.

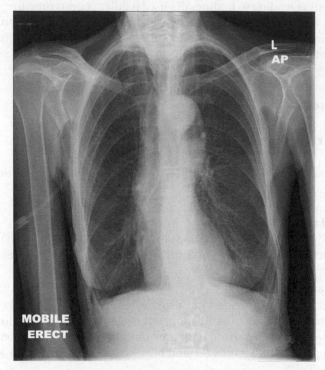

Figure 6.1 Hyperinflated lungs in chronic obstructive pulmonary disease.

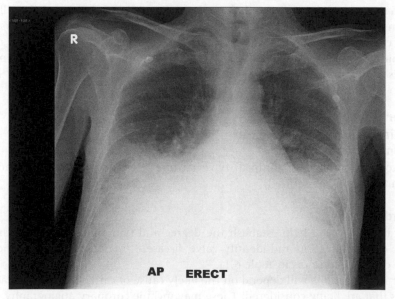

Figure 6.2 Acute pulmonary oedema.

KEY POINT: The prevalence of diastolic dysfunction rises in the older population with a history of chronic hypertension (8). Over half of patients with heart failure over 70 years old have a preserved left ventricular systolic function on echocardiography (9). The distinction between systolic and diastolic failure may not alter acute management, but has implications for prognosis and ongoing management.

If an exacerbation of asthma or COPD is suspected
Additional blood tests
Check theophylline levels in patients taking theophylline-containing medications.

Blood cultures
Blood cultures should be taken if there is clinical suspicion of infection (e.g. a history of rigors, or high or low temperature). Consider sending sputum samples for microscopy and culture if an atypical organism is suspected or the patient is not responding to treatment.

Peak expiratory flow measurements
They are useful in younger asthmatics, but are of limited use in older patients who may have difficulty using the peak flow meter due to reduced manual dexterity and coordination.

Bedside ultrasound
This is increasingly undertaken by Emergency Physicians and may identify respiratory and cardiac conditions such as pneumothoraces, pleural and pericardial effusions, consolidation or right ventricular dilatation in acute massive PE.

Management

Management of the dyspnoeic patient will depend on the likely aetiology or aetiologies. Acute dyspnoea is a frightening sensation and reassuring the patient is important.

Oxygen
In patients with acute respiratory distress, high flow oxygen should be applied whilst the initial assessment is being undertaken.

Oxygen therapy may lead to carbon dioxide retention and respiratory acidosis in some COPD patients. Clinically, this may be manifest by the patient becoming drowsy and/or delirious. In known or suspected COPD, oxygen should be provided via a fixed rate delivery device (e.g. Venturi mask) to target an oxygen saturation of 88–92% (7). In other patients, oxygen should be provided to maintain saturation of 94–98%.

The patient should be closely monitored following initiation of oxygen therapy and repeat arterial blood gas measurements taken if necessary.

KEY POINT: Oxygen is a treatment for hypoxaemia, not breathlessness (7).

Management of suspected exacerbation of COPD and asthma

Box 6.5 Treatments to consider in obstructive airway disease in the older patient.

Bronchodilators	Be aware that systemic complications from nebulised beta 2 agonists are increased in older patients and include tachyarrhythmias, hypertension, hypokalaemia and headache
Systemic corticosteroids	A short course of steroids is often advocated for an exacerbation of obstructive airways disease. However, side effects include delirium, disrupted glycaemic control, peptic ulceration and a risk of osteoporosis and adrenal insufficiency in frequent or prolonged courses
Antibiotics	Worsening dyspnoea with increased sputum purulence often indicates infection, and antibiotic therapy should be considered. Antibiotic choice will depend on illness severity, previously documented sputum pathogens and local resistance patterns. Local microbiology guidance should be followed. Viral infections are common and viral swabs should be sent if viral infection is suspected. *Haemophilus Influenza* accounts for 30–70% of all exacerbations, along with *Streptococcus pneumonia* and *Moraxella catarrhalis*. Consider that older patients have greater risk of infection with multi-resistant and gram-negative organisms
Intravenous magnesium, IV beta 2 agonists or IV theophylline	Although lacking in evidence base, these treatments should be considered in severe obstructive airways disease unresponsive to initial treatment. Serious effects and the potential for drug interactions may limit use in older patients
Chest physiotherapy	May assist with sputum clearance and relieve distressing symptoms

---

Type 2 respiratory failure in older patients

Older patients with COPD are at increased risk of developing respiratory failure, as a result of limited reserve, loss of muscle mass, nutritional deficiencies and associated comorbidities.

Non-invasive ventilation (NIV)

NIV should be considered in AECOPD with persistent hypercapnic respiratory failure despite optimal medical therapy. NIV may reduce the need for endotracheal intubation, decrease mortality and shorten duration of hospital stay. Patients started on NIV should have a clearly documented plan covering ceilings of therapy and actions in the event of deterioration. See Chapter 3 for further discussion.

Older patients are more likely to develop nasal pressure injuries during use of a tight-fitting NIV mask. The present of delirium or dementia may make compliance with NIV more difficult. Requirement for NIV is generally associated with a poor prognosis: survival at 2 and 5 years was 52% and 26%, respectively, in one study (10).

Contraindications for NIV in older patients include those who should proceed immediately to invasive ventilation, vomiting, excess secretions, recent oesophageal surgery and those in whom palliative treatment should be the prime focus.

Invasive ventilation

Intubation and mechanical ventilation should be considered if NIV is contraindicated, poorly tolerated or unsuccessful in improving hypoxaemia or hypercapnia. Invasive ventilation in AECOPD is associated with a risk of ventilator-associated pneumonia and failure to wean from the ventilator. Clinicians may be overly negative when approaching this decision; however, and age alone is not a reliable predictor of survival for COPD patients undergoing mechanical ventilation (11). Patients mechanically ventilated with an acute exacerbation of COPD have been shown to have a lower mortality rate than patients receiving mechanical ventilation due to respiratory failure of another aetiology (12). A subset of older patients with a reversible cause of deterioration may benefit from a short period of mechanical ventilation (13).

Factors to consider when contemplating intubation and ventilation include the patient's wishes, previous functional status, comorbidities, body mass index, long-term oxygen therapy and previous ICU admissions. Further discussion on intensive care treatment in the older patient can be found in Chapter 3.

Recurrent presentations with COPD 'the revolving door patient'

Older age in COPD is an independent risk factor for acute exacerbations and hospitalisation. Frequent exacerbations are associated with a more rapid decline in lung function and a substantially poorer quality of life (14).

AECOPD is a frequent presentation in older patients, and many hospitals have tried to reduce admission rates by encouraging community-based or 'hospital at home' schemes. In certain circumstances as in Box 6.6, hospitalisation is recommended.

Box 6.6 Factors indicating a need for hospital admission in exacerbation of COPD.

History	*Examination*	*Functional status*
• Significant comorbidity – particularly cardiac failure and insulin-dependent diabetes	• Severe breathlessness • Cyanosis • Worsening peripheral oedema	• Poor or deteriorating general condition • Limited mobility or bedbound
• Long-term oxygen therapy		• Unable to cope at home
Investigation results	*Mental status*	
• Arterial pH <7.35 • Arterial PaO$_2$ <7 kPa • Changes on CXR	• Impaired level of consciousness • Delirium	

Source: Adapted from NICE guidelines (15).

Discharging older patients with COPD

When considering discharging patients from the emergency department, consider the factors outlined in Chapter 2. In patients with COPD, important additional points include:

- *Check inhaler technique*: Impaired inhaler technique in the older patient may result from impaired cognitive function, impaired vision and fine motor skills, and decreased inspiratory flow generation. Try an alternative device or a spacer.
- *Immunisations*: Ensure pneumococcal and annual influenza vaccines have been given.
- *Smoking cessation*: Even in advanced years, the potential benefits of stopping smoking are well-established. Care should be taken with nicotine replacement therapy or pharmacotherapy in older patients due to potential drug interactions or other side effects.
- *Optimise medication*, which in some cases may mean simplifying medication regime. Consider also whether home oxygen may be indicated.
- *Pulmonary rehabilitation* may improve function and quality of life.

Management of end-stage lung disease

Lung diseases such as COPD and pulmonary fibrosis cause a progressive decline in lung function. Historically, these patients received poor palliative care provision due to the unpredictable course of deterioration compared to malignant disease.

There is now a greater awareness of the needs of this patient population; however, identification of those with advanced lung disease is a key part of this process. Box 6.7 illustrates features suggestive of end-stage lung disease.

Box 6.7 Features suggestive of advanced lung disease

- Cachexia and low body mass index. Poor or deteriorating performance status.
- Increased hospital admissions for infective exacerbations or respiratory failure.
- Severe airways obstruction or restrictive deficit (FEV1 < 30%; vital capacity < 60%)
- Persistent hypoxia (PaO_2 < 7.3 kPa), on long-term oxygen therapy.
- Persistent, severe symptoms despite optimal treatment.
- Breathlessness limiting daily activities between exacerbations, at rest or on minimal effort.
- Symptomatic right heart failure.

Patients with end-stage lung disease may present to an emergency department in the terminal stages of their illness. Dyspnoea is a frightening sensation for patients and their relatives, and they may seek urgent medical attention despite the most thorough community palliative care plan.

If it is clear that further treatment is not appropriate or would not be successful, the priority should be providing symptom management and comfort care. Careful discussion with the patient or their proxy decision maker should take place.

If there is time, hospice admission should be arranged. Box 6.8 highlights actions that can be of assistance in the emergency department. See Chapter 3 for more general information on palliative care emergencies.

Management of cardiac failure

The prevalence of heart failure increases with age and it is the most common reason for hospital admission in those aged over 65 years (16). Acute cardiac failure in the older patient is associated with a high inpatient mortality (17).

Box 6.8 End-of-life care in the emergency setting for patients with advanced lung disease.

- Support the patient in a comfortable position.
- Provide a flow of fresh air, e.g. open window or a fan.
- Keep the patient cool.
- Ensure mouth care and adequate hydration, avoiding fluid overload.
- Trial small amount of opioids, intravenously or subcutaneously if the patient is unable to take medication orally, to relieve symptoms of dyspnoea and cough.
- Providing oxygen may help alleviate other symptoms of hypoxia, but has not been shown to improve breathlessness.
- If increasing dyspnoea does not improve with opioids, benzodiazepines or tricyclic antidepressants may assist with symptoms of anxiety and panic.
- Glycopyrroneum or hyoscine subcutaneously can reduce respiratory secretions. Suctioning may cause more distress than benefit.
- Delirium is common in dying patients and should be screened for routinely. Small doses of antipsychotic drugs may help with psychotic symptoms or severe distress.

Acute cardiac failure in the older patient frequently presents with other co-existing diseases, making diagnosis and management more complex.

Acute pulmonary oedema

The aim in the management of acute pulmonary oedema is to relieve respiratory congestion and breathlessness, optimise cardiac output and identify and treat the likely precipitating cause. Specialist advice from cardiology should be sought, particularly in older patients whose presentation may be complicated by comorbidities.

Box 6.9 Treatments to consider in acute cardiac failure in the older patient (18).

High flow oxygen	May provide symptomatic benefit in hypoxic patients
Opioids	Small doses of opioids, e.g. morphine titrated in 1 mg increments may relieve distress, and help abate the adrenergic response which may be worsening symptoms. They should be avoided in patients who are drowsy. Consider giving an antiemetic simultaneously.
Non-invasive ventilation (NIV)	Continuous positive airways pressure (CPAP) decreases left ventricular afterload and reduces work of breathing. Early NIV may relieve dyspnoea and improve hypercarbia and acidosis, optimising oxygen delivery to vital organs. Contraindications include hypotension, vomiting and depressed consciousness
Vasodilators	Vasodilators such as nitroglycerine reduce preload and afterload and increase stroke volume. They should be avoided in patients with a systolic blood pressure of less than 110 mmHg and in aortic or mitral stenosis
Loop diuretics	Intravenous loop diuretics may provide symptomatic relief and relieve pulmonary congestion. Monitor the response carefully as diuresis may cause acute kidney injury, electrolyte disturbance and orthostatic hypotension, particularly in the older patient

In the patient with poorly controlled atrial fibrillation and acute cardiac failure, rate control with digoxin, amiodarone or other agents is often the most appropriate option (Chapter 5).

Initial treatment may not be effective and repeat drug doses are often required. Close monitoring of the patient's condition is required throughout, until stability is achieved. Specialist advice may be required.

Cardiac failure with acute or chronic kidney injury

Over 70% of older patients with acute decompensated cardiac failure experience a deterioration in renal function (19), likely due to a complex interplay of factors. Worsening renal function correlates with higher mortality in older patients with cardiac failure (20). Diuretics are less effective in the failing kidney, and high doses may be required, with the risk of further worsening renal function. An individual approach to managing the balance between pulmonary oedema and renal function is required, and specialist advice should be sought early.

In cases of acute kidney injury and severe cardiac failure where a clearly reversible cause of the deterioration is identified, referral to critical care for renal replacement therapy or inotropic support may be indicated (Chapter 3). In many patients, this may not be appropriate.

Prognosis

Patients with chronic cardiac failure can oscillate between good functional status and near-fatal exacerbations. Up to 50% of patients will be readmitted within just 3–6 months of discharge from hospital due to decompensated heart failure. Prognosis may be difficult to predict, but advanced care planning and palliative care provision should be arranged for those with adverse features.

Take home messages

- Dyspnoea is a distressing symptom and significantly impacts the quality of life in community dwelling, hospitalised and dying patients
- Dyspnoea is the presenting symptom in many systemic diseases in older patients; it is frequently multi-factorial, and requires careful assessment
- Patients with airways disease and cardiac failure require multidisciplinary input in primary and secondary care to maintain function, reduce readmission rates and prevent rapid decline
- Increasing numbers of patients are dying of end-stage lung disease and may present to the Emergency Department requiring palliation of their symptoms
- Cardiac failure in older patients has a high mortality, and management strategies may be complicated by other comorbidities, especially renal failure.

References

1 Imperato J, Sanchez LD. Pulmonary emergencies in the elderly. *Emerg Med Clin North Am.* 2006;24(2):317–338, vi.

2 Parshall MB, Schwartzstein RM, Adams L, Banzett RB, Manning HL, Bourbeau J, et al. An official American Thoracic Society statement: update on the mechanisms, assessment, and management of dyspnea. *Am J Respir Crit Care Med*. 2012;185(4):435–452.

3 Torres M, Moayedi S. Evaluation of the acutely dyspneic elderly patient. *Clin Geriatr Med*. 2007;23(2):307–325, vi.

4 Reed CE. Asthma in the elderly: diagnosis and management. *J Allergy Clin Immunol*. 2010;126(4): 681–687; quiz 688–689.

5 Braman SS. Asthma in the elderly. *Clin Geriatr Med*. 2003;19(1):57–75.

6 Gibson PG, McDonald VM, Marks GB. Asthma in older adults. *Lancet*. 2010;376(9743):803–813.

7 O'Driscoll BR, Howard LS, Davison AG. BTS guideline for emergency oxygen use in adult patients. *Thorax*. 2008;63 Suppl 6(October):vi1–vi68.

8 McDonald K. Diastolic heart failure in the elderly: underlying mechanisms and clinical relevance. *Int J Cardiol*. 2008;125(2):197–202.

9 Thomas S, Rich MW. Epidemiology, pathophysiology, and prognosis of heart failure in the elderly. *Clin Geriatr Med*. 2007;23(1):1–10.

10 Chung LP, Winship P, Phung S, Lake F, Waterer G. Five-year outcome in COPD patients after their first episode of acute exacerbation treated with non-invasive ventilation. *Respirology*. 2010;15(7):1084–1091.

11 Wakatsuki M, Sadler P. Invasive mechanical ventilation in acute exacerbation of COPD: prognostic indicators to support clinical decisions. *JICS*. 2012;13.3:238–243.

12 Esteban A, Anzueto A, Frutos F, Alía I, Brochard L, Stewart TE, et al. Characteristics and outcomes in adult patients receiving mechanical ventilation: a 28-day international study. *JAMA*. 2002;287(3):345–355.

13 Nevins ML, Epstein SK. Predictors of outcome for patients with COPD requiring invasive mechanical ventilation. *Chest*. 2001;119(6):1840–1849.

14 Albertson TE, Louie S, Chan AL. The diagnosis and treatment of elderly patients with acute exacerbation of chronic obstructive pulmonary disease and chronic bronchitis. *J Am Geriatr Soc*. 2010;58(3):570–579.

15 Chronic obstructive pulmonary disease. National Institute for Health and Care Excellence (NICE) Guideline. 2010.

16 Chan M, Tsuyuki R. Heart failure in the elderly. *Curr Opin Cardiol*. 2013;28(2):234–241.

17 Komajda M, Hanon O, Hochadel M, Lopez-Sendon JL, Follath F, Ponikowski P, et al. Contemporary management of octogenarians hospitalized for heart failure in Europe: Euro Heart Failure Survey II. *Eur Heart J*. 2009;30(4):478–486.

18 McMurray JJ V, Adamopoulos S, Anker SD, Auricchio A, Böhm M, Dickstein K, et al. ESC Guidelines for the diagnosis and treatment of acute and chronic heart failure 2012: the task force for the diagnosis and treatment of acute and chronic heart failure 2012 of the European Society of Cardiology. Developed in collaboration with the heart. *Eur Heart J*. 2012;33(14):1787–1847.

19 Zhou Q, Zhao C, Xie D, Xu D, Bin J, Chen P, et al. Acute and acute-on-chronic kidney injury of patients with decompensated heart failure: impact on outcomes. *BMC Nephrol*. 2012;13:51.

20 Shirakabe A, Hata N, Kobayashi N, Shinada T, Tomita K, Tsurumi M, et al. Prognostic impact of acute kidney injury in patients with acute decompensated heart failure. *Circ J*. 2013;77(3):687–696.

CHAPTER 7

Infection and sepsis

Introduction

At least 1 in 10 deaths in the older population are caused by infectious disease. Susceptibility to infection increases due to changes in the immune system, exposure to pathogens in hospitals and care institutions, frailty and decreased physiological reserve. Infection often presents with a change in mental and functional status rather than signs of localised infection. This diagnostic challenge sometimes necessitates empirical treatment, because delayed antibiotic therapy is associated with a higher risk of systemic sepsis, multi-organ dysfunction and death. However, inappropriate antibiotics in the older adult are associated with drug side effects, drug interactions, antibiotic resistance and *Clostridium difficile* infection.

Background

Immunosenescence describes the changes in the ageing immune system that contribute to an increased risk of infection (Figure 7.1). These changes lead to atypical presenting signs and symptoms, delayed or absent fever, delayed or absent rise in inflammatory markers such as white cell count (WCC) or CRP (C-reactive protein) and reduced effectiveness of treatment (1). Impaired adaptive immunity predisposes to the reactivation of tuberculosis or herpes zoster. Vaccination may be less effective in the older adult due to impaired ability to respond to foreign antigens.

Specific causes of infection

The commonest infections in the older person are urinary tract infections, pneumonia and cellulitis, and these will be addressed specifically in this chapter.

Urinary tract infection (UTI)

UTI is the most frequent infection in the older adult. It is also the commonest hospital-acquired infection, often associated with urinary catheters (2). A number of factors predispose to the development of UTI in the older adult (Box 7.1). UTI may be mistakenly diagnosed in 40% of hospitalised older patients (3), due to the high incidence of asymptomatic bacteriuria.

Geriatric Emergencies, First Edition.
Iona Murdoch, Sarah Turpin, Bree Johnston, Alasdair MacLullich and Eve Losman.
© 2015 John Wiley & Sons, Ltd. Published 2015 by John Wiley & Sons, Ltd.

Causes	Consequences
Compromised skin and mucosal barriers Indwelling lines and catheters Exposure to pathogens in care homes and hospital environment	Increased susceptibility to infection
Impaired innate immunity • Reduced macrophage activity and complement activation	
	Delayed, potentially inadequate response to infection
Comorbidities, especially: • Diabetes and cardiorespiratory disease • Frailty and malnutrition • Reduced cardiopulmonary reserve • Immunosuppressant medications	
	Atypical presenting features causing delayed diagnosis and higher morbidity and mortality
Impaired adaptive immunity • Altered T and B cell activity • Reduced antibody production and response to new antigens • Reduced cytokine production • Absent or delayed fever due to reduced hypothalamic response	

Figure 7.1 Immunosenescence in the older person.

Box 7.1 Factors increasing the possibility of urinary tract infection in the older patient (4).

• Increased post-void bladder volume due to prostatic hypertrophy, cystocoele or weak detrusor muscle function.
• Reduced ability of the kidney to concentrate and acidify the urine.
• Post-menopausal atrophy of the urothelium and shortening of the urethra. Less effective urethral closure in women, with increased incontinence.
• Increased prevalence of faecal incontinence causing contamination of the perineum with bowel organisms.

Lower urinary tract infections
Lower urinary tract infections include infection of the bladder (cystitis) or prostate (prostatitis).

Upper urinary tract infections
Upper urinary tract infections affect the kidneys (pyelonephritis) or ureters and are more often associated with systemic illness.

Asymptomatic bacteriuria
Asymptomatic bacteriuria refers to a positive urine culture in a patient without symptoms suggestive of UTI. It represents colonization of the urinary tract rather than infection and occurs in approximately 20% of women and 10% of men over 80, rising

to 40–50% of older adults in care institutions (5). Asymptomatic bacteriuria is a risk factor for subsequent development of a UTI, but there is no evidence that prophylactic treatment with antibiotics is of benefit.

 KEY POINT: Almost all catheterized patients will have bacteria in their urine within 3–4 days of insertion (6).

An attempt must be made to distinguish asymptomatic bacteriuria from active infection in the older patient, to avoid the complications of unnecessary antibiotic therapy.

Older adults who are hospitalised or in care homes, in particular those with indwelling urinary catheters, are more prone to UTIs from pseudomonas, gram-positive organisms and antibiotic-resistant bacteria including *methicillin-resistant Staphylococcus aureus* (MRSA) and extended spectrum beta lactamase (ESBL)-producing *Escherichia Coli*. Fungal infections with *candida* species may also occur.

Respiratory tract infections

Respiratory tract infections are the seventh leading cause of death in the United States (7). Risk factors include increasing age, alcohol excess, chronic respiratory or cardiac disease, reduced mobility and neuromuscular weakness. Residents of long-term care facilities are at particularly high risk.

Pneumonia is the presence of symptoms and signs consistent with acute lower respiratory tract infection, in association with new consolidation visible on chest radiograph (8).

Streptococcus pneumoniae is the commonest cause of community-acquired pneumonia, accounting for over 50% of cases in the older person (9). *Haemophilus influenzae, Staphylococcus aureus* and respiratory viruses make up the majority of other cases. Gram-negative bacilli predominate in patients in hospital and care homes, and in those with comorbid respiratory disease and recent antibiotic use. Patients at risk of aspirating oropharyngeal or gastric contents due to swallowing difficulties, reduced conscious level (commonly seen in the context of delirium or stroke) or impaired mobility may develop pneumonia due to anaerobes or gram-negative organisms.

Influenza is a contagious viral respiratory tract infection caused by influenza A, B or C virus. Outbreaks of influenza are common in care homes and hospitals during the winter months. Most infected persons experience a self-limiting febrile illness with myalgia, headache and fatigue. However, in the older adult, it is frequently complicated by superimposed bacterial infection, often S*taphylococcus aureus, Streptococcus pneumoniae* or *H. influenzae*, leading to higher morbidity and mortality (10).

Cellulitis

Cellulitis is an infection of the skin and subcutaneous tissues. It commonly affects the lower leg in the older patient, where chronic ulcers, tinea pedis (athlete's foot) and other wounds can provide a route of entry for bacteria. The majority of cases are caused by *Streptococcus pyogenes* or *Staphylococcus aureus*. In the presence of chronic ulceration or pressure sores, organisms such as MRSA and *Pseudomonas* may be involved.

Initial assessment

Sepsis

Sepsis is defined as the presence (probable or confirmed) of infection together with one or more systemic manifestations of infection such as tachycardia, tachypnoea, altered temperature or raised WCC or CRP (11).

Assessment of the older patient with potential sepsis should begin with a rapid survey with the aim of identifying any life-threatening features requiring immediate intervention (Box 7.2). In addition, it is important to determine the patient's goals of care promptly so that the patient does not receive unwanted or inappropriate treatments (Chapter 3).

KEY POINT: Signs of sepsis may be subtle in the older patient and it is easy to underestimate severity.

Box 7.2 Initial assessment in the older patient with sepsis.

Airway and Breathing	Assess respiratory rate, oxygen saturations and work of breathing and apply high flow oxygen in the first instance. *Tachypnoea* (respiratory rate over 20 bpm) may be the first sign of systemic illness
Circulation	Measure heart rate and blood pressure and peripheral capillary refill time. Obtain IV access. Draw bloods (including blood cultures) and give antibiotics and fluids. *Tachycardia* may be absent due to cardiac medication, reduced response to sympathetic stimulus with ageing or conduction abnormalities. Patients who are usually hypertensive may have a blood pressure in the normal range. Hypotension can be considered as a systolic blood pressure more than 40 mmHg below the patient's baseline. Systolic blood pressures of 110 or less are often indicative of relative hypotension in older people
Disability	Note conscious level according to the AVPU (alert, response to voice, response to pain, unresponsive) scale. Measure blood sugar. *Loss of glycaemic control may be an early sign of sepsis in an older patient.* Analgesia should be provided if pain is a feature of the presentation
Exposure	Measure temperature and examine for sources of infection including wounds, rashes, joint swelling and abdominal tenderness *Fever* may be absent in up to one-third of older patients with sepsis (12). *Hypothermia* may occur and is associated with a poorer prognosis

---

In suspected sepsis, *broad-spectrum antibiotics should be given urgently*, following blood cultures if possible. In the presence of severe sepsis, each hour delay in administration of effective antibiotics increases mortality (11). In suspected influenza, anti-viral agents should be given within the first 48 hours of the illness to those over 65 years old, and have been shown to reduce severity and duration of the illness (13). Local guidance on antibiotic choice and anti-viral therapy should be referred to.

A more detailed history and examination can take place following the primary assessment and initial treatment.

History

Infection in older adults may present with delirium, falls and reduced mobility, fatigue, vomiting, anorexia and lethargy, rather than specific complaints.

It is important to identify medications in the drug history which may interact with planned antibiotic therapy, particularly those with a narrow therapeutic window such as warfarin, digoxin or phenytoin.

In suspected urinary tract infection

New onset frequency, incontinence, urinary retention, urgency or dysuria may be an indication of UTI. Offensive smelling, cloudy or blood-stained urine may be present. Care should be taken to distinguish acute from chronic symptoms. Ask about risk factors such as prostatic disease. A higher UTI may present with loin or back pain, fevers or rigors.

Abdominal pain should not be attributed to an UTI without first excluding more serious pathology (Chapter 15).

 KEY POINT: Carers or emergency medical services will often report unpleasant smelling urine. This may be associated with incontinence and is not a reliable indicator of infection (14).

In patients with long-term urinary catheters, clinical judgement is required. Fever without any localising signs is a common occurrence in catheterised patients and UTI appears to be responsible for about a third of these episodes (15). Box 7.3 highlights some of the history and examination findings which may suggest UTI when a catheter has been in situ for longer than 7 days and there is no obvious alternative source of infection.

Box 7.3 Factors suggestive of possible catheter-associated UTI (15).

- New costovertebral tenderness
- Rigors
- New onset delirium
- Fever greater than 37.9 °C or 1.5 °C above baseline on two occasions over 12 hours.

In suspected pneumonia

Typical symptoms such as a productive cough, shortness of breath and fever are much less common in the older patient.

In suspected cellulitis

Determine symptom onset, as slowly progressive symptoms with chronic skin changes are less likely to represent acute cellulitis.

Examination

General examination may reveal fever, tachycardia, tachypnoea, malaise and vomiting. Non-specific findings such as delirium or generalised weakness may predominate.

In suspected urinary tract infection

Examination may reveal suprapubic, abdominal or costovertebral tendernesss. Palpation and percussion may reveal urinary retention. Examine the external genitalia for features of epididymo-orchitis and candida infection. Per rectal examination can elicit an enlarged prostate or faecal impaction which may lead to retention or inadequate voiding, precipitating UTI.

In suspected pneumonia

Tachypnoea and hypoxia are sensitive indicators for pneumonia in the older patient, and should be carefully looked for. Chest signs on auscultation may be absent or subtle.

In suspected cellulitis

Cellulitis usually presents as a hot, tender, erythematous and poorly demarcated area of skin. The skin is usually smooth and shiny. Blisters, vesicles, oedema and associated lymphangitis and lymphadenopathy may be present. There may be signs of systemic illness. The calves, soles of the feet and between the toes should be carefully inspected for skin wounds offering a port of entry to bacteria. In lower limb cellulitis, inspect the other leg to look for evidence of chronic oedema or skin changes. Peripheral vascular disease and peripheral neuropathy should be excluded and pulses and sensation checked.

Cellulitis has a wide differential diagnosis and is misdiagnosed in up to 28% of cases (16). Other diagnoses (Table 7.1) may need to be considered as contributory or alternative causes.

Table 7.1 Alternative diagnoses to cellulitis (17, 18).

Stasis dermatitis (venous or varicose eczema)	The commonest mimic of cellulitis
	Erythematous, scaling, itchy, exudative skin due to venous insufficiency
	May be unilateral or bilateral
	Pain or fever is absent. Cellulitis may be superimposed, however
Deep vein thrombosis	Examination findings may include tenderness along the deep venous system and dilated superficial veins
Thrombophlebitis	Tender, firm superficial vein with overlying redness. Consider co-existing DVT
Allergic contact dermatitis	Owing to creams, dressings or a drug reaction
Acute oedema due to heart failure or low protein state	Usually bilateral
	New onset peripheral oedema may be associated with a localized inflammatory reaction causing erythema
	There may be associated contact or stasis dermatitis or superimposed infection

DVT, deep vein thrombosis.

KEY POINT: Cellulitis is rarely bilateral. Stasis dermatitis is the most common mimic of cellulitis.

In an older adult with signs of systemic infection but with no obvious focus, a thorough physical examination to include the areas in Figure 7.2 should take place.

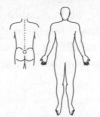

Check for tenderness in the vertebra and intervertebral spaces suggestive of *osteomyelitis* or *discitis*

Palpate costovertebral angles for signs of tenderness due to *pyelonephritis*

Auscultate the heart for murmurs and examine for peripheral stigmata of *bacterial endocarditis*

Abdominal examination may demonstrate tenderness suggestive of cholecystitis, appendicitis or diverticulitis (Chapter 15)

Perform per rectum examination for evidence of recent diarrhoea or perianal abscess

Figure 7.2 Examining for alternative sources of infection in the older patient.

Check for tenderness, swelling and range of movement in all joints for evidence of *septic arthritis* or *osteomyelitis*

Look for signs of central nervous system infections such as photophobia, neck stiffness, or focal neurology. A change in conscious level or cognition may be due to delirium as a result of sepsis or due to meningitis, encephalitis or cerebral abscess

Carefully examine skin creases under breasts, and in any abdominal and groin skin folds for evidence of cellulitis. Examine the sacrum for evidence of infected pressure areas. Remove any dressings and inspect wounds and ulcers carefully

Investigations

Blood tests
Routine blood tests along with blood cultures should be taken. In suspected sepsis, an arterial or venous blood gas may reveal raised lactate, hypoxia or metabolic acidosis. Inflammatory markers and WCC may remain unchanged acutely despite infection.

In suspected urinary tract infection
UTI is a clinical diagnosis based on symptoms or signs of inflammation in the urinary tract, and investigations are of limited use.

Urinalysis
Point-of-care urine dipstick testing is readily available but false positive and false negative results are frequent. A positive dipstick does not distinguish between acute UTI and asymptomatic bacteriuria. Dipstick testing has traditionally supported a clinical diagnosis of UTI if both bacteria (nitrites) and pus (leukocyte esterase) are present in the urine. However, nitrites may be absent in infections with organisms such as *Streptococcus pneumonia*, *Enterococcus* or *Pseudomonas*, which do not express nitrate reductase. High urine output, inadequate dietary nitrate or a low urine pH may also cause false negative nitrite results. Urine positive for leukocytes in the absence of UTI – sterile pyuria – may be due to the presence of a catheter, renal stone, tumour or prior treatment with antibiotics.

Blood or protein in the urine are non-specific findings, and do not assist with diagnosis of infection.

Urine dipstick should not be performed on catheterised patients, as bacteriuria is almost universally present.

> **KEY POINT: UTI is a clinical diagnosis. Point-of-care urinalysis has little role in the diagnosis of UTI in the older patient.**

Urine microscopy, culture and sensitivity

In cases of suspected UTI, urine should be sent for culture, to identify any causative pathogen along with its sensitivity to antibiotic therapy. Urine testing for culture should be a clean-catch midstream urine (MSU) specimen. If this is not possible due to urinary incontinence, the most reliable method is in-out catheterisation using an aseptic technique (6). In a catheterised patient, the catheter should ideally be removed and a urine sample acquired from a freshly inserted catheter before commencing antimicrobials (6). Growth of a pathogen on culture may represent asymptomatic bacteriuria rather than acute infection and careful clinical correlation should always be applied.

Urinary tract imaging

An ultrasound of the urinary tract, particularly in upper UTIs, may reveal obstruction or a collection requiring intervention.

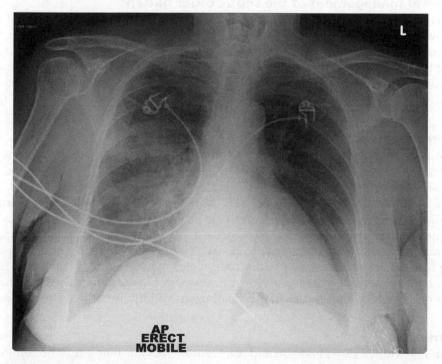

Figure 7.3 Right-sided pneumonia.

In suspected pneumonia
Chest radiograph
This may reveal an area of consolidation, atelectasis or pleural effusion but may also be normal, particularly early in the presentation. Any historical images should be viewed, as changes may be chronic. Malignancy or tuberculosis may be an underlying cause of pneumonia (Figure 7.3).

Arterial blood gases
Arterial blood gases should be considered if oxygen saturations are <94% or if hypoventilation is suspected (19).

Sputum culture
This should be performed for all patients with severe pneumonia, where possible (8). Consider testing for pneumococcal urine antigen or atypical organisms if suspected.

In suspected cellulitis
Wound swabs
Swabs of wounds and ulcers should be sent for culture, but results may represent colonisation rather than acute infection.

Management

General management of the septic older patient
Management of the septic older patient includes antibiotic therapy and general supportive care. This includes maintenance of oxygen delivery to tissues and organs with adequate fluid resuscitation, nutritional support and preventing complications such as drug interactions, delirium, acute kidney injury and complications of reduced mobility such as venous thromboembolism and pressure ulcers. It is important to consider escalation strategy and resuscitation status following careful discussion (Chapter 3).

Antibiotic therapy
Choice of antibiotic type and route will depend on the likely causative pathogen, severity of illness and regional patterns of antibiotic resistance. Local antibiotic prescribing guidelines should be consulted. Aim for the narrowest spectrum possible, with early de-escalation to oral antibiotics after 48 hours if there is clinical improvement. Consider, however, the increasing prevalence of healthcare-associated infections and multi-resistant organisms in the older patient requiring specific antibiotic therapy. Depending on the geographical region, 20–40% of patients in hospital or in long-term care facilities are colonised with MRSA (20), which may be implicated in a new infection. Meticulous hand hygiene, surveillance strategies and eradication therapies may be required to reduce transmission of these pathogens within the hospital environment.

Admission
A patient with localised infection and few signs of systemic illness may be considered for discharge to their place of residence. Various severity scores may be useful in

determining patient disposition, but deterioration may be more rapid and unpredictable in the older patient, and clinical judgement remains equally important. Poor social support or other comorbidities may necessitate hospital admission. See Chapter 2 for further discussion on safe discharge.

Critical care referral

Infection in the older patient is more often complicated by *severe sepsis*. Referral to critical care may be considered in patients who do not improve with ward-based management or in the scenarios mentioned in Box 7.4.

Box 7.4 Indications for admission to critical care in the patient with severe sepsis.

- Septic shock requiring vasopressor or inotropic support to maintain a perfusing blood pressure.
- Respiratory failure due to pneumonia or acute respiratory distress syndrome (ARDS) requiring intubation and mechanical ventilation (Chapter 6).
- Acute kidney injury with indications for renal replacement therapy such as hyperkalaemia, worsening acidosis, fluid overload or uraemic delirium (Chapter 17).

In general, older patients have worse outcomes following intensive care unit admission, although age alone is not a reliable predictor of prognosis. The decision to refer a patient for critical care should be based on patient wishes, severity of the acute illness, comorbid conditions and previous functional ability including mobility and exercise tolerance. Further discussion on the role of intensive care in the older adult is covered in Chapter 3.

Management of specific infections
Urinary tract infection

In suspected UTI in a catheterised patient, the catheter should be changed and a fresh urine sample sent for culture, ideally before antibiotics are given.

Duration of catheterisation is strongly associated with the risk of infection, and attempts should be made to remove urinary catheters as soon as they are no longer clinically necessary. In routine catheter changes, some centres advocate giving a single dose of antibiotics before the change.

Asymptomatic bacteriuria does not require treatment and inappropriate antimicrobials promotes antibiotic resistance and exposes patients to adverse effects of antibiotic therapy. If a diagnosis of UTI is uncertain, it may appropriate to adopt a 'watch and wait' strategy and monitor closely before giving any antibiotic treatment (15).

Respiratory tract infections

Oxygen therapy should be administered if the patient is hypoxic with the aim to maintain oxygen saturations of 94–98%, unless the patient is known to have COPD (chronic obstructive pulmonary disease) or other chronic lung disease where a target of 88–92% may be appropriate (19)

Chest physiotherapy encourages mucous clearance and prevents atelectasis. Saline nebulisers can be useful to loosen secretions and facilitate expectoration.

Cellulitis

The area of cellulitis should be delineated with a marker pen to allow progress to be assessed. The leg should be elevated and analgesia provided.

Oral antibiotics with both staphylococcal and streptococcal cover are appropriate if the patient is otherwise well. Admission for intravenous antibiotics is necessary if the patient is systemically unwell or if there is evidence of spreading lymphangitis. Intravenous antibiotics may be given once daily as an outpatient in some centres if the patient is otherwise well but failing to respond to oral treatment.

Imaging to investigate for an underlying collection or osteomyelitis, or consideration of an alternative diagnosis (Table 7.1), may be necessary if the patient does not improve.

Take home messages

- Symptoms and signs of infection may be subtle and non-specific in the older patient. Blood tests and other investigations are often limited in their ability to confirm a diagnosis
- Older patients may deteriorate rapidly and unpredictably. Each hour of delay in antibiotic therapy is associated with increased mortality in sepsis
- Cellulitis is frequently over-diagnosed due to numerous mimics in the older patient
- Urinary tract infections and cellulitis are diagnosed largely on the basis of history and examination. Although the older adult is at increased risk of UTI, asymptomatic bacteriuria is very common. Think twice before ascribing a UTI as the cause of delirium, reduced mobility or falls in an older person
- Antibiotic stewardship is particularly important in the older patient who is at higher risk of complications from antibiotic therapy, particularly *C. difficile* infection. Use the narrowest spectrum antibiotic and shortest course possible

References

1 Wordsworth D, Dunn-Walters D. The ageing immune system and its clinical implications. *Rev Clin Gerontol.* 2010;21(02):110–124.
2 Beveridge LA, Davey PG, Phillips G, McMurdo ME. Optimal management of urinary tract infections in older people. *Clin Interv Aging.* 2011;6:173–180.
3 Woodford HJ, George J. Diagnosis and management of urinary tract infection in hospitalized older people. *J Am Geriatr Soc.* 2009;57(1):107–114.
4 Benton TJ, Nixon-Lewis B. The aging urinary tract and asymptomatic bacteriuria. *Clin Geriatr.* 2007;15(2):17–22.
5 Nicolle LE. Urinary infections in the elderly: symptomatic of asymptomatic? *Int J Antimicrob Agents.* 1999;11(3–4):265–268.
6 Beveridge LA, Davey PG, Phillips G, McMurdo ME. Optimal management of urinary tract infections in older people. *Clin Interv Aging* 2011;6:173–180.
7 Mandell LA, Wunderink RG, Anzueto A, Bartlett JG, Campbell GD, Dean NC, et al. Infectious Diseases Society of America/American Thoracic Society consensus guidelines on the management of community-acquired pneumonia in adults. *Clin Infect Dis.* 2007;44(Suppl 2):S27–S72.
8 Lim WS, Baudouin S V, George RC, Hill AT, Jamieson C, Le Jeune I, et al. BTS guidelines for the management of community acquired pneumonia in adults: update 2009. *Thorax.* 2009;64 Suppl 3(October):iii1–iii55.

9 Kaplan V, Angus DC. Community-acquired pneumonia in the elderly. *Crit Care Clin*. 2003;19(4): 729–748.

10 Harper SA, Bradley JS, Englund JA, File TM, Gravenstein S, Hayden FG, et al. Seasonal influenza in adults and children–diagnosis, treatment, chemoprophylaxis, and institutional outbreak management: clinical practice guidelines of the Infectious Diseases Society of America. *Clin Infect Dis*. 2009; 48(8):1003–1032.

11 Dellinger RP, Levy MM, Rhodes A, Annane D, Gerlach H, Opal SM, et al. Surviving sepsis campaign: international guidelines for management of severe sepsis and septic shock: 2012. *Crit Care Med*. 2013;41(2):580–637.

12 Liang SY, Mackowiak PA. Infections in the elderly. *Clin Geriatr Med*. 2007;23(2):441–456, viii.

13 Health Protection Services. HPA guidance on use of antiviral agents for the treatment and prophylaxis of influenza. Version 3. Health Protection Agency, October 2012.

14 Midthun SJ, Paur R, Lindseth G. Urinary tract infections. Does the smell really tell? *J Gerontol Nurs*. 2004;30(6):4–9.

15 SIGN (Scottish Intercollegiate Guidelines Network). Management of suspected bacterial urinary tract infection in adults. 2012.

16 David C V, Chira S, Eells SJ, Ladrigan M, Papier A, Miller LG, et al. Diagnostic accuracy in patients admitted to hospitals with cellulitis. *Dermatol Online J*. 2011;17(3):1.

17 Keller EC, Tomecki KJ, Alraies MC. Distinguishing cellulitis from its mimics. *Cleve Clin J Med*. 2012; 79(8):547–552.

18 Phoenix G, Das S, Joshi M. Diagnosis and management of cellulitis. *BMJ*. 2012;345(aug07_2):e4955.

19 O'Driscoll BR, Howard LS, Davison AG. BTS guideline for emergency oxygen use in adult patients. *Thorax*. 2008;63 Suppl 6(October):vi1–vi68.

20 Horner C, Parnell P, Hall D, Kearns A, Heritage J, Wilcox M. Meticillin-resistant *Staphylococcus aureus* in elderly residents of care homes: colonization rates and molecular epidemiology. *J Hosp Infect*. 2013; 83(3):212–218.

CHAPTER 8

Falls and immobility

Part 1: Falls

Introduction

'This patient was found on the floor, exact circumstances unclear'

Many older people present to the ED having been found on the floor in their place of residence. Some are unable to recollect the exact circumstances of the event and even those who are cognitively intact may be too tired, distressed or unwell to give a clear history when they first present.

Differentiating between a fall due to a slip or trip and a fall complicated by transient loss of consciousness can be challenging, but early differentiation between these phenomena is essential in directing further investigation and management.

Definition

A fall is an unexpected event that results in a person coming to rest on the ground or other lower surface (1).

Background

One in three people over the age of 65 will fall each year (2), rising to one in two people over the age of 80 (3); half of those who fall will fall again in the following year. Falls are the leading cause of accidental death in the United Kingdom and the United States for people aged over 65 (2).

Falls are a common presenting symptom to the ED with over 2.3 million non-fatal falls treated in United States EDs in 2010 (2) and over 90,000 hospital admissions per year in the United Kingdom (3). The number of hospital admissions relating to falls is rising, and it is estimated that in the next 10–20 years, falls and fall-related injuries will cost the US Healthcare system $54.9 billion (4) and the UK National Health Service will spend over £6 billion on hip fractures alone (3).

Geriatric Emergencies, First Edition.
Iona Murdoch, Sarah Turpin, Bree Johnston, Alasdair MacLullich and Eve Losman.
© 2015 John Wiley & Sons, Ltd. Published 2015 by John Wiley & Sons, Ltd.

Box 8.1 Why do older people fall? (4, 5)

The ageing process	Modifiable risk factors	Key risk factors
Decreased sensory input:	Medication (see Table 8.1)	Lower limb weakness
Visual impairment	Orthostatic hypotension	History of falls
Degeneration of	Acute illness (atypical presentation)	Gait/balance problem
semicircular canals	Delirium	Visual impairment
Decreased proprioception	Carotid sinus hypersensitivity	Cognitive Impairment
	Neurological	Decreased functional
Decreased central processing:	disease – Parkinson's/stroke	status
Cognitive impairment	Lower limb disease – peripheral	Polypharmacy and/or
Decreased reaction time	neuropathy/peripheral vascular	sedative use
	disease (PVD)	Use of walking aid
Decreased response:	Arthropathy	Depression
Decreased muscle	Visual impairment	Arthritis
activation time	Urinary incontinence	
Decreased movement time	Environmental hazards	
Muscle weakness		

Table 8.1 Medications increasing the risk of falls (9–12).

Drug class	Mechanism of action
Benzodiazepines and hypnotics	Reduce reaction time
	Reduce proprioception
	Balance disturbance/ataxia
Antidepressants & antipsychotics	Sedation with psychomotor retardation
TCAs	Orthostatic hypotension
SSRIs	
Antipsychotics	
Anti-convulsants	Sedation
	Dizziness
	Balance disturbance/ataxia
Digoxin	Proven association with falls but causal mechanism remains
Type 1 antiarrythmics	unclear
Diuretics	
ACE inhibitors	Systematic reviews have identified no formal association;
Nitrates	however, they are likely to contribute to orthostatic hypotension
Ca channel blockers and β-blockers	Frequently feature in polypharmacy (i.e. heart failure) which
	increases falls risk
Levodopa	Orthostatic hypotension
Opioids	Sedation

TCA, tricyclic antidepressant; SSRI, selective serotonin reuptake inhibitor; ACE, angiotensin-converting-enzyme.

History

When undertaking the initial assessment of the patient found on the floor think: *Before, During and After.*

Box 8.2 highlights a few questions that should help clarify important aspects of the event.

Box 8.2 Questions to ask a patient who has been found on the floor.

Before   What was the patient doing?
            How did they feel?
During   Do they remember falling through the air?
            Do they remember hitting the ground?
After   How did they feel when they were on the ground?
            What did they land on?
            Could they get up? (If not, why not?)
            How did they summon help?

If they are unable to answer any of the above questions either:
(a) They have cognitive impairment or delirium (or both)
(b) They lost consciousness: this should prompt an additional work-up for transient loss of consciousness/syncope.

In any case where the patient is unable to give a complete history, a witness history from a care giver, bystander or paramedic is very important and should be obtained at the earliest opportunity.

The exact details surrounding a fall can be difficult to establish. The questions above will help distinguish a fall from transient loss of consciousness; however, the acronym SPLATT (symptoms, previous falls, location, activity, time, and trauma) (6) can be helpful in obtaining a focused history from a patient who has fallen, which, combined with a *targeted examination* is a solid foundation for further assessment and management.

Symptoms around time of fall
Previous falls
Location of fall and length of lie
Activity at time of fall
Timing of the fall
Trauma (physical or psychological) resulting from the fall.

Box 8.3 Fear of falling (7, 8).

This is reported by 20–55% of community dwelling older people and is related to an increased risk of falling, conscious decreasing of activity, worsened mobility and loss of independence. Fear of falling is an independent risk factor for admission to a care home.

History should also encompass a systemic screen for symptoms of recent illness, and environmental considerations such as trip hazards or the use of restraints.

KEY POINT: A fall can be the presentation of acute illness in an older person: why did they fall *today*?

Examination

General

The first objective of examination is to establish whether there is significant injury or medical complication resulting from the fall and if there is any underlying acute illness responsible. See Chapter 11 for a more detailed discussion on initial assessment following trauma.

All patients should then receive a general physical examination with particular focus on the locomotor system and neurological assessment.

A gait assessment should also take place in the ED. This may take the form of the 'get up and go test', where the patient is asked to stand up from a chair, walk a short distance, turn around, return and sit down again (13).

Specific areas of focus on examination

See Figure 8.1.

Investigations

Initial investigations

Blood tests: Full blood count, urea and electrolytes, glucose
ECG: 12 lead ECG
Imaging: will be directed by the history and presentation but a low threshold for chest, hip and pelvic radiographs should be adopted, in addition to plain films of any area that is significantly bruised or tender.

Further investigations

Consider CT head and neck in patients with suspected head injury (see Chapter 14).

In patients with severe hip or groin pain and normal plain films, consider CT or MR hip to identify more subtle fractures; this is discussed further in Chapter 12.

There is a role for tilt table testing, 24 hour ECG and detailed vestibular assessment in older patients who have recurrent or unexplained falls; however, these are usually undertaken at a later stage (14).

Management

General

The management of patients who fall depends on the underlying cause and resulting complications. Acute illnesses such as pneumonia or urinary tract infection should

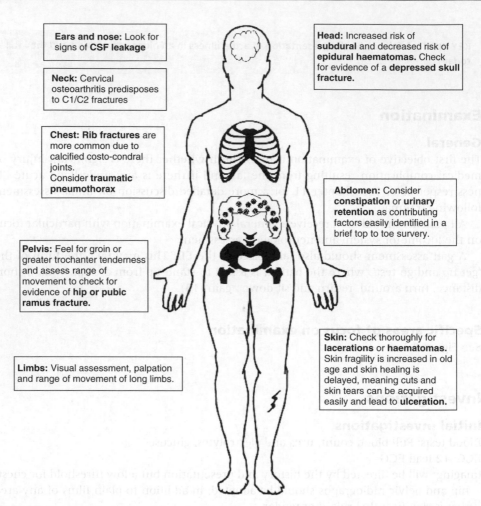

Ears and nose: Look for signs of **CSF leakage**

Neck: Cervical osteoarthritis predisposes to C1/C2 fractures

Chest: Rib fractures are more common due to calcified costo-condral joints.
Consider **traumatic pneumothorax**

Pelvis: Feel for groin or greater trochanter tenderness and assess range of movement to check for evidence of **hip or pubic ramus fracture.**

Limbs: Visual assessment, palpation and range of movement of long limbs.

Head: Increased risk of **subdural** and decreased risk of **epidural haematomas.** Check for evidence of a **depressed skull fracture.**

Abdomen: Consider **constipation** or **urinary retention** as contributing factors easily identified in a brief top to toe survery.

Skin: Check thoroughly for **lacerations** or **haematomas.** Skin fragility is increased in old age and skin healing is delayed, meaning cuts and skin tears can be acquired easily and lead to **ulceration.**

Figure 8.1 Head to toe assessment for minor trauma post fall: considerations when examining an older patient.

be treated promptly and complications such as fractures or pneumothorax should be referred to the appropriate specialty.

For the management of falls resulting in major trauma, head injury, skin tears and fractures in older patients, see Chapters 11–14.

Patients presenting to the ED with recurrent falls who do not require hospital admission should be directed to their primary care provider or local falls multi-disciplinary clinic where they can be appropriately assessed. There is evidence that multi-disciplinary input from physiotherapy, occupational therapy, nursing and specialist medical staff reduces the incidence and prevalence of falls in community dwelling adults (17).

Specific management considerations in older patients

Soft tissue injury
Thirty to fifty percent of falls result in soft tissue injuries such as lacerations and bruising (15). Whilst many of these injuries are relatively minor and easily managed in the ED, in some cases, skin tears can be a major cause of morbidity requiring hospital admission, plastic surgery input and prolonged follow-up by specialist tissue viability (wound care) nurses. For more information on managing skin tears, see Chapter 13.

Fractures
Falls are the commonest cause of fractures in older people, Chapter 12 covers fracture management in further details.

Head injury
Many older people are on anticoagulants and this alters the management of traumatic head injury. For specific information on managing head injury in older patients, see Chapter 14.

Prolonged immobility
A *'long lie'* can lead to multiple complications associated with prolonged immobility; these include rhabdomyolysis, dehydration, pneumonia and pressure ulcers. The management of these conditions is covered later in this chapter under the section Immobility.

Overview of an approach to a patient with a fall
If major injury and medical complications have been excluded, a decision should be made regarding the need for discharge or follow-up; this will often depend on a number of factors including mental state, ability to walk safely and social circumstances (Figure 8.2).

Part 2: Immobility

Introduction
There are three types of immobile older patient:
1 The patient who presents with a gradual decline in mobility which may be transiently worsened by an intercurrent illness or event.
2 The patient who presents following a 'long lie'.
3 The patient who presents with normal or near normal mobility, who becomes immobile whilst in hospital.

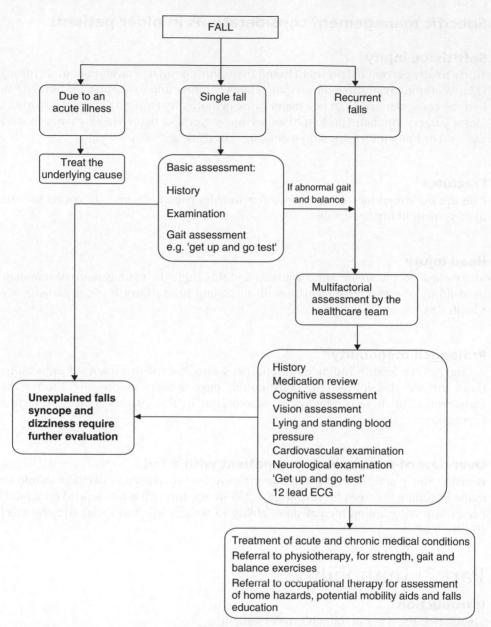

Figure 8.2 Overview of an approach to a patient with a fall. Source: Adapted from 'Falls' in ABC of Geriatric Medicine, Cooper N et al, 2009, with permission from Wiley & Sons.

Immobility is a complex phenomenon in older adults, often born of an interconnecting series of medical, psychological and social factors.

The causes and consequences of immobility will be reviewed in this section, with advice on validated tools for assessing mobility and managing the medical complications associated with prolonged immobility and in patients presenting following a 'long lie'.

Definition
Immobility
It has no single definition although for the purposes of this chapter, we will consider that immobility can be absolute, e.g. bed-bound and unable to mobilise, and relative, e.g. less mobile than normal but still able to mobilise with encouragement and/or assistance as necessary (16).

A 'long lie'
This is defined as remaining on the ground for greater than 1 hour after a fall.

Background
Immobile older patients can lose up to 5% of their muscle strength per day, are six times more likely to be discharged to institutional care and 34 times more likely to die than their mobile counterparts (17–19). Multiple studies have shown that even short periods of bed rest, for example as little as 2 or 3 days, in healthy older adults can be associated with loss of lower limb strength and significant decline in their ability to carry out key activities of daily living (20, 21). When combined with the catabolic process of intercurrent illness and background comorbid conditions, the consequences of immobility are severe and can be fatal (22) (Figure 8.3).

History

The focus of history-taking in immobile patients should be establishing the timescale of immobility and whether the decline has been gradual or sudden. Baseline function should be sought and a history of falls and the use of walking aids should be established. Recent changes in social circumstances such as bereavement or a move to different housing can interrupt well-established routines and lead to reduced mobility.

Immobility in older patients is often multi-factorial and a review of the patient's medical history can often identify many contributing medical conditions. A relatively minor medical condition such as a broken finger affecting the hand used to hold a walking stick can lead to major problems with mobility. Pain and a fear of falling should also be documented.

In patients who present following a 'long lie', history-taking should include an exploration of risk factors for pressure injuries, along with other factors such as diabetes and steroid medication which may impair wound healing. Previous pressure ulcers and the treatment they required may provide useful information.

A thorough systemic enquiry should be taken to identify any intercurrent illness that may contribute to a recent decline in mobility (Table 8.2).

> **KEY POINT:** A seemingly minor medical or social problem can lead to a major reduction in mobility.

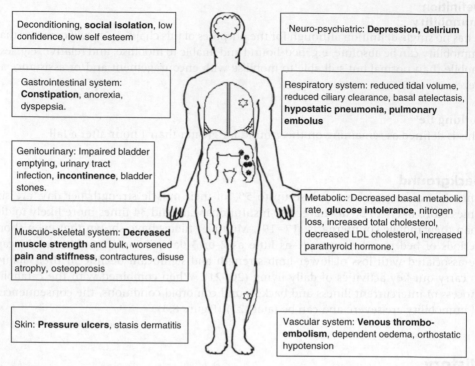

Figure 8.3 Consequences of immobility in older people.

Table 8.2 Causes of immobility in older people (23, 24).

Cause	Example
Physical	Pain: arthritis, severe angina, peripheral vascular disease, back pain
	Breathlessness: COPD, cardiac failure, chronic thromboembolism
	Neurological: Parkinson's disease and related conditions, stroke, peripheral neuropathy, advanced dementia
	Intercurrent infection
	Delirium
Iatrogenic	Hospital admission
	Inappropriate bed rest
	Restraint
	Sedative drugs
Environmental	Inappropriate or insufficient mobility aids
	Cluttered environment
Social	Fear of falling
	Embarrassment at slowness/unsteadiness of gait
	Lack of purposeful social activity
Psychological	Depression
	Anxiety

COPD, chronic obstructive pulmonary disease.

Examination

General examination

All immobile patients should be examined thoroughly, identifying chronic disease and signs of focal illness or injury which could contribute to a recent decline in mobility. Particular attention should be paid to the locomotor and neurological systems, similar to when examining a patient with recurrent falls.

Specific conditions to check for include:

- Osteoarthritis
- Gout and pseudogout
- Joint, bone and skin injuries
- Delirium
- Pneumonia
- Constipation
- Urinary retention
- Pressure ulcers
- Thromboembolic disease.

Examining pressure ulcers
Definition

A pressure ulcer is defined as an area of localised damage to the skin and underlying tissue caused by pressure, shear, friction and/or a combination of these (25).

Examination should establish the surface area, depth, anatomical location and grade of the pressure ulcer, as this will determine management strategy (Table 8.3).

Further examination should include assessment of neurovascular status; the presence and type of exudate; signs of infection in the surrounding soft tissues and the presence or absence of a sinus or fistula. Medical photography is essential in documenting ulcer grade and assessing healing.

Investigations

Initial investigations

Since immobility is often multi-factorial, specific initial investigations vary depending on individual patients. The aim of investigation is to identify an acute cause for presentation and check for evidence of complications such as pneumonia, dehydration or fractures; routine evaluation should include blood tests and a 12 lead ECG.

Further investigations

Investigation of immobile patients is guided by the initial history. However, if a reduction in mobility is unexplained, then actively searching for mechanical causes such as fractures or spinal cord compression should be considered. See Chapter 12 for a discussion on appropriate investigations.

Table 8.3 European and US pressure ulcer staging criteria (26).

Grade 1	Non-blanchable erythema of intact skin
	Discolouration of the skin, warmth, oedema, induration or hardness may also be used as indicators, particularly on individuals with darker skin
Grade 2	Partial thickness skin loss involving epidermis or dermis. The ulcer is superficial and presents clinically as an abrasion or blister
Grade 3	Full thickness skin loss involving damage to or necrosis of subcutaneous tissue that may extend down to, but not through, underlying fascia
Grade 4	Extensive destruction, tissue necrosis or damage to muscle or bone with or without full thickness skin loss
Unstageable (additional US stage)	Full thickness tissue loss in which actual depth of the ulcer is completely obscured by slough (yellow, tan, grey, green or brown) and/or eschar (tan, brown or black) in the wound bed. Until enough slough and/or eschar are removed to expose the base of the wound, the true depth cannot be determined, but it will be either a category/stage III or IV. Stable (dry, adherent, intact without erythema or fluctuance) eschar on the heels serves as 'the body's natural (biological) cover' and should not be removed
Suspected deep tissue injury (additional US stage)	Full thickness tissue loss in which actual depth of the ulcer is completely obscured by slough (yellow, tan, grey, green or brown) and/or eschar (tan, brown or black) in the wound bed. Until enough slough and/or eschar are removed to expose the base of the wound, the true depth cannot be determined, but it will be either a category/stage III or IV. Stable (dry, adherent, intact without erythema or fluctuance) eschar on the heels serves as 'the body's natural (biological) cover' and should not be removed

Management

General management

The management of immobility in older patients focuses on supportive care and addressing the consequences of multi-organ deconditioning.

Physiotherapists and nursing staff play a huge role in both the prevention of iatrogenic immobility and the rehabilitation of older patients who present with multi-factorial immobility.

Pressure ulcers in older patients
Background

Pressure injuries occur in up to 10% in hospital inpatients and are common in residents of long-term care institutions.

Risk factors for pressure ulcers include advancing age; immobility due to neurological disease, intercurrent illness or sedative drugs; malnutrition and dehydration; obesity; peripheral vascular disease; incontinence and major surgery or trauma.

A number of different risk scoring systems, such as the Waterlow score or Braden scale, are available to assess the overall risk of pressure ulcers in a particular patient on admission to hospital. Preventative strategies are key to reducing the incidence of pressure injuries.

A pressure injury may develop within 2 hours in a patient placed on an inappropriate surface such as an ED trolley or operating theatre.

There may be a significant delay between the ischaemic insult and the appearance of a pressure ulcer.

> **KEY POINT: The first principle of pressure ulcer management is preventing further pressure injuries.**

A local tissue viability expert can provide valuable input and access to specialist equipment for both prevention and management of pressure injuries.

Box 8.4 Prophylaxis of pressure injuries.

S – Support surface	Utillise a pressure-reducing foam mattress, or pressure-reducing cushion if sitting in a chair. Alternating pressure or continuously low pressure systems may be required
K – Keep moving	Regular repositioning, every 2 hours for bed-bound patients
I – Incontinence	Patients should be kept dry and clean. Catheterisation or bowel management system may be an option, but the benefits and risks should be carefully considered
N – Nutrition and hydration	Avoid undernutrition and keep skin adequately moisturised

---

Intercurrent illness may significantly delay wound healing. Ensure adequate tissue oxygenation by optimising cardiac output and treating anaemia, glycaemic control should also be optimised. Associated pain should be identified and treated. Antimicrobial therapy should be considered in the presence of local or systemic signs of infection.

The ulcer should be carefully dressed with a hydrocolloid, foam or soft silicone dressing depending on the ulcer site and grade.

In higher grade pressure injuries, specialist management such as debridement, vacuum dressings, skin grafting or flaps may be required.

Patients with Parkinson's disease

It is essential that patients with Parkinson's disease receive their medications on time. Medication omissions can result in a rapid and significant decrease in mobility and an increase in the frequency of aspiration pneumonia.

If there are concerns about swallowing, then alternative methods of administration such as a nasogastric tube should be strongly considered. Expert help should be sought early (within 24 hours of admission) if there are concerns about the availability or route of administration of specific Parkinson's disease medications.

Thromboembolism

All immobile patients should be assessed for the risk of developing deep vein thromboses or pulmonary emboli and active efforts made to prevent these. The best way to prevent thromboembolism is early ambulation. If early ambulation is not possible, other options include:

- Lower limb exercises whilst seated or in bed.
- Intermittent external pneumatic pressure devices
- Compression stockings
- Subcutaneous low molecular weight heparin, heparin or in some cases other anticoagulants.

Complications of a 'long lie'

Rhabdomyolysis

Patients who have fallen are at risk of developing rhabdomyolysis secondary to prolonged muscle compression associated with a 'long lie' – defined as remaining on the ground for greater than 1 hour after a fall (27–29). The commonest muscle groups affected are the calves and lower back. Rhabdomyolysis results in the leakage of potassium, phosphate, myoglobin and creatine kinase (CK) into the circulation and is a clinical syndrome ranging from isolated raised CK to acute kidney injury (AKI), hyperkalaemia and death. CK levels rise in rhabdomyolysis within 12 hours of the onset of muscle injury, peak in 1–3 days, and decline 3–5 days after the cessation of muscle injury.

Myoglobinuria can be screened for in the ED with simple urinalysis which reads positive for haemoglobin if myoglobinuria is present. True myoglobinuria can be identified via formal laboratory testing.

In any patient who has been found on the floor, the possibility of rhabdomyolysis should be considered, particularly in those with signs of pressure damage, compartment syndrome or other musculoskeletal injuries. The classical triad of 'muscle pain, weakness and dark urine' is seen in less than 10% of patients.

Its complications include:

1 *Acute kidney injury (AKI)*: this occurs secondary to myoglobin causing renal tubular obstruction; the level of CK is not directly related to the likelihood of AKI developing, and is more common in patients with renal comorbidity. Treatment is prompt aggressive IV rehydration, bladder catheterisation and monitoring of urine output aiming for 200–300 ml/h. In patients with known cardiac failure, fluid resuscitation must be carefully balanced against signs of cardiac decompensation and admission to a high dependency environment (critical care or step-down unit) for advanced monitoring may need consideration. The longer it takes for fluid resuscitation to be started, the more likely it is that AKI will develop. Patients who develop AKI in the context of rhabdomyolysis have an overall mortality of approximately 20% and in patients whose renal function is not responding to IV rehydration, a period of renal replacement therapy in ICU or a renal unit should be considered. See Chapter 17 for further discussion on AKI.
2 *Hyperkalaemia*: This is due to direct release of potassium into the circulation; addressing the underlying cause and optimising rehydration are essential to the management of hyperkalaemia; however, it may also require emergency treatment with calcium gluconate and an insulin-dextrose infusion. Arrhythmias are more common in patients with cardiac comorbidity.

3 *Hypocalcaemia*: This is often asymptomatic but parenteral calcium replacement should be administered if there is signficiant derangement.

   Patients with rhabdomyolysis should be admitted for IV rehydration, sequential monitoring of blood profiles and management of potential complications. Patients with renal or cardiac comorbidities and frail older patients with multiple comorbidities may require a monitored bed for 24–48 hours due to their increased risk of developing life-threatening arrhythmias.

> **KEY POINT: The level of CK does not always predict the likelihood or severity of complications in rhabdomyolysis (27).**

Hypothermia

Categorised as mild (<35 °C), moderate (<32 °C) and severe (<28 °C), the pathophysiology and management of hypothermia in older patients is described in Chapter 16.

> **KEY POINT: Falls and reduced mobility can be a presentation of sepsis in older people, and hypothermia in this context may indicate severe sepsis (30, 31).**

Take home messages

- Falls are the leading cause of accidental death in people aged over 65 in the United Kingdom and the United States
- The causes and consequences of falls and immobility are complex and require careful assessment
- Falls and reduced mobility can be the presenting feature of an acute illness in older people
- Gait assessment is an essential part of assessing a patient presenting with a fall or reduced mobility
- Multi-disciplinary intervention significantly improves outcomes for falling or immobile patients.

References

1 World Health Organisation (WHO). *Falls.* http://www.who.int/mediacentre/factsheets/fs344/en/ [cited 2013 Feb 13].
2 Centers for Disease Control and Prevention (CDC). *Older Adult Falls – Falls Among Older Adults: An Overview – Home and Recreational Safety – Injury Center.* http://www.cdc.gov/homeandrecreational-safety/falls/adultfalls.html [cited 2013 Jan 19].
3 Department of Health. *Better Care to Prevent Falls and Fractures will Improve Lives and Save the NHS Billions.* http://mediacentre.dh.gov.uk/2012/02/23/better-care-to-prevent-falls-and-fractures-will-improve-lives-and-save-the-nhs-billions/ [cited 2013 Feb 9].
4 Rubenstein LZ, Josephson KR. The epidemiology of falls and syncope. *Clin Geriatr Med.* 2002;18(2): 141–158.
5 Department of Health. *Standard Six – Fall.* 2004. http://webarchive.nationalarchives.gov.uk/+/www.dh.gov.uk/en/SocialCare/Deliveringadultsocialcare/Olderpeople/OlderpeoplesNSFstandards/DH_4002294 [cited 2013 Feb 13].

6 Howard MF, Rockwood K, Woodhouse K. Brocklehurst's Textbook of Geriatric Medicine and Geron-tology. 7th Revised ed. Saunders; 2010. 1152 p.

7 Painter JA, Allison L, Dhingra P, Daughtery J, Cogdill K, Trujillo LG. Fear of falling and its relationship with anxiety, depression, and activity engagement among community-dwelling older adults. *Am J Occup Ther*. 2012;66(2):169–176.

8 Viljanen A, Kulmala J, Rantakokko M, Koskenvuo M, Kaprio J, Rantanen T. Fear of falling and coexisting sensory difficulties as predictors of mobility decline in older women. *J Gerontol A Biol Sci Med Sci*. 2012;67(11):1230–1237.

9 Boyle N, Naganathan V, Cumming RG. Medication and falls: risk and optimization. *Clin Geriatr Med*. 2010;26(4):583–605.

10 Huang AR, Mallet L, Rochefort CM, Eguale T, Buckeridge DL, Tamblyn R. Medication-related falls in the elderly: causative factors and preventive strategies. *Drugs Aging*. 2012;29(5):359–376

11 Woolcott JC RK. MEta-analysis of the impact of 9 medication classes on falls in elderly persons. *Arch Intern Med*. 2009;169(21):1952–1960.

12 Daal JO, van Lieshout JJ. Falls and medications in the elderly. *Neth J Med*. 2005;63(3):91–96.

13 Mathias S, Nayak US, Isaacs B. Balance in elderly patients: the 'get-up and go' test. *Arch Phys Med Rehabil*. 1986;67(6):387–389.

14 National Institute for Health and Care Excellence (NICE). *Falls*. http://www.nice.org.uk/ [cited 2013 Feb 13].

15 Meldon S, Ma OJ, Woolard R. Geriatric Emergency Medicine. 1st ed. McGraw-Hill Medical; 2003. 585 p.

16 Emed JD, Morrison DR, Rosiers LD, Kahn SR. Definition of immobility in studies of thrombopro-phylaxis in hospitalized medical patients: A systematic review. *J Vasc Nurs*. 2010;28(2):54–66

17 Stall N. Tackling immobility in hospitalized seniors. *CMAJ*. 2012;184(15):1666–1667.

18 Brown CJ, Friedkin RJ, Inouye SK. Prevalence and Outcomes of Low Mobility in Hospitalized Older Patients. *J Am Geriatr Soc*. 2004;52(8):1263–1270.

19 English KL, Paddon-Jones D. Protecting muscle mass and function in older adults during bed rest. *Curr Opin Clin Nutr Metab Care*. 2010;13(1):34–39.

20 Boyd CM, Landefeld CS, Counsell SR, Palmer RM, Fortinsky RH, Kresevic D, et al. Recovery of activities of daily living in older adults after hospitalization for acute medical illness. *J Am Geriatr Soc*. 2008;56(12):2171–2179.

21 Gill TM, Allore H, Guo Z. The deleterious effects of bed rest among community-living older persons. *J Gerontol A Biol Sci Med Sci*. 2004;59(7):755–761.

22 Rousseau P. Immobility in the aged. *Arch Fam Med*. 1993;2(2):169–177; discussion 178.

23 Mobily PR, Skemp Kelley LS. Iatrogenesis in the elderly. Factors of immobility. *J Gerontol Nurs*. 1991;17(9):5–11.

24 The Resource Center On Healthy Ageing: The SOHO Center of Gerontology and Geriatrics. *Immobility*. http://healthyageing.sphpc.cuhk.edu.hk/immobility_en.htm [cited 2013 Oct 24].

25 European Pressure Ulcer Advisory Panel (EUPAP). http://www.epuap.org/ [cited 2013 Nov 4].

26 The National Pressure Ulcer Advisory Pane (NPUAP). *NPUAU Pressure Ulcer Stages/Categories*. http://www.npuap.org/resources/educational-and-clinical-resources/npuap-pressure-ulcer-stages-categories/ [cited 2014 May 7].

27 Clinical Geriatrics. *Torso Trauma in the Elderly*. http://www.clinicalgeriatrics.com/articles/Torso-Trauma-Elderly?page=0,6&mobify=0 [cited 2013 Feb 13].

28 Huerta-Alardín AL, Varon J, Marik PE. Bench-to-bedside review: rhabdomyolysis – an overview for clinicians. *Crit Care*. 2005;9(2):158–169.

29 Lord SR, Sherrington C, Menz HB. Falls in Older People: Risk Factors and Strategies for Prevention. Cambridge University Press; 2007. 388 p.

30 Mallet ML. Pathophysiology of accidental hypothermia. *QJM*. 2002;95(12):775–785.

31 Muszkat M, Durst RM, Ben-Yehuda A. Factors associated with mortality among elderly patients with hypothermia. *Am J Med*. 2002;113(3):234–237.

CHAPTER 9
Syncope

Introduction

Definition
Syncope is a temporary loss of consciousness due to transient global cerebral hypoperfusion, characterised by rapid onset, short duration and spontaneous complete recovery (1).

Background
Syncopal events account for approximately 3% of ED visits and up to 6% of hospital admissions (2). Up to 25% of syncopal events in older people present as unexplained falls, and the morbidity and mortality of syncope in older patients is greater than in the general population due to the higher frequency of resulting trauma such as fractures or significant head injuries (2). Syncope in geriatric patients can be a complex phenomenon: younger patients tend to develop syncope due to a single cause, whereas geriatric patients often experience multifactorial syncope (3, 4). In addition to this, there is significant overlap between falls, syncope and other disorders of consciousness; many patients, both with and without cognitive impairment, will have difficulty detailing the exact events surrounding their presentation.

Why are older patients predisposed to syncope?
A number of physiological changes, particularly to the autonomic nervous system, predispose older patients to syncope (4):
- Reduction in β-adrenergic vasodilatory response
- Reduction in α-adrenergic vasoconstrictive responses
- Decreased β-adrenergic–mediated cardioacceleratory response to sympathetic activation
- Reduced parasympathetic tone leading to reduced heart rate variability
- Decreased baro-reflex sensitivity leading to reduced heart rate augmentation with low blood pressure
- Reduced numbers of sinoatrial cells
- Increased rate of salt and water loss by the kidneys
- Reduced thirst response

Geriatric Emergencies, First Edition.
Iona Murdoch, Sarah Turpin, Bree Johnston, Alasdair MacLullich and Eve Losman.
© 2015 John Wiley & Sons, Ltd. Published 2015 by John Wiley & Sons, Ltd.

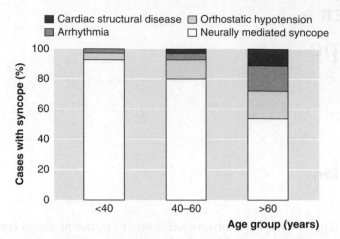

Figure 9.1 Causes of syncope by age. Source: From Parry SW, Tan MP. An approach to the evaluation and management of syncope in adults. *BMJ*. 2010 Feb 19;340(feb19 1):c880–c880.

Types of syncope in the older population

Neurally mediated syncope, otherwise termed reflex syncope, remains the commonest cause of syncope in older patients; however, proportionally, older patients have higher rates of orthostatic hypotension, arrhythmias and structural cardiac causes (5). The cause of syncope in older patients is not always clear, and in studies of older patients presenting with and being investigated for syncope, between 10.4% and 47.5% remained undiagnosed (6) (Figure 9.1).

> **KEY POINT: Cardiac causes of syncope are disproportionately represented in the older population and have high morbidity and mortality (6).**

History

History-taking provides the diagnosis in 50% of cases where the cause of syncope can be established (7).

It is important to ask about specific triggers and associated symptoms before, during and after the event. A general systems enquiry may identify potential causes of decreased intravascular volume, such as diarrhoea, vomiting or internal and external haemorrhage (Table 9.1).

Conditions that may be mistaken for syncope, e.g. causing loss of consciousness or loss of postural tone or both but in the absence of cerebral hypoperfusion, include (but are not limited to) the following (1):

- Epilepsy
- Metabolic disturbance, e.g. hypoglycaemia
- Cataplexy
- Drop attacks
- Psychogenic or functional causes
- Falls

Table 9.1 Types of syncope with associated triggers and symptoms (1, 2, 8).

Types	Triggers	Associated features
Reflex/neurally mediated	Orthostatic stress/emotional	Prodrome of
Neurocardiogenic (vasovagal)	distress/pain/noxious stimuli	Pallor
		Sweating
		Nausea
Situational	Cough/sneeze	Tunnel vision
	Micturation	
	Defaecation	
	Swallow	
	Post prandial	
Carotid sinus		
Cardioinhibitory	Activities involving pressure over the	
Vasodepressive	neck: e.g. shaving/head turning/tight	
	collar	
Orthostatic hypotension	Rapid postural change	Typical prodrome with documented
	Hypovolaemia	blood pressure drop
	Haemorrhage	
	Medication induced: particularly	
	recent dose changes or new drugs	
Cardiac		
Electrical	Tachyarrhythmias/bradyarrhythmias/	Lack of prodrome should raise
	AV blocks	suspicion of cardiac cause
		Abnormal ECG
		Chest pain, palpitations, SOB,
Structural	Valvular disease/MI/	sweating
	Cardiomyopathy/pulmonary	
	hypertension/tumour	
Neurological		
Posterior circulation stroke	No trigger	Dysarthria, diplopia, vertigo, nausea
Subclavian steal	Activities involving arms being raised	
	for prolonged time: painting, hair	
	combing etc	
SAH	No trigger	Headache
Rare causes	Pulmonary embolism/	Associated symptoms depend on
	Hyperventilation/	underlying cause
	Psychiatric	

SOB, shortness of breath.

Examination

General examination

General aspects of the examination should include skin and mucous membrane assessment for hydration status, consideration of rectal examination to check for melaena, a search for evidence of sepsis and focal infection and any signs of traumatic injury sustained during the collapse.

Examination can identify the cause of syncope in 20% of cases where the cause can be established (7). However, patients presenting with syncope can have a normal examination even with a potentially life-threatening cause for their collapse.

Specific areas of focus on examination

Cardiovascular

Look for jugular venous distension or other signs of cardiac failure, listen for heart murmurs and bruits and feel for the cardiac apex, central and peripheral pulses and note their rate, rhythm and character, and check for signs of abdominal aortic aneurysm (AAA).

Neurological

Examine for focal weakness, eye movement abnormalities or speech disturbance which may be associated with a neurological cause of syncope, or signs of parkinsonism associated with autonomic nervous system dysfunction.

Investigations

Initial investigation

In conjunction with a careful history and examination, all patients must have the following (1):

- 12-lead ECG
- Blood sugar measurement
- Erect and supine (orthostatic) blood pressure monitoring
- Baseline blood screen including full blood count and urea and electrolytes to assess renal function and hydration status. Troponin measurement is appropriate only in cases where there is concern about possible cardiac syncope (9).

Further investigation

Specific further investigations should be directed by the results of a careful history, examination and initial investigations.

Suspected neurally mediated/Reflex syncope

If there is clear evidence from the history of a precipitating factor (e.g. sight of blood or prolonged standing in a warm room) in combination with an isolated event and unremarkable initial assessment, further assessment may not be required (6, 8).

Carotid sinus massage (CSM) is indicated in patients aged over 40 who present with a history suggestive of carotid sinus hypersensitivity. Cases that are recurrent or associated with a high risk profile may require further evaluation using a tilt table in a specialist syncope or cardiology clinic (1).

Box 9.1 How to perform carotid sinus massage (11).

Firmly massage the anterior margin of the sternocleomastoid muscle at the level of the cricoid cartilage (the site where the common carotid artery bifurcates) for 5–10 seconds. Perform first on the right hand side, and then, if no response is obtained, repeat on the left hand side.

Observe for either

1 a fall in systolic BP of 50 mmHg or more
2 a ventricular pause lasting 3 seconds or more.

Perform the above in both the supine and erect positions: a tilt table may be necessary for this.

Perform this maneuver only when there is continuous ECG and non-invasive blood pressure monitoring so that a drop in blood pressure (vasodepressor response) or ventricular pause (cardio-inhibitory response) can be reliably identified.

Contraindications to CSM include patients who have had a TIA (transient ischaemic attack) within 3 months or have bruits audible on examination (unless Doppler has excluded carotid stenosis), myocardial infarction within 6 months, or history of ventricular arrhythmias (1).

Suspected orthostatic hypotension

Provide an orthostatic challenge in the form of active stand or tilt table (the latter should usually be performed and analysed in specialist syncope clinics). The drug history should include enquiring about new medications or recent dosage changes, to identify any possible contributing medications (1).

Suspected cardiovascular syncope

Continuous ECG monitoring should be initiated at presentation if the history, ECG or examination suggests a cardiac cause (7).

The European Society of Cardiology suggests that features highlighted in Box 9.2 are short-term high-risk criteria that require prompt hospitalisation or intensive evaluation.

Box 9.2 ESC features suggesting life threatening causes of syncope.

Severe structural or coronary artery disease

Clinical or ECG features suggestive of cardiac syncope:

Syncope on exertion or while supine
Palpitations at the time of syncope
Family history of SCD (sudden cardiac death)
Non-sustained VT (ventricular tachycardia)
Bifascicular block or other interventricular conduction delay and QRS > 120 s
Inadequate sinus bradycardia (<50 bpm) or sinoatrial block in the absence of negative chronotropic medications or physical training
Pre-excited QRS
Prolonged or short QTc
RBBB (right bundle branch block) with ST elevation in V1–V3 (Brugada pattern)
Negative T waves in inferior leads, epsilon waves, or ventricular late potentials suggestive of ARVC (arrhythmogenic right ventricular cardiomyopathy)

Severe anaemia

Electrolyte disturbance.

Source: From Moya A, Sutton R, Ammirati F, Blanc J-J, Brignole M, Dahm JB, et al. Guidelines for the diagnosis and management of syncope (version 2009). The Task Force for the Diagnosis and Management of Syncope of the European Society of Cardiology (ESC). *Eur Heart J.* 2009;30(21):2631–2671. With permission.

Echocardiogram to assess for evidence of structural heart disease and LV ejection fraction should be undertaken as an urgent inpatient investigation if unexplained cardiogenic syncope is suspected (3).

Suspected neurological syncope

A detailed neurological assessment should be undertaken by an appropriate specialist and consideration given to brain imaging. CT and MRI imaging should be avoided in cases where the underlying diagnosis appears to be uncomplicated neurally mediated/reflex syncope, and where there is no suggestion of head or neck injury (1).

If other rare causes are suspected, further investigations are determined by the suspected cause.

> **KEY POINT: An underlying cause of syncope cannot be found in a significant proportion of patients.**

Management

General management

Aside from making a causative diagnosis, an essential part of syncope assessment is to risk stratify the possibility of cardiac syncope and identify the need for further assessment and monitoring to identify a life-threatening cause (9).

Patients with uncomplicated neurally mediated/reflex syncope may not require admission, and patients with confirmed orthostatic hypotension may not require admission if there has been a clear precipitant that can be rectified by simply adjusting a medication dose or rehydrating the patient.

Over 50% of patients aged over 80 are admitted to hospital following a syncopal episode.

Specific management considerations in older patients

Older patients are at higher risk of having cardiac syncope, and some patients presenting with syncope may give a less explicit history due to cognitive impairment. These patients are especially vulnerable to misdiagnosis, and risk stratification plays an important role in their further management and investigation.

Risk stratification in syncope

No scoring system or screening test is perfect, and none can replace the clinical judgment of assessing clinicians or expert opinion. They are, however, useful for identifying high-risk patients.

The EGSYS score

This is a simple screening test based on the Evaluation of Guidelines in Syncope Study trial (10). It is drawn from information based on history and general (non-specialist) clinical assessment and validated in an unselected patient population presenting urgently to a general hospital. It is designed to help differentiate between patients at

Table 9.2 Risk stratification tools for patients presenting with syncope.

Study	Risk factors	Score	Endpoints	Results
San Francisco syncope rule	Abnormal ECG Congestive heart failure Shortness of breath Haematocrit < 30% Systolic BP < 90 mmHg	No risk = 0 item Risk≥1 item	Serious events at 7 days	98% sensitive and 56% specific
Martin et al.	Abnormal ECG History of ventricular arrhythmia History of congestive heart failure Age > 45 years	0–4 1 point each item	1 year severe arrhythmias or arrhythmic death	0% score 0 5% score 1 16% score 2 27% score 3 or 4
OESIL score	Abnormal ECG History of cardiovascular disease Lack of prodrome Age > 65 years	0–4 1 point each item	1 year total mortality	0% score 0 0.6% score 1 14% score 2 29% score 3 53% score 4
EGSYS score	Palpitations before syncope (+4) Abnormal ECG and/or heart disease (+3) Syncope during effort (+3) Syncope whilst supine (+2) Autonomic prodrome (−1) Predisposing and/or precipitating factors (−1)	Sum of + and − points	2 year mortality Cardiac syncope probability	2% score <3 21% score ≥3 2% score <3 13% score 3 33% score 4 77% score >4

Source: From Moya A, Sutton R, Ammirati F, Blanc J-J, Brignole M, Dahm JB, et al. Guidelines for the diagnosis and management of syncope (version 2009) The Task Force for the Diagnosis and Management of Syncope of the European Society of Cardiology (ESC). *Eur Heart J.* 2009 Jan 11;30(21):2631–71. Reproduced with permission of Oxford University Press.

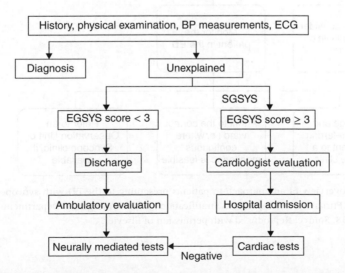

Figure 9.2 EGSYS risk stratification flow chart. Source: From Moya A, Sutton R, Ammirati F, Blanc J-J, Brignole M, Dahm JB, et al. Guidelines for the diagnosis and management of syncope (version 2009) The Task Force for the Diagnosis and Management of Syncope of the European Society of Cardiology (ESC). *Eur Heart J.* 2009 Jan 11;30(21):2631–71. Reproduced with permission of Oxford University Press.

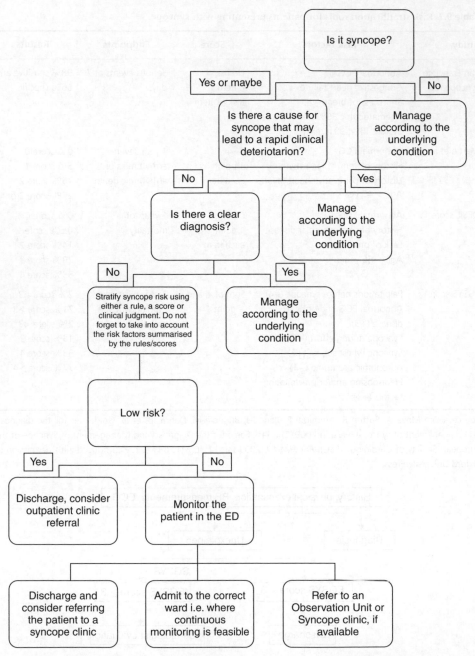

Figure 9.3 An overview of an approach to patients presenting to the ED with syncope. Source: From Costantino G, Furlan R. Syncope Risk Stratification in the Emergency Department. *Syncope*. 2013 Feb;31(1):27–38. Source: Reproduced with permission of Elsevier.

high risk and low risk of cardiac syncope and provide guidance on when it is appropriate to admit.

The EGSYS is currently the preferred screening tool for health professionals in the United Kingdom; however, other screening tools also exist, and all are summarised in Table 9.2.

Figure 9.2 presents a suggested risk stratification flow diagram for patients presenting to the ED with syncope.

Overview of an approach to a patient presenting with syncope

See Figure 9.3.

Take home messages

- Syncope can masquerade as recurrent or unexplained falls in older patients
- A careful history can help establish the cause of syncope in 50% of cases where the diagnosis of syncope can be established
- Multifactorial syncope is commonly present in older patients and can pose a diagnostic challenge
- Older patients are at higher risk of life-threatening causes of syncope
- The morbidity and mortality associated with syncope is greatest in older patients
- Risk stratification is an essential part of initial assessment of a patient presenting with syncope.

References

1 Moya A, Sutton R, Ammirati F, Blanc J-J, Brignole M, Dahm JB, et al. Guidelines for the diagnosis and management of syncope (version 2009) The Task Force for the Diagnosis and Management of Syncope of the European Society of Cardiology (ESC). *Eur Heart J*. 2009;30(21):2631–2671.
2 Grubb BP, Karabin B. Syncope: evaluation and management in the geriatric patient. *Clin Geriatr Med*. 2012;28(4):717–728.
3 Mappilakkandy R, Edwards I. Update on syncope in the older person – a clinical review. *Rev Clin Gerontol*. 2013;23(01):15–31.
4 Forman DE, Lipsitz LA. Syncope in the elderly. *Cardiol Clin*. 1997;15(2):295–311.
5 Parry SW, Tan MP. An approach to the evaluation and management of syncope in adults. *BMJ*. 2010;340(feb19 1):c880.
6 Marrison VK, Fletcher A, Parry SW. The older patient with syncope: practicalities and controversies. *Int J Cardiol*. 2012;155(1):9–13.
7 Meldon S, Ma OJ, Woolard R. Geriatric Emergency Medicine. 1st ed. McGraw-Hill Medical; 2003. 585 p.
8 National Institute for Health and Care Excellence (NICE). *CG109 Transient Loss of Consciousness in Adults and Young People: NICE Guideline*. http://publications.nice.org.uk/transient-loss-of-consciousness-blackouts-management-in-adults-and-young-people-cg109 [cited 2013 Feb 13].
9 Costantino G, Furlan R. Syncope risk stratification in the emergency department. *Cardiol Clin*. 2013;31(1):27–38

10 Del Rosso A1, Ungar A, Maggi R, Giada F, Petix NR, De Santo T, Menozzi C, Brignole M. Clinical predictors of cardiac syncope at initial evaluation in patients referred urgently to a general hospital: the EGSYS score. *Heart*. 2008 Dec;94(12):1620–6.

11 Brignole M1, Alboni P, Benditt DG, Bergfeldt L, Blanc JJ, Bloch Thomsen PE, van Dijk JG, Fitzpatrick A, Hohnloser S, Janousek J, Kapoor W, Kenny RA, Kulakowski P, Masotti G, Moya A, Raviele A, Sutton R, Theodorakis G, Ungar A, Wieling W. Guidelines on Management (Diagnosis and Treatment) of Syncope – Update 2004. The Task Force on Syncope, European Society of Cardiology. *Europace*. 2004;6(6):467–537.

CHAPTER 10
Dizziness

Introduction

Definition
Dizziness has typically been divided into four subtypes (Box 10.1). In practice, however, older people frequently report symptoms that suggest more than one subtype (1). In addition to this, patients may use the term 'dizziness' to describe sensations of weakness, lethargy or lassitude.

Box 10.1 Drachman and Hart dizziness subtypes (2).

Vertigo: A sense of the room spinning, rotatory symptoms.
Presyncope: Lightheaded, 'about to pass out'.
Disequilibrium: General unsteadiness felt when walking, rather than in the head.
Others: Other non-specific symptoms including giddiness or floating.

Background
Dizziness is a common symptom in older people, with studies suggesting a prevalence of 21–29% in people aged over 65 in the community in the United Kingdom and the United States. It is responsible for 3.3% of ED visits (3).

The causes of dizziness are varied, ranging from the benign and self-limiting to life-threatening conditions and time-sensitive emergencies (Figure 10.1).

History

A detailed history is very helpful in directing further investigations and identifying potentially life-threatening conditions that may necessitate more timely management (Table 10.1).

What is the nature of the dizziness?
Is there a sensation of movement or spinning, a feeling of light-headedness, or feeling of being about to faint? Is there a sensation of being on a boat or merry-go-round?

Geriatric Emergencies, First Edition.
Iona Murdoch, Sarah Turpin, Bree Johnston, Alasdair MacLullich and Eve Losman.
© 2015 John Wiley & Sons, Ltd. Published 2015 by John Wiley & Sons, Ltd.

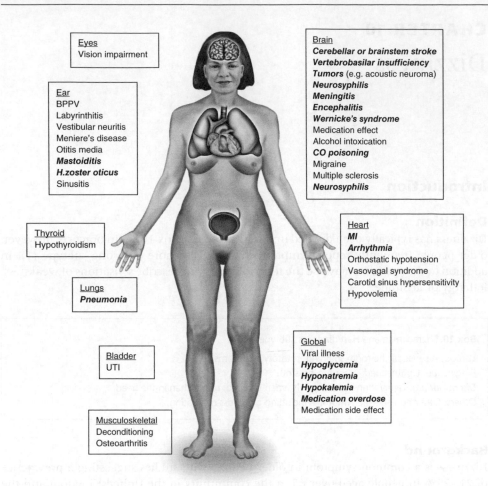

Eyes
Vision impairment

Ear
BPPV
Labyrinthitis
Vestibular neuritis
Meniere's disease
Otitis media
Mastoiditis
H.zoster oticus
Sinusitis

Thyroid
Hypothyroidism

Lungs
Pneumonia

Bladder
UTI

Musculoskeletal
Deconditioning
Osteoarthritis

Brain
Cerebellar or brainstem stroke
Vertebrobasilar insufficiency
Tumors (e.g. acoustic neuroma)
Neurosyphilis
Meningitis
Encephalitis
Wernicke's syndrome
Medication effect
Alcohol intoxication
CO poisoning
Migraine
Multiple sclerosis
Neurosyphilis

Heart
MI
Arrhythmia
Orthostatic hypotension
Vasovagal syndrome
Carotid sinus hypersensitivity
Hypovolemia

Global
Viral illness
Hypoglycemia
Hyponatremia
Hypokalemia
Medication overdose
Medication side effect

Figure 10.1 Causes of dizziness in older patients. Conditions requiring rapid diagnosis in the ED are shown in bold italic type. Source: From Lo AX, Harada CN. Geriatric dizziness: evolving diagnostic and therapeutic approaches for the emergency department. *Clin Geriatr Med*. 2013 Feb;29(1):181–204. Reproduced with permission of Elsevier.

Precipitants of the dizziness

Is dizziness experienced when the patient stands up, or moves from lying to sitting or standing? Is it precipitated by the patient turning their head or whilst turning over in bed?

Timescale

The causes of abrupt onset vertigo are different from the causes of chronic unsteadiness or light-headedness, and a careful distinction should be made.

Frequency of attacks

The number and frequency of attacks should be established, along with tempo and duration.

Symptom	Subtype	Likely cause	Comment
Vertigo	Position induced	Benign paroxysmal positional vertigo (BPPV)	If nystagmus does not match BPPV (it should rotational with the fast phase towards the affected side), consider central pathologies; if induced by neck rotation, consider cervical vertigo
	Acute onset persistent with neurologic signs	Stroke/tumour/neuro-degenerative disease	Acute ischaemia involving vestibular structures can mimic vestibular neuronitis
	Acute onset persistent without neurologic signs	Labyrinthitis Vestibular neuronitis	Differential diagnosis is based on the presence of hearing loss
	Recurrent with no neurologic signs	Ménière's disease Migraine	Late onset Ménière's disease is possible but not common. Migraines lack progressive auditory symptoms. Transient ischaemic attacks (TIA) should be considered in patients with risk factors
Disequilibrium	Acute or rapidly progressive	Stroke	Autoimmune post-infectious diseases should also be considered; may also include severe occulomotor problems
	Worse in the absence of other sensory inputs	Bilateral vestibular loss	Check for ototoxicity. Hearing loss or oscillopsia may be present
	Worse in the absence of vision with numbness/weakness	Proprioception and somatosensory loss	Often associated with peripheral neuropathy from metabolic, renal failure, toxic or diabetic causes
	With bradykinesia/rigidity/tremor	Parkinsonism	Frontal lobe or other basal ganglia disorders
	With speech disorder/incoordination/intention tremor	Cerebellar lesion	The imbalance is usually the same with and without vision
	Isolated disequilibrium/gait difficulty/light-headedness	Disequilibrium of ageing	Often accompanied by borderline diffuse central findings but no other specific complaints
Presyncope	With BP drop on standing	Postural hypotension	Associated with reduced blood volume, autonomic disorders or chronic use of antihypertensives
	Abnormal cardiac examination	Heart valve disease, arrhythmia	Warrants consideration of 24-hour ECG
	Introduced by fear or anxiety	Vasovagal	Decline in heart rate and blood pressure leads to decrease in cerebral blood flow
Light-headedness (nonspecific)	Associated with fear, anxiety or depression	Psychogenic	Often accompanied by autonomic symptoms

Source: From Barin K, Dodson EE. Dizziness in the elderly. *Otolaryngol Clin North Am.* 2011 Apr;44(2):437–454, x. Reproduced with permission of Elsevier.

Table 10.2 Examination of a dizzy patient.

Physical examination	
Vital signs	Bradycardia or hypotension may point to underlying cause
Erect and supine blood pressures	Rule out orthostatic hypotension as cause of dizziness
Head, eyes, ears, nose and throat	
Ear examination	Rule out otitis media, mastoiditis; test hearing
Vestibular examination	Dix–Hallpike test for BPPV or other tests of vestibular dizziness (see text)
Neurological examination	
Eye examination	Evaluate for nystagmus or vision changes (may suggest stroke)
Speech/language	Dysarthria or aphasia suggests stroke
Motor examination	Focal weakness suggests stroke; global weakness suggests deconditioning
Sensory examination	Focal sensory deficit suggests stroke
Cerebellar	Cerebellar signs (dysmetria, ataxia) suggests posterior stroke
Cardiac examination	Evaluate for arrhythmia, diaphoresis, signs of tamponade, orthostatic vital signs
Respiratory examination	Pneumonia, asthma or COPD exacerbation may cause dizziness/hyperventilation
Remainder of general examination	Helps with broad differential for dizziness

Source: From Lo AX, Harada CN. Geriatric dizziness: evolving diagnostic and therapeutic approaches for the emergency department. *Clin Geriatr Med*. 2013 Feb;29(1):181–204. Reproduced with permission of Elsevier.

Past medical history
The patient's medical history should be explored with particular focus on previous conditions causing dizziness such as Ménière's disease, falls, malignancy, previous head trauma, and cardiac or vascular risk factors that may place the patient at increased risk of stroke.

Medication and alcohol history
Alcohol excess can cause dizziness by either direct cerebellar toxicity or chronic cerebellar damage Cardiovascular medication, particularly antihypertensives, may result in postural hypotension leading to presyncopal dizziness.

Examination

General examination
A comprehensive physical examination is important for evaluating a dizzy patient (Table 10.2).

Specific areas of focus on examination
Differentiation of central from peripheral vertigo
Patients presenting with 'acute vestibular syndrome' (Box 10.2) are most likely to have a self-limiting or viral cause such as BPPV (benign paroxysmal positional vertigo) or labyrinthitis. A small proportion will have more serious pathology such as a brain stem or cerebellar stroke. CT brain scans are not very sensitive (~16%) for identifying acute

infarction in these regions and so rapid differentiation between central and peripheral vertigo is important early in the clinical assessment (4).

Box 10.2 Features of acute vestibular syndrome.

Rapid onset (over seconds to hours)
Vertigo
Nausea/vomiting
Gait unsteadiness
Head motion intolerance
Nystagmus

The Dix-Hallpike test

The Dix–Hallpike test and the supine roll test can aid in identifying peripheral vertigo (originating from posterior and horizontal semi-circular canals respectively) (5).

1 The patient sits upright while the examiner rotates the patient's head 45° to one side.
2 With their eyes open, the patient lies back with their head hanging slightly below the level of the examination table while the examiner observes for nystagmus and inquires about subjective vertigo. Latency, duration, and direction of any nystagmus should be noted.
3 If negative, repeat the manoeuvre with patient's head rotated to the opposite side.

Interpreting the Dix-Hallpike test

A positive result is when rotational nystagmus occurs approximately 5–10 seconds after the patient is placed in the horizontal position; this usually also reproduces the patient's symptoms. The fast phase of the nystagmus will beat towards the affected ear, which is the ear closest to the ground.

Note: if rotational nystagmus does not occur but up- or down-beating nystagmus is observed, a central cause should be considered.

Cautions and contraindications to canalith repositioning manoeuvres

Note that there are some contraindications and cautions to performing this procedure, and also the Epley manoeuvre, which is discussed later in this chapter Figure 10.2; these are as follows (6):

Contraindications:

- Odontoid peg fracture or other recent cervical spine fracture
- Atlanto-axial subluxation
- Cervical disc prolapse
- Known vertibro-basilar insufficiency
- Recent neck trauma that restricts rotational movement.

Cautions:

- Carotid sinus syncope
- Severe back pain
- Recent stroke
- Cardiac bypass within the last 3 months
- Rheumatoid arthritis affecting the neck

- Recent neck surgery
- Cervical myelopathy
- Severe orthopnoea.

Investigations

Initial investigations
All dizzy patients should have:
- erect and supine blood pressures
- baseline blood screen: FBC (full blood count), U&Es (urea and electrolytes), LFTs (liver function tests) and consideration of troponin and toxicology screens if history suggests these tests may be relevant
- ECG.

Further investigations
If a central cause of dizziness is suspected, CT or MRI brain should be considered.

If a peripheral cause of dizziness is suspected, the Dix–Hallpike test should be performed to help establish the diagnosis Table 10.3.

Table 10.3 Differentiating between central and peripheral vertigo.

	Peripheral cause			Central cause	
	Labyrinthitis	BPPV	Ménière's	Stroke/TIA	Migraine
Tempo/duration	Acute (<3 days)	Episodic Lasts seconds	Epsiodic Lasts hours	Constant (stroke) Hours/minutes (TIA)	Episodic Minutes to days
Clues from history	Unlikely if >1 episode Spontaneous Worsened by head movement Auditory symptoms if labyrinthitis	Triggered by change in position, e.g. lying down or turning over in bed	Unilateral tinnitus, hearing loss, sense of ear fullness	Spontaneous and continuous	Precipitated by movement
Dix Hallpike or supine roll test	Negative	Positive	Negative	Negative	Negative
Spontaneous nystagmus	Horizontal	Horizontal	Horizontal if present	Purely vertical Purely tortional Gaze evoked and bidirectional	May be present, direction varies
Head thrust	Positive	Normal	Normal	Normal	May be positive
Gait	Wide based, slow, cautious	Normal	Unknown	Often impaired	Normal
Romberg	Negative	Negative	Negative	Positive if cerebellar lesion	Negative

Source: Reproduced with permission of Elsevier. Lo AX, Harada CN. Geriatric dizziness: evolving diagnostic and therapeutic approaches for the emergency department. *Clin Geriatr Med*. 2013 Feb;29(1):181–204.

If a cardiac cause of dizziness is a possibility, based on either concerning features in the history or abnormal resting ECG then further cardiac monitoring should be considered, either in the form of inpatient monitoring or a ambulatory recording e.g. 24 hour tape.

Management

General management
The main priority when initially assessing a dizzy patient is to differentiate the life-threatening from the benign and self-limiting. An appropriate history and examination, as detailed above, should provide adequate information to direct management accordingly.

Specific management considerations in older patients
Attempting to establish the underlying cause is essential for initiating appropriate management.

Medications
Vestibular suppressants are overprescribed and all are noted to be poorly tolerated in older patients as well as reducing the brain's ability to compensate for vertigo over time. Disease-specific therapies and vestibular rehabilitation are the preferred strategy.

If symptoms are very severe and life-threatening causes have been excluded, patients should be counselled on the risks associated with vestibular suppressants, and therapy should be prescribed at the lowest possible dose for the shortest possible time (1, 3). Long-term use of vestibular suppressants for symptomatic management of non-specific dizziness is not recommended.

Benign paroxysmal positional vertigo
Canalith repositioning methods such as the Epley manoeuvre (Figure 10.2) are the first-line treatment for patients presenting with BPPV; this simple procedure is effective and takes less than 5 minutes. Studies have shown that its use in the ED is effective (3) and it can also be performed in primary care (7). Videos of the Epley manoeuvre to supplement the explanation in Figure 10.2 are available online.

Box 10.3 How to perform the Epley manoeuvre (8).

- Begin by performing the same sequence used in the Dix–Hallpike test:
  - the patient is seated upright
  - the head is turned towards the affected side (say the left)
  - with the head still turned, the patient is reclined past the horizontal
  - hold for 30 seconds
- in the reclined position the head is turned to the right
  - hold for 30 seconds
- the patient is rolled onto the right side
  - the head is still turned to the right (the patient is now looking towards the floor)
  - hold for 30 seconds
- the patient is sat upright, still looking over the right shoulder
  - hold for 30 seconds
- the patient turns the head to the midline with the neck flexed and chin downwards
  - hold for 30 seconds

The same contraindications to the Dix-Hallpike test also apply to the Epley manoeuvre. Vestibular suppressants should be avoided in BPPV unless symptoms are very severe.

Vestibular neuronitis

Steroids for days 1–3 of suspected vestibular neuritis (prednisolone 1 mg/kg) can help speed up symptom resolution; however, they often resolve spontaneously.

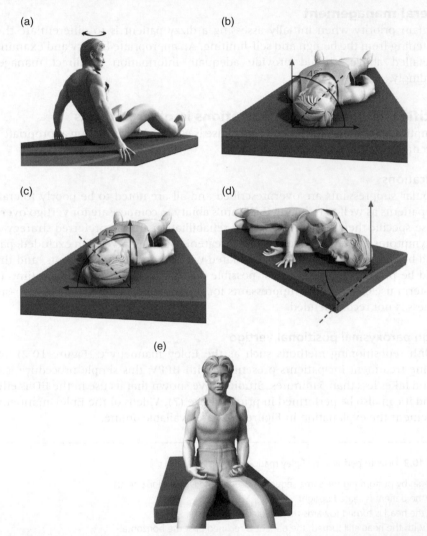

Figure 10.2 The Epley Manoeurve (a) Position patient on the bed and turn their head 45° to the right (symptom site). (b) Keep their head turned to the side and lie the patient down for 5 minutes. (c) Turn the patient's head to the opposite side, lying still for a further 5 minutes. (d) Roll the patient's body onto their side in the direction they are facing; now they are pointing their head nose down. Stay in this position for another 5 minutes. (e) Swing the patient's legs and feet over the side of the bed and sit them upright, keeping their head straight, and remain in place for a further 5 minutes. Source: Reproduced with permission of John Wiley and Sons. Daniel W. K. Kao. *Clinical Maxillary Sinus Elevation Surgery*. Copyright © 2014, John Wiley and Sons.

Ménière's disease

The management of Ménière's disease is based on a low salt diet (<1–2 g/day) and diuretics. Vestibular suppressants can be of benefit but should not be used unless symptoms are severe and debilitating and should ideally be avoided long term.

Vestibular rehabilitation

Vestibular rehabilitation can take place on an outpatient basis in centres staffed by specialist physiotherapists and geriatricians and with access to 'virtual' and physical rehabilitation exercises.

Criteria for admission of a dizzy patient

- Suspicion of or confirmed brainstem or cerebellar stroke
- Patients who are unable to safely walk
- Severe refractory symptoms (regardless of cause) rendering an older person unable to perform their usual activities of daily living.

Take home messages

- Dizziness is a common presenting symptom in older patients with a wide range of differential diagnoses
- 'Dizziness' may mean different things to the patient and the clinician
- Careful and detailed history taking is the cornerstone for establishing a diagnosis
- Brain imaging is of limited value unless a brain stem or cerebellar stroke is suspected
- The Dix–Hallpike test and Epley manoeuvres are effective in diagnosis and treatment, respectively, but are under-used
- Vestibular suppressants should only be prescribed on a short-term basis.

References

1 Barin K, Dodson EE. Dizziness in the elderly. *Otolaryngol Clin North Am*. 2011;44(2):437–454.
2 Drachman DA, Hart CW. An approach to the dizzy patient. *Neurology*. 1972;22(4):323–334.
3 Lo AX, Harada CN. Geriatric dizziness: evolving diagnostic and therapeutic approaches for the emergency department. *Clin Geriatr Med*. 2013;29(1):181–204.
4 Kattah JC, Talkad AV, Wang DZ, Hsieh Y-H, Newman-Toker DE. HINTS to diagnose stroke in the acute vestibular syndrome three-step bedside Oculomotor examination more sensitive than early MRI diffusion-weighted imaging. *Stroke*. 2009;40(11):3504–3510.
5 Tusa RJ. Vertigo. *Neurol Clin*. 2001;19(1):23–55.
6 British Society of Audiology. Recommended Procedure for Hallpike Manoeuvre. 2001.
7 Cranfield S, Mackenzie I, Gabbay M. Can GPs diagnose benign paroxysmal positional vertigo and does the Epley manoeuvre work in primary care? *Br J Gen Pract*. 2010;60(578):698–699.
8 Swartz R, Longwell P. Treatment of vertigo. *Am Fam Physician*. 2005;71(6):1115–1122.

CHAPTER 11
Major trauma

Introduction

Beyond the age of 70 years, mortality after a traumatic injury significantly increases in comparison to that in younger patients (1). Older persons account for 28% of deaths due to trauma while representing only 12% of the overall trauma population (2).

Mechanisms of injury differ in the older patients with 60% of trauma due to falls, and 25% from motor vehicle accidents. Falls occur due to a multitude of factors such as gait instability, leg weakness, postural hypotension, and acute illness (Chapter 8). Slower reaction times, cognitive decline, reduced visual acuity, hearing impairment, physical disabilities, and slower ambulation are contributing factors to motor vehicle accidents in older drivers and pedestrians. The presence of comorbidities and polypharmacy in older adults has been shown to increase the risk of motor vehicle collision (3). Loss of control at the wheel may be triggered by an acute cardiac or cerebrovascular event.

 KEY POINT: Always look for an acute change in medical condition preceding a traumatic injury in the older patient.

Definition

Major trauma describes serious and often multiple injuries resulting from an external source or impact and where there is a strong possibility of death or disability (4).

Background

A lower transmitted kinetic injury results in more severe injuries due to reduced bone density and other degenerative changes. Around one quarter of older patients in motor vehicle accidents sustain chest trauma such as rib fractures. Fractures of the cervical spine, hip and pelvic ring are common. There is a higher incidence of fatal injuries such as intracranial haemorrhage.

Geriatric Emergencies, First Edition.
Iona Murdoch, Sarah Turpin, Bree Johnston, Alasdair MacLullich and Eve Losman.
© 2015 John Wiley & Sons, Ltd. Published 2015 by John Wiley & Sons, Ltd.

The high mortality rate reflects comorbidities, decreased physiological reserve and medications such as anticoagulants or antihypertensives rather than chronological age alone. For example, trauma patients with heart failure have more than double the risk of death; if they are also taking β-blockers or warfarin this risk is even higher (5). Despite the increased mortality rate, geriatric trauma is frequently under-triaged to local hospitals rather than major trauma centres, potentially delaying access to expert care and definitive treatment (6). Reasons for this may include delayed recognition of shock; an under-appreciation amongst emergency medial services of the increased susceptibility of the older population to minor injury mechanisms; and reduced representation of the older patient in trauma triage guidelines.

A large proportion of older trauma patients return to independent living (7), and an initial aggressive approach to resuscitation should be pursued. In an older patient with catastrophic injuries, a decision in consultation with family and the trauma team to switch to palliative treatment may sometimes be appropriate.

Initial Approach

Management of an older person with a traumatic injury should begin with a *primary survey* to identify and treat any life-threatening issues, according to Advanced Trauma Life Support® (ATLS®) Guidelines (8). Vital signs can be falsely reassuring and increased mortality has been shown in older patients with heart rates greater than 90 beats/min

Disability
- Cerebral atrophy increases the likelihood of subdural haematoma
- Dementia or delirium may affect assessment of pain or GCS

Cervical spine
- Osteoporosis, osteoarthritis and cervical spondylosis increase the risk of fractures, cord syndromes or diagnostic difficulties on imaging

Breathing
- Increased vulnerability to rib and sternal fractures due to calcification of costochondral cartilage and a more 'brittle' chest wall
- Weaker respiratory muscles, which are more susceptible to fatigue when faced with increased work of breathing
- Presence of COPD or other chronic lung disease
- Reduced effectiveness of cough and mucociliary clearance

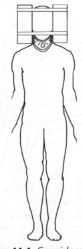

Figure 11.1 Considerations in the primary survey in an older adult.

Circulation
- Higher baseline systolic pressure means patients may be hypovolaemic with a blood pressure in the 'normal' range
- Decrease in maximum heart rate
- Reduced catecholamine response leading to absence of tachycardia despite shock
- Presence of heart failure, valve disease or coronary artery disease: trauma may trigger ischaemia or decompensation

Exposure
- Increased risk of hypothermia due to loss of subcutaneous fat and impaired thermoregulation
- Increased risk of fractures after minimal energy mechanism due to reduced bone mineral density
- Increased risk of skin tears or pressure injuries resulting from transfers or prolonged immobility

and a systolic blood pressure less than 110 mmHg (9). Older patients report less pain for the same injury than do younger trauma patients, also potentially falsely reassuring clinicians that an injury is less severe (10). Figure 11.1 illustrates particular considerations when evaluating the older trauma patient.

Airway and cervical spine immobilisation

Assess airway patency while immobilising the cervical spine.

Provide high-flow oxygen.

Inspect the airway for foreign bodies, loose teeth, dentures or facial injuries.

In an obstructed airway perform a jaw-thrust and insert an oropharyngeal airway. Prepare for intubation or a surgical airway if necessary.

Anatomical changes in the airway of an older adult can make airway maintenance and tracheal intubation more difficult (Figure 11.2).

Brittle or loose teeth may fracture easily during airway manoeuvres

Bag-valve mask ventilation may be difficult in edentulous patients with loss of maxillary subcutaneous tissue. Malfitting or displaced dentures may contribute to this

Reduced mouth opening secondary to microstomia or temporomandibular arthritis

Airway bleeding may occur during insertion of airway adjuncts or laryngoscopy due to friable nasal and pharyngeal tissue

Airway patency may be lost earlier due to decreased oropharyngeal reflexes

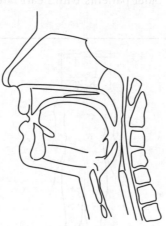

Figure 11.2 Factors that may lead to difficult airway management in the geriatric patient.

Increased risk of aspiration as a result of decreased oropharyngeal reflexes and slower gastric emptying

Decreased cervical spine and atlanto-occipital joint mobility makes intubation potentially difficult even if the cervical spine has been cleared

The atlanto-occipital joint may be unstable due to rheumatoid arthritis or degenerative changes

Maintenance of in-line cervical stabilisation is necessary unless the cervical spine has been cleared

Endotracheal intubation should be considered early in patients with an unprotected airway due to reduced level of consciousness or in significant chest trauma. Rapid sequence induction is associated with increased complications in the older person such as hypotension and hypoxia (11). Reduced doses of induction agents are required to avoid post-induction hypotension.

> **KEY POINT:** In edentulous patients leaving dentures in place may help maintain airway patency and facemask seal during pre-oxygenation or bag-mask ventilation.

Breathing

Expose the neck, chest and axillae and inspect and palpate for visible injuries, tracheal deviation, chest movement, and subcutaneous emphysema.
Feel for tenderness along the ribs, clavicle and sternum.
Percuss the chest to elicit any dullness or hyper-resonance.
Listen for bilateral air entry.

The older patient has a reduced or delayed response to hypoxia and hypercapnia. Arterial blood gases are useful to assess adequacy of oxygenation and ventilation. Asking the patient to take a deep breath in and cough can provide a good indication of respiratory function.

Chest injuries including rib fractures, pneumothoraces and pulmonary contusions are poorly tolerated and associated with a much higher rate of complications, including atelectasis and pneumonia.

Circulation with haemorrhage control

Identify any external haemorrhage, and apply direct pressure. Simple scalp lacerations or facial injuries may bleed profusely

Assess pulse rate, volume and regularity. Measure blood pressure. Assess skin colour and capillary refill. Attach cardiac monitoring and obtain an ECG

Examine the abdomen, pelvis and thighs for signs of internal bleeding due to blunt injury or fractures. Consider application of a pelvic binder or splint

Perform a FAST (focused assessment with sonography for trauma) or eFAST ultrasound scan at the bedside to identify free fluid in the abdomen, pericardial fluid or pneumothorax

Insert two large-bore IV lines and take a blood sample including for cross-match. Give IV fluid or blood products depending on findings and likely injuries

Medications such as β-blockers or antihypertensives, or the presence of a pacemaker, may reduce the patient's compensatory response to haemorrhage and mask hypovolaemic shock. Pre-existing conditions, such as cardiac failure, may confuse the clinical picture. Serial base deficit and blood lactate measurements may identify impaired perfusion due to occult haemorrhage. Anti-coagulation may need to be urgently reversed (Box 14.5).

> **KEY POINT:** Normal vital signs may be falsely reassuring. A trauma patient with a normal blood pressure who is known to be hypertensive should be assumed to be bleeding until proven otherwise (12).

Abdominal injuries occur at a similar rate to that in younger patients, but splenic injuries are less common due to involution of the spleen with ageing (12). Abdominal examination is less reliable in older patients (Chapter 15), and a low threshold for CT should be adopted.

Significant pelvic fractures in patients aged over 60 have a high likelihood of retroperitoneal bleeding (13). Lateral compression fractures are five times more common than anterior compression fractures in the older adult (14), and these are more likely to cause significant haemorrhage with a greater need for angiography, despite the same being considered a more benign fracture in younger patients (15). Mortality in patients suffering pelvic fracture has been reported to be between 12% and 21% (12). Occult bleeding into the pelvis may be detected by performing serial full blood count, lactate and base deficit. Repeat imaging or angiography may be necessary (16).

Disability

Establish the level of consciousness using the Glasgow coma scale (GCS)
Assess the pupils: size, reactivity and equality
Measure a bedside blood sugar

Head injury is discussed in Chapter 14.

KEY POINT: The older trauma patient is at increased risk of pressure injuries resulting from prolonged immobility. Aim to remove the spinal backboard or pre-hospital scoop as early as possible.

Exposure and environmental control

Undress the patient to assess for other life-threatening injuries.
Measure temperature and instigate warming measures to prevent or treat hypothermia.
Assess pain and administer analgesia.

Pain management is discussed in Chapter 3.

History

After the primary survey has excluded any life-threatening injuries, a brief initial (AMPLE) history is important as comorbidities and medication may affect immediate management (Table 11.1).

Investigations

Table 11.2 highlights investigations to be considered in the geriatric trauma patient.

Table 11.1 AMPLE history in older trauma patients.

Allergies	Especially to antibiotics, analgesics and anaesthetic drugs
Medication	Particularly note anticoagulants, antiplatelet agents, β-blockers, antihypertensives and steroids
Past medical history	Especially record coronary artery disease, respiratory disease and liver disease.
Last food or drink	Trauma results in delayed gastric emptying
Events	A brief outline of events, and any preceding symptoms such as chest pain or dizziness (see Chapter 8)

Table 11.2 Investigations in the older trauma patient.

Full blood count, coagulation, urea and electrolytes, cross-match	Baseline blood tests are required, especially if the patient is taking anticoagulants, where reversal of coagulation may be necessary. Consider point-of-care PT/INR or haemoglobin if available. Cardiac enzymes may be elevated in cases of cardiac contusion, or when trauma has been precipitated by an acute myocardial infarction
Arterial or venous blood gas	Arterial blood gases are useful to assess for adequacy of oxygenation and ventilation, and demonstrate signs of tissue hypoxia such as raised base deficit and lactic acid
Electrocardiogram	Perform a 12-lead ECG to assess for ischaemia or arrhythmia as a cause or consequence of trauma
Chest radiograph, pelvic radiograph	Useful as part of the primary survey to detect complications of chest trauma or pelvic fractures. Plain radiographs have a lower sensitivity compared to CT, however
Bedside ultrasound (FAST exam)	FAST or eFAST is undertaken to identify free fluid, assumed to be blood in the case of trauma, in the abdomen, pelvis or pericardium; or a pneumothorax. Older patients with heart failure or liver disease may have a false-positive FAST scan due to pre-existing ascites, but this should be assumed to be due to haemorrhage until proven otherwise
Trauma CT with intravenous contrast	CT should be considered the imaging of choice in the older trauma patient. Trauma centres are increasingly adopting a low threshold for trauma CT (head, neck, chest, abdomen, pelvis) due to the prevalence of occult injuries, even in cases with a relatively minor mechanism. This is especially relevant for the older patient where clinical signs may be absent. Use of intravenous contrast may precipitate acute kidney injury in patients with pre-existing renal failure or hypovolaemia, and this should be considered when imaging strategies are being considered. In an unstable patient with evidence of abdominal free fluid immediate transfer to the operating theatre without an initial CT scan may be necessary

PT, prothrombin; INR, international normalized ratio.

General management

Management of the major trauma patient will depend on the injuries, degree of haemodynamic compromise and investigation findings. Considerations for the older trauma patient include the following:

- Aim for early transfusion of blood products in the unstable trauma patient. Deliberate maintenance of a lower blood pressure in patients with severe haemorrhage, termed *permissive hypotension*, may limit bleeding and allow clot stabilisation prior to definite control of a bleeding source. Anti-fibrinolytics (tranexamic acid) should be administered in cases of traumatic bleeding.
- Serial lactate and base deficit measurements may assist with the diagnosis of occult bleeding (7) and should be repeated within the first hour in the emergency department (12).
- In centres with interventional radiology capability, angiography with or without embolisation should be considered in older patients with major pelvic fractures, even if they are haemodynamically stable (17), due to the risk of significant retroperitoneal bleeding. Similarly, consider angiographic embolisation in the non-operative management of splenic lacerations, if urgent laparotomy is not deemed to be required (15).
- If operative intervention such as laparotomy or surgical fixation of fractures is required this should be undertaken promptly to facilitate early mobilisation.

Secondary survey and tertiary survey

Once the primary survey has been completed and the patient confirmed to be stable, a full examination from head to toe should take place to detect any other injuries such as fractures, skin tears or burns. A logroll should be performed to examine the back for signs of injury and to perform a rectal examination if indicated. In major trauma, logrolling may worsen bleeding associated with pelvic or abdominal injuries and it is often appropriate to await the results of CT imaging. Further investigations such as limb radiographs may be required following the secondary survey.

A tertiary survey should be undertaken within 24 hours of admission to identify any injuries that may have been missed during the initial emergency department assessment. It should include a general physical examination, assessment of vital signs and a review of all imaging and blood results. It is particularly important in the older patient due to reduced reporting of pain or cognitive impairment.

Rib fractures

Half of adults who sustain rib fractures do so following falls from a standing position, often from hitting a piece of furniture or step while falling to the ground (18). Older adults are more susceptible to rib and sternal fractures due to seatbelts in low- and medium-speed road traffic collisions, with an incidence of sternal fractures of 11% in those aged over 65 compared to 1.5% in a younger age group (15). Rib fractures may also occur following coughing in those with severe osteoporosis.

Pain following thoracic trauma causes hypoventilation and a reluctance to cough. Atelectasis and retained bronchial secretions, combined with reduced respiratory muscle strength in the older adult, can quickly lead to pneumonia and respiratory failure. Rib fractures are associated with twice the mortality than in younger patients, with 12% mortality in patients sustaining one to two fractures, to nearly 40% in patients with seven or more fractures (18). Thirty-five percent of patients develop pulmonary contusions or pneumonia following rib fractures, complicating any pre-existing cardiorespiratory disease (19). This risk is higher the greater the number of rib fractures. Rib fractures are also associated with an increase in hepatic and splenic injury in the older patient.

Rib fractures are diagnosed clinically based on a history of trauma with musculoskeletal pain and localised chest wall tenderness on palpation. A chest radiograph should be performed to detect early complications such as haemothorax or pneumothorax, and is useful as a baseline if the patient is being admitted to hospital. However, chest radiograph is often insensitive for detecting rib fractures and associated complications, and CT of the thorax, or whole body trauma CT if indicated, is preferable.

Admission for analgesia, monitoring and chest physiotherapy is recommended if the patient is known to have cardiopulmonary comorbidities, has two or more rib fractures, is in significant pain and is unable to cough, or if investigations have revealed inadequate ventilation or other complications.

Epidural anaesthesia should be considered the first-line analgesia for patients with four or more rib fractures. Other options for analgesia include a paravertebral or intercostal catheter, or patient controlled intravenous analgesia. Patients should be admitted to an intensive care unit or other high dependency area where they can receive close monitoring, regular chest physiotherapy to encourage deep ventilation and clearance of secretions, and optimisation of analgesia. Regular incentive spirometry can detect early decompensation before physiological parameters become deranged. Early mechanical ventilation or non-invasive ventilation may be necessary, particularly in flail chest or severe pulmonary contusion causing hypoxia.

Cervical spine injuries

Cervical spine fractures following blunt trauma are twice as likely in patients over the age of 65. Cervical spondylosis, narrowing of the cervical canal, ligamentous laxity and osteoporosis predispose to fractures and spinal cord injury following low-energy trauma. Morbidity and mortality following these injuries is higher in the older patient as with all trauma.

Falls from standing height are associated with a risk of upper cervical fractures, at the atlanto-axial complex, whereas motor vehicle accidents are more likely to result in lower cervical vertebrae pathology. Relatively minor extension injuries may result in central cord syndromes without bony injury. Assessment of the cervical spine in the older trauma patient is more time consuming, resulting in prolonged immobilisation with associated complications.

Initial assessment
Patients at risk of cervical spine injury should be immobilised initially in a hard collar, on a backboard with blocks and tape. Patients with known cervical spine disease such as ankylosing spondylitis should be immobilised in a position of comfort, due to the risk of worsening an injury by forcing them into an ill-fitting collar. Restraining patients with agitation due to delirium or dementia may worsen an injury and careful evaluation of the risk and benefits of sedation is necessary.

> **KEY POINT:** Immobilisation in suspected cervical spine injury may worsen outcome in agitated patients or those with pre-existing cervical spine disease.

Following completion of the primary survey, history should include the mechanism of injury, presence or absence of neck pain, weakness or sensory changes in the upper and lower limbs, and bowel and bladder disturbance. Clarify previous cervical spine pathology such as rheumatoid arthritis or ankylosing spondylitis and the patient's usual range of movement.

The upper and lower limb nerve roots should be examined for power, sensation, and reflexes. While maintaining immobilisation of the cervical spine, assess for midline tenderness from the occiput down to the upper thoracic spine. Carefully logroll the patient and examine for tenderness in the thoracic and lumbar spine, performing a rectal examination to assess for anal tone and perianal sensation.

> **KEY POINT:** Cervical spine fractures in the older patient are associated with a second fracture of the thoracic or lumbar spine in 10% of cases. Be sure to examine the whole spine for tenderness and consider extended imaging.

Imaging

In adults with potential cervical spine injury, validated decision rules such as the Canadian C-Spine rule and the NEXUS criteria are widely utilised to risk stratify patients and determine in whom imaging is required.

The Canadian C-Spine rule excludes patients over 65 years old (20), viewing older age as a marker of high risk that necessitates imaging. The NEXUS rule has been validated in the older adult, suggesting that the cervical spine can be cleared clinically in the presence of other low-risk features, including the absence of cervical spine tenderness, distracting injury, intoxification or reduced consciousness level, and a normal neurological examination (21). However, a number of older patients will not have cervical spine tenderness in the presence of a significant spinal cord injury. Clinical judgement is required but a low threshold for imaging is recommended.

> **KEY POINT:** CT should be considered the primary imaging modality for the cervical spine in older patients (22).

Adequate plain radiographs are more difficult to obtain and interpret due to pre-existing degenerative disease in the older patient. Upper cervical spine fractures are more likely to be missed on plain radiography, and these are the most common sites of injury in the older adult. CT imaging is superior to plain radiography in detecting injuries of the cervical spine and is therefore advocated as the preferred first-line imaging. This is especially the case if the patient is undergoing CT imaging to assess for head injury or chest or abdominal trauma. Proceeding straight to CT imaging will, if normal, potentially reduce the period of immobilisation in a hard collar with associated risks of pressure sores, brachial plexus injuries as well as pulmonary atelectasis. A normal CT does not exclude an unstable ligamentous injury or a spinal cord injury such as central cord syndrome (see below). Full examination of the neck should take place before the immobilisation is discontinued and if movement is limited or there are other concerns, further imaging, usually magnetic resonance imaging (MRI), should be requested.

If, on initial assessment, there are neurological signs of symptoms referable to the cervical spine, MRI is indicated to evaluate for a spinal cord injury. CT or MRI angiography may be indicated if there is a suspicion of vascular injury such as a fracture causing disruption of the vertebral artery.

Odontoid peg fractures

Degenerative changes in the cervical spine reduce mobility of the lower cervical spine region, resulting in increased movement at C1/C2 and increased vulnerability following minor trauma, either flexion or extension. Fractures of the odontoid peg, especially type II fractures through the base of the dens, are the most common cervical spine fracture in older patients (Figure 11.3). They are associated with a high risk of non-union. They may present with minimal or absent symptoms with a normal appearance on plain radiographs.

Due to the increased width of the spinal column in the high cervical spine, odontoid peg fractures are infrequently associated with neurological deficit due to cord impingement. Management options include surgical fixation, use of external fixation devices or a hard collar. Patients with failure of conservative management, grossly unstable fractures and neurological deficits should be considered for surgical fixation. Use of external

Type I

Type II

Type III

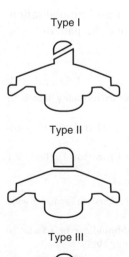

Figure 11.3 Anderson D'Alonso Classification of Odontoid Peg fractures. Type II is the commonest occurring in older patients (23). Source: From Lewis E, Liew S, Dowrick A. Risk factors for non-union in the non-operative management of type II dens fractures. *ANZ J Surg.* 2011;81(9):604–607. Reproduced with permission of Wiley and Sons.

fixation devices, such as the halo vest, can be associated with respiratory failure, pneumonia and swallowing difficulties. Careful multidisciplinary discussion is required when making management decisions in these patients.

Central cord syndrome

Central cord syndrome occurs due to hyperextension in the neck causing compression of the cervical spinal cord. A typical mechanism is a fall down stairs with an impact to the face or forehead and extension of the neck, but it may result from more trivial trauma. It is the commonest cause of incomplete spinal cord injury and frequently occurs in the older patient who has narrowing of the cervical canal (cervical stenosis) due to degenerative disease. The central part of the spinal cord is most damaged, leading to greater weakness in the upper limbs compared to the lower limbs. There is often no associated fracture or acute ligamentous injury of the cervical spine, with CT only demonstrating degenerative changes. MRI will identify the cord injury and exclude an acute disc herniation or a ligamentous injury requiring surgical fixation. Most patients with central cord syndrome will achieve some improvement in neurological impairment with conservative treatment. Surgical decompression or fixation may be considered.

Take home messages

- Geriatric trauma is associated with a high mortality but is commonly under-triaged. Minor mechanisms of trauma may be associated with significant injuries that may be missed on initial assessment. Normal observations may be falsely reassuring. *Always assume the worst-case scenario in the older trauma patient until proven otherwise*
- Consider an acute medical condition that may have precipitated a traumatic injury in the older patient
- Early CT scanning helps identify occult injury and limits prolonged immobilisation, which is associated with a risk of significant complications in the older patient

References

1 Caterino JM, Valasek T, Werman HA. Identification of an age cutoff for increased mortality in patients with elderly trauma. *Am J Emerg Med*. 2010;28(2):151–158.
2 Koval KJ, Meek R, Schemitsch E, Liporace F, Strauss E, Zuckerman JD. An AOA critical issue. Geriatric trauma: young ideas. *J Bone Joint Surg Am*. 2003;85-A(7):1380–1388.
3 Multiple Medications and Vehicle Crashes: Analysis of Databases. National Highway Traffic Safety Administration 2008.
4 Major Trauma Care in England. National Audit Office. 2010.
5 Ferraris VA, Ferraris SP, Saha SP. The relationship between mortality and preexisting cardiac disease in 5,971 trauma patients. *J Trauma*. 2010;69(3):645–652.
6 Shifflette VK, Lorenzo M, Mangram AJ, Truitt MS, Amos JD, Dunn EL. Should age be a factor to change from a level II to a level I trauma activation? *J Trauma*. 2010;69(1):88–92.
7 Calland JF, Ingraham AM, Martin N, Marshall GT, Schulman CI, Stapleton T, et al. Evaluation and management of geriatric trauma: an Eastern Association for the Surgery of Trauma practice management guideline. *J Trauma Acute Care Surg*. 2012;73(5 Suppl 4):S345–S350.
8 American College of Surgeons Committee on Trauma. Advanced Trauma Life Support Program for Doctors, 9th ed. American College of Surgeons: Chicago, IL; 2012.

9 Heffernan DS, Thakkar RK, Monaghan SF, Ravindran R, Adams CA, Kozloff MS, et al. Normal presenting vital signs are unreliable in geriatric blunt trauma victims. *J Trauma*. 2010;69(4): 813–820.

10 Gibson SJ, Helme RD. Age-related differences in pain perception and report. *Clin Geriatr Med*. 2001;17(3):433–456, v–vi.

11 Theodosiou CA, Loeffler RE, Oglesby AJ, McKeown DW, Ray DC. Rapid sequence induction of anaesthesia in elderly patients in the emergency department. *Resuscitation*. 2011;82(7):881–885.

12 Aschkenasy MT, Rothenhaus TC. Trauma and falls in the elderly. *Emerg Med Clin North Am*. 2006;24(2):413–432, vii.

13 Kimbrell BJ, Velmahos GC, Chan LS, Demetriades D. Angiographic embolization for pelvic fractures in older patients. *Arch Surg*. 2004;139(7):728–732; discussion 732–733.

14 Henry SM, Pollak AN, Jones AL, Boswell S, Scalea TM. Pelvic fracture in geriatric patients: a distinct clinical entity. *J Trauma*. 2002;53(1):15–20.

15 Callaway DW, Wolfe R. Geriatric trauma. *Emerg Med Clin North Am*. 2007;25(3):837–860, x.

16 Bonne S, Schuerer DJE. Trauma in the older adult: epidemiology and evolving geriatric trauma principles. *Clin Geriatr Med*. 2013;29(1):137–150.

17 Cullinane DC, Schiller HJ, Zielinski MD, Bilaniuk JW, Collier BR, Como J, et al. Eastern Association for the Surgery of Trauma practice management guidelines for hemorrhage in pelvic fracture – update and systematic review. *J Trauma*. 2011;71(6):1850–1868.

18 Bergeron E, Lavoie A, Clas D, Moore L, Ratte S, Tetreault S, et al. Elderly trauma patients with rib fractures are at greater risk of death and pneumonia. *J Trauma*. 2003;54(3):478–485.

19 Ziegler DW, Agarwal NN. The morbidity and mortality of rib fractures. *J Trauma*. 1994;37(6): 975–979.

20 Stiell IG, Wells GA, Vandemheen KL, Clement CM, Lesiuk H, De Maio VJ, et al. The Canadian C-spine rule for radiography in alert and stable trauma patients. *JAMA*. 2001;286(15):1841–1848.

21 Hoffman JR, Mower WR, Wolfson AB, Todd KH, Zucker MI. Validity of a set of clinical criteria to rule out injury to the cervical spine in patients with blunt trauma. National Emergency X-Radiography Utilization Study Group. *N Engl J Med*. 2000;343(2):94–99.

22 Greenbaum J, Walters N, Levy PD. An evidenced-based approach to radiographic assessment of cervical spine injuries in the emergency department. *J Emerg Med*. 2009;36(1):64–71.

23 Lewis E, Liew S, Dowrick A. Risk factors for non-union in the non-operative management of type II dens fractures. *ANZ J Surg*. 2011;81(9):604–607.

CHAPTER 12

Fractures and back pain

Fractures

Introduction

Five percent of falls in the older adult will result in a fracture. About 40–50% of older women and 13–22% of older men will experience a hip, vertebral or forearm fracture in their lifetime (1). The high risk of morbidity and mortality after an osteoporotic fracture demands a multidisciplinary approach to prevent fracture complications, assess and address the reasons for the initial injury and rehabilitate to pre-injury function. This process should commence as soon as possible after the older patient arrives in the emergency department.

Definition and background

A *fragility fracture* results from mechanical forces that would not ordinarily result in a fracture, known as *low-energy trauma* (2), such as falling from a standing height or less. Fragility fractures occur most commonly in the proximal femur, vertebrae and distal radius, as well as the humerus, ankle, pelvis and ribs. Fractures are more common in the older population due to the increased incidence of falls (Chapter 8) and osteoporosis.

Osteoporosis is the reduction in bone density and disruption in bone architecture that renders the bone more fragile and liable to break. Diagnosis is made clinically, with the presentation of a typical fracture, such as hip, vertebra or distal radius or with bone density (DEXA) scanning. Risk factors for osteoporosis include age, family history, steroid use, alcohol and smoking, immobility, renal failure and endocrine disorders.

Other risk factors for fractures include osteomalacia due to vitamin D deficiency, Paget's disease and primary and secondary malignancy.

Initial assessment

The initial priorities in the management of a patient with a suspected fracture are highlighted in Box 12.1.

Geriatric Emergencies, First Edition.
Iona Murdoch, Sarah Turpin, Bree Johnston, Alasdair MacLullich and Eve Losman.
© 2015 John Wiley & Sons, Ltd. Published 2015 by John Wiley & Sons, Ltd.

Box 12.1 Priorities in the management of an older patient with a suspected fracture.

- Identify life- and limb-threatening complications of trauma (ATLS®) – see Chapter 11.
- Provide analgesia.
- Identify fractures and other injuries and prevent any secondary injuries due to immobilisation; remove backboards and cervical collars as soon as safe to do so.
- Reduce the fracture to enable as close to normal anatomical alignment as possible, e.g. closed reduction in the emergency department or operating theatre, or open reduction.
- Fix or immobilise the fracture, e.g. plaster cast, ±internal fixation.
- Prevent complications resulting from the fracture itself and associated reduction in mobility.
- Facilitate early mobilisation.

Hip fractures

A fracture of the proximal femur is the commonest fracture in the older adult, with huge implications for the individual patient and health services alike.

Hip fracture is associated with a mortality rate of 10% at 1 month and 30% at 1 year, and up to 30% of those admitted from their homes subsequently require institutional care. This often reflects comorbidities resulting in a fall and post-operative medical and functional complications, and is less often due to the fracture or the operative process itself.

Hip fractures occur between the edge of the femoral head and 5 cm below the lesser trochanter, and can be classified into intracapsular, intertrochanteric and subtrochanteric (Figure 12.1). This distinction influences operative management but basic emergency care is unchanged. Prompt operative fixation is associated with reduced mortality, decreased post-operative pain, early mobilisation, and reduced length of hospital stay and major complications (3). Surgical intervention is the best form of analgesia and is undertaken in the vast majority of patients, even in cases of severe frailty or terminal illness. Surgery should ideally take place on the day of or day after the fracture.

KEY POINT: Initial history and examination should be focused around identifying and treating comorbidities that may delay surgery.

History and examination

Hip fractures can result from relatively minor trauma and in some cases no history of injury is provided, especially in patients with delirium or dementia. A high index of suspicion should be assumed in any older person with new immobility or who is 'found on the floor'. Patients may not volunteer experiencing pain in the hip: pain may only be present on movement or may radiate to the knee, groin or lower back.

On examination, the leg may be shortened and externally rotated. There may be tenderness over the greater trochanter or in the groin. Remember that a fall may result in multiple injuries and the initial approach should be similar to that described in Chapter 11.

KEY POINT: Range of movement and even weight bearing may be preserved in patients with an undisplaced intracapsular fracture so a low threshold of suspicion should be adopted.

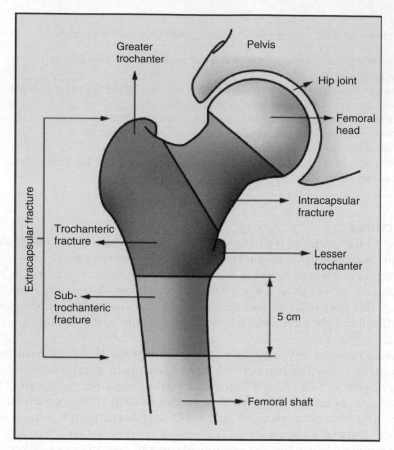

Figure 12.1 Classification of hip fractures. Source: From Parker M, Johansen A. Hip fracture. *BM J.* 2006 Jul 1;333(7557):27–30. Reproduced with permission of BMJ Publishing Group Ltd.

Investigations
Radiographs
Standard imaging is an anterior–posterior and lateral radiograph. If the proximal femur appears normal, check for pubic rami, acetabular or sacral fractures. Radiographs should be inspected closely for disrupted trabeculae and breaches in cortical continuity, Shenton's line and the neck-shaft angle. Shenton's line is formed by the medial edge of the femoral neck and the inferior edge of the superior pubic ramus and lack of contour is suggestive of a fractured neck of femur. The neck-shaft angle should be 120–130°, determined by measuring the angle of the lines drawn through the centres of the femoral shaft and the femoral neck.

If the radiograph appears normal
An undisplaced intracapsular fracture occurs in 15% of cases and may not be visible on plain radiographs. An AP film centred on the hip may confirm a fracture, but if it appears normal and there is still a clinical suspicion of fracture further imaging is required. MRI (magnetic resonance imaging) is the most sensitive imaging modality for detecting

occult hip fractures, and it also identifies alternative pathology such as pelvic fractures, psoas abscess, haematoma, and significant soft tissue injuries (4). If MRI is not available promptly or is contraindicated, CT (computed tomography) is recommended (5).

Chest radiograph

This is usually requested simultaneously to hip radiographs to screen for chest pathology as a cause or consequence of fall and to assist pre-operative anaesthetic assessment.

Blood tests

Full blood count, urea and electrolytes, liver function and blood typing and coagulation should be requested.

Table 12.1 'HEADACHES': factors to consider pre-operatively in fractured neck of femur.

H	Heart	Consider an urgent echocardiogram if there are signs or symptoms of severe aortic stenosis or severe undiagnosed left ventricular failure. Avoid delaying surgery where possible If the patient has a pacemaker, get this checked if there is any evidence that failure might have been the cause of the fall
E	ECG	Observe for concerning features requiring intervention or urgent cardiology review: • Poorly controlled AF • Complete heart block • Trifascicular block • Multiple ectopics, bigemini or trigemini
A	Anaemia	Note haemoglobin and platelet count and arrange transfusion if required
D	Drugs	Withhold ACE inhibitors, angiotensin receptor blockers, oral diuretics and oral hypoglycaemics prior to surgery. Intravenous diuretics can be used as required. Consider stopping or reducing antihypertensives. Stop NSAIDs. Maintain any chronic corticosteroids, adding a stress dose peri-operatively. Continue anti-Parkinson's drugs, antidepressants and beta-blockers (unless the blood pressure is low)
A	Anticoagulation	If the patient is taking anticoagulants, consider whether the patient is at high risk (e.g. valve replacement) or lower risk (e.g. recurrent DVT, AF). Reverse INR with vitamin K and consider an IV heparin infusion or SC low molecular weight heparin. Consult with haematology if necessary
C	Chest	Examine for signs of chest infection or lung disease, which may complicate anaesthetic management. Look at the chest radiograph for these features
H	Hyperglycaemia	A dextrose infusion and insulin sliding scale may be necessary pre-operatively in diabetic patients normally on insulin. Blood glucose should be monitored closely and the patient placed at the start of the theatre list
E	Electrolytes and fluid balance	Exclude severe hypokalaemia, acute hyponatraemia or acute kidney injury Patients are usually dehydrated on admission: check volume status and give intravenous fluids. Exclude urinary retention
S	Mental status	Assess for pre-existing dementia, delirium and decision-making capacity

ACE, angiotensin-converting-enzyme; NSAID, non-steroidal anti-inflammatory drug; AF, atrial fibrillation; INR, international normalized ratio.

Electrocardiogram

An ECG may identify a trigger for the injury such as ischaemia or complete heart block, and will identify any issues requiring intervention prior to anaesthesia.

Echocardiogram

An echocardiogram may be required if the patient demonstrates signs of valvular heart disease but in many cases will not change management and should not result in a delay to surgery.

See Table 12.1 for further discussion on investigations in hip fracture patients.

> **KEY POINT: If plain radiographs are normal, further imaging is required if the patient is not weight bearing or is in significant pain.**

Management

Management in the ED should be in accordance with the general management of fractures highlighted in Box 12.1, with a focus on relieving pain and preparing for surgery.

Pain should be assessed immediately on presentation to the ED and within 30 minutes of analgesia being given, and then at hourly intervals or more frequently as indicated (5).

To avoid reliance on opioids with their frequent side effects in the older patient, consider providing regional anaesthesia as the first-line method of pain control in patients presenting with a fractured neck of femur (6, 7). The most common procedure offered is a fascia iliaca compartment block (FICB) described below.

Contraindications to FICB include patient refusal, anticoagulation, previous femoral bypass surgery, inflammation or infection over the injection site, or an allergy to local anaesthetics. If any of these contraindications is present; there is no appropriately skilled clinician available or pain is still poorly controlled; intravenous opioids, e.g. IV morphine, are usually required in small doses, repeated if required. (See Chapter 3 for a discussion about analgesia in the older patient.) Ensure that regular and as required analgesia is prescribed.

Fascia iliaca compartment block (FICB)

FICB is an effective, safe and easy-to-learn procedure, which can be performed at the bedside in the ED without a need for a nerve stimulator. It may be undertaken with or without ultrasound guidance.

Box 12.2 How to perform a fascia iliaca compartment block (Landmark technique).

Draw a line on the skin joining the pubic tubercle to anterior superior iliac spine, and divide into three equal parts.

The site of injection is 1–2 cm below the junction of the lateral third with the medial two-thirds. Palpate the femoral artery to ensure that the point of injection is at least 2 cm lateral to this.

A semiblunt needle is used to penetrate the skin so that its tip lies immediately subcutaneously.

The needle is advanced and two distinct 'pops' of loss of resistance are experienced as the fascia lata and then the fascia iliaca are pierced.

The tip of the needle is now in the fascia iliaca compartment.

Inject approximately 30 ml of local anaesthetic. Consult local protocols for the type of local anaesthetic and be cautious with maximum doses in the older patient.

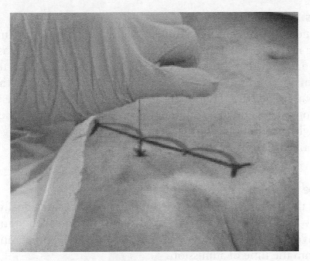

Figure 12.2 Surface anatomy of FICB. Source: From Fujihara Y, Fukunishi S, Nishio S, Miura J, Koyanagi S, Yoshiya S. Fascia iliaca compartment block: its efficacy in pain control for patients with proximal femoral fracture. *J Orthop Sci*. 2013 Sep 1;18(5):793–7 (9). Reproduced with permission of Springer.

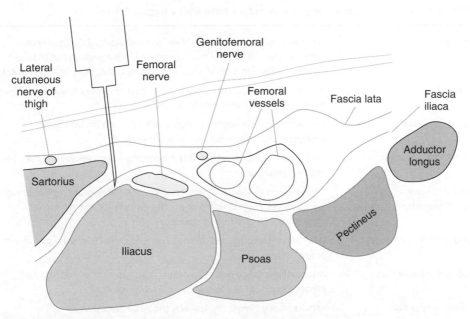

Figure 12.3 Anatomy of the fascia iliaca compartment block. Source: From Shiv Kumar Singh and S. M. Gulyam Kuruba. The Loss of Resistance Nerve Blocks. ISRN Anesthesiol. 2011. (10) Reproduced under the Creative Commons Attribution Licence.

An injection of local anaesthetic into the fascia iliaca compartment aims to block the femoral nerve, lateral cutaneous nerve of the thigh and obturator nerve, and provides effective analgesia in proximal femoral fractures (8). See Box 12.2 and Figures 12.2 and 12.3 for further explanation.

Facilitating surgery

Hip fracture patients are medically complex. Nearly half of hip fracture patients have dementia, and a majority will develop significant complications such as delirium, acute kidney injury, and lower respiratory tract infection. Evidence suggests that early (ideally pre-operative) involvement of a geriatric medicine team specialising in orthogeriatrics improves outcomes. The NICE (National Institute for Health and Care Excellence) provides guidance on management of hip fractures from admission to discharge (5).

Table 12.1 highlights important aspects to consider when preparing a patient with a hip fracture for theatre from the ED.

Ongoing care

Postoperatively, the patient should receive multidisciplinary care, ideally on a designated ortho-geriatric ward. Table 12.2 lists areas of focus in the rehabilitation process. It is important to have awareness of these issues in the ED, as the preparation for discharge should begin from the time of admission.

Table 12.2 Considerations in the ongoing care of a patient with a fragility fracture (2).

Analgesia	Prescribe regular non-opioid and PRN opioid analgesia. NSAIDs are not recommended. Oxycodone may be preferred over morphine and codeine because of the high rates of acute and chronic kidney injury in these patients
Mobilisation	Aim to mobilise as soon as possible postoperatively with physiotherapy input if there are no orthopaedic contraindications
Prevent surgical site infections	Give antibiotics immediately preoperatively and for a limited duration postoperatively. Inspect the wound as per protocol
Protect pressure areas	See Chapter 8. Ensure regular skin inspections, a pressure-relieving mattress and heel protection
Prevent of venous thromboembolism	If there are no contraindications, prescribe pharmacological prophylaxis with low molecular weight heparin or a factor Xa inhibitor and mechanical prophylaxis with compressive stockings
Rationalise drug treatment	Eliminate unnecessary medications to prevent complications associated with polypharmacy
Protect the urinary tract	Avoid catheterisation if at all possible – it increases risk of infection and impairs mobility. Check frequently for urinary retention
Prevent constipation	Regular stool softeners and laxatives should be prescribed
Prevent delirium	Monitor closely to detect any postoperative complications early. Optimise environmental factors, e.g. surroundings, orientation and lighting, hearing and visual aids. See Chapter 18
Assess cause of original fall	See Chapter 8
Treat osteoporosis	Most patients should be treated with a bone protection agent, calcium and vitamin D to prevent further fractures
Provide nutritional support	Assess risk of malnutrition, and use supplements if indicated

Pelvic insufficiency fractures

Pelvic fractures account for 7% of all fragility fractures (11) and carry a mortality risk similar to that of hip fractures at 1 year post injury (12). They are associated with significant loss of independence, with only 39% returning to their pre-injury level of function at 1 year in one study (13).

Pelvic fractures commonly present with a lateral compression type fracture pattern, resulting from a fall from standing onto the side. In two-thirds of cases this results in stable fractures of the pubic rami (14). However, 50% of pubic rami fractures are associated with an additional fracture of the posterior pelvic ring, such as an iliac wing fracture or sacral insufficiency fracture, which is often missed on plain radiography. Most of these remain stable, and heal well with non-operative treatment but the time for recovery of symptoms may be much longer than expected. A small proportion of these posterior pelvic ring fractures are unstable and may require operative intervention (15). Fractures of the lumbar vertebrae or acetabulum may also be missed.

History, examination and investigations

Radiographs of the hip and pelvis will often be performed immediately following arrival in the ED, and it is important to review these initially, as approach to examination may be different if there is any sign of an unstable injury. A description of the type and location of pain is important. Patients with pubic rami fractures will usually complain of hip or groin pain, but may also report sacral, lumbar or buttock pain in the case of an associated posterior fracture. Tenderness may be elicited over the groin or pubic symphysis. Carefully examine the sacroiliac joint and lumbosacral spine to identify additional sites of tenderness, and assess range of movement in the hip joint. Hip flexion may be particularly painful.

Perform a neurological examination of the lower legs, particularly looking for any signs of nerve root compression or cauda equina syndrome, which may occur following displaced lumbar or sacral fractures associated with a pelvic injury (16).

Plain radiographs often identify pubic ramus fractures but have a low sensitivity for detecting additional fractures in the sacrum, iliac wing or acetabulum, often due to overlying bowel gas. CT imaging may be indicated in patients with a suspected unstable injury, posterior tenderness with a high suspicion for an additional fracture, inability to weight bear following analgesia or at a later time in patients with prolonged pain (17). Routine CT in the work-up of all pubic rami fractures is not currently advocated, however (16) (Figure 12.4).

> KEY POINT: Occult posterior pelvic ring fractures are easily missed in patients with pubic rami fractures occurring after a simple fall. Always examine the back and posterior pelvic ring. A CT scan of the pelvis may be necessary.

Management

Unstable pelvic injuries and acetabular fractures may require surgical fixation, and advanced imaging should be obtained and a discussion held with the orthopaedic team.

Uncomplicated pubic rami fractures are stable and allow full weight bearing. They are managed non-operatively but often require hospital admission for analgesia,

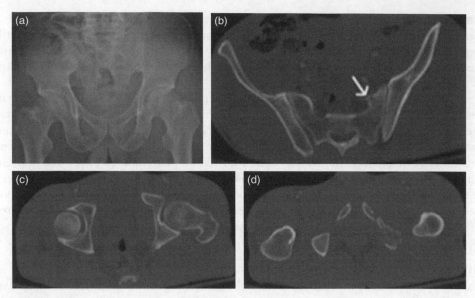

Figure 12.4 Radiographic series of an older patient who fell onto her left side. (a) AP projection of the pelvis clearly illustrates left superior and inferior rami fractures but no obvious posterior pelvic injury is identified. (b–d) Axial CT cuts from the same patient taken at the level of the sacrum (b), superior ramus (c) and inferior ramus (d). The arrow demonstrates the left sacral buckle fracture. Source: From Humphrey CA, Maceroli MA. Fragility fractures requiring special consideration: pelvic insufficiency fractures. *Clin Geriatr Med.* 2014 May;30(2):373–86. Reproduced with permission of Elsevier.

physiotherapy and arrangement of additional social support. Low energy pelvic fractures are associated with a small risk of significant haemorrhage in the older patient, especially those on anticoagulants. All the aspects of care highlighted in Table 12.2 should be instigated. The length of hospital admission for patients with acetabular fractures or other pelvic fracture types is significantly longer than in patients with pubic rami fractures (18).

If the patient is being discharged, it should be explained that the injury may be painful for a number of weeks. This duration will be increased if there is an additional posterior fracture. It is useful to advise the patient to reattend if pain is worsening or not improving, to consider further imaging to rule out an additional fracture, if this was not undertaken initially. Some centres may routinely repeat pelvic radiographs at intervals to check for fracture healing or complications (16).

Distal radial fractures
Otherwise known as Colles' fractures, fractures of the distal radius are the second most common fracture in the older patient. They frequently result from low-energy falls, and have a lifetime risk of 15% (19) among women.

Distal radius fractures in osteoporotic bone have greatly diminished stability due to bone impaction and fragmentation (20). Fractures are highly likely to displace after manipulation, more so with increasing age, although functional outcomes are often good despite this (21). Complications of distal radial fractures are listed in Box 12.3. Management in the ED is summarised in Box 12.4.

There is a lack of clear consensus on which older patients should undergo surgical management. More marked deformity on initial radiographs such as radial shortening over 6 mm, articular step and dorsal angulation over 10° have been associated with worse functional outcomes (22). Operative intervention to restore articular alignment and pre-injury anatomy should be considered in these cases. However, operative management is made more difficult by reduced bone quality for attachment of fixation devices (23). Considerations such as the patient's physiological age and level of functioning are important (22). In patients who are sedentary, bedbound or otherwise dependent, functional outcomes with conservative management are good despite the presence of deformity. Active patients, who are independent in their activities of daily living (ADLs), mobile with or without a walking aid or have particular hobbies, may benefit from fracture stabilisation with internal or external fixation.

Box 12.3 Specific complications of distal radial fractures.

Persistent pain and/or deformity
Reduced function: difficulty with ADLs and walking, especially if using a walking aid
Complications due to cast: muscle atrophy and joint stiffness, especially in fingers
Nerve damage, e.g. median nerve or carpal tunnel syndrome
Tendon damage, e.g. extensor pollicis longus rupture, often delayed
Infection secondary to operative intervention

Box 12.4 Managing a distal radius fracture in the older adult.

- Consider the cause of the fall and other injuries requiring more urgent attention (e.g. head or neck injuries, bleeding lacerations).
- Ask about hand dominance and social circumstances: discuss discharge plans early. Extra support may be required for the patient to be discharged to their usual place of residence.
- Examine the arm to ensure there is no neurovascular compromise and to exclude an open fracture.
- Provide analgesia and evaluate the patient's radiographs.
- Displaced fractures require closed manipulation followed by application of a plaster of Paris backslab and elevation in a sling. Options for performing this in the emergency department include
  - Haematoma block ±nitrous oxide
  - Bier's block or other regional anaesthesia technique
  - Procedural sedation (see below).

  Consider the potential contraindications and complications of each of these options. Particular care should be taken to avoid skin tears in the older adult when manipulating fractures (Chapter 13).
- If there is an open fracture, marked displacement, instability or failed manipulation, the patient is likely to require operative intervention or manipulation under general anaesthesia. Liaise with the orthopaedic team.

  In other cases, provide analgesia, a broad arm sling and a follow-up appointment with orthopaedics, and inform about possible complications (Box 12.3).

Back pain in the older adult

Immediate assessment

Thirty percent of those over 65 years report back pain as a significant complaint (24). Acute back pain may be a presentation of ruptured abdominal aortic aneurysm or aortic dissection (Chapter 15). All older adults who present to the ED with acute back pain should have a full set of vital signs recorded and have a prompt initial assessment. Examine the abdomen and assess peripheral pulses. Consider bedside ultrasound to exclude aortic aneurysm as a cause of the presentation.

Differential diagnosis

Acute back pain in the older adult may be due to

*   abdominal or retroperitoneal pathology: leaking aortic aneurysm, pancreatitis, renal colic, cholecystitis, duodenal ulcer.
*   thoracic cause: aortic dissection, myocardial infarction, pulmonary embolism.
*   vertebral compression fractures, usually as a result of osteoporosis. Other injury patterns may occur following higher energy trauma.
*   osteoarthritis, particularly of facet joints.
*   disc disease.
*   metastatic malignancy: especially breast, prostate and myeloma.
*   osteomyelitis of the vertebrae or discitis.

KEY POINT: Ruptured abdominal aortic aneurysm should be considered in every older adult presenting with acute back pain.

History

Establish whether there was a clear precipitant for the pain, such as a fall, prolonged period of immobility or episode of heavy lifting. Onset of pain in cases of vertebral fractures can be sudden or insidious, and pain may be worse when standing or sitting up. Particularly important in the past medical history is previous chronic back pain or osteoporotic fractures of the vertebrae, hip or wrist.

In addition to the standard pain history (SOCRATES; site, onset, character, radiation, associated features, timing; exacerbating features, severity) other important features include associated limb weakness, sensory loss or bladder or bowel problems. Symptoms such as fever, general malaise and weight loss are also concerning. A past history of malignancy may indicate pain due to metastatic disease. Risk factors for osteoporosis (as above) should be explored.

KEY POINT: There may not be a history of injury in osteoporotic vertebral compression fractures.

Examination

Expose the patient adequately to assess for bruising, pressure areas or deformities such as kyphosis.

Apply gentle pressure down each vertebral level to assess for tenderness. Palpate the paraspinal and gluteal muscles, sacroiliac joints and renal angles for tenderness.

Perform a full neurological examination including rectal examination to assess for perianal tone and sensation. In men, note the size and consistency of the prostate gland. Assess the lower limbs for muscle wasting and examine tone, power, reflexes and sensation. Assess for the presence of a sensory level.

Examine the abdomen for masses, organomegaly or a distended bladder due to urinary retention. Vertebral fractures may lead to ileus so note any tenderness in the abdomen and listen for bowel sounds. Malignancy may be associated with palpable lymphadenopathy. Breast examination is often forgotten, but is very important in older women.

Back pain may result from osteoarthritis in the hips and knees: palpate for tenderness and assess range of movement. Perform a straight leg raise if lumbar nerve root irritation is suspected and record the angle that reproduces pain. Assess gait if possible.

Investigations
Blood tests
Routine bloods tests should be taken including bone profile, including ALP (alkaline phosphatase) and calcium, and prostate-specific antigen (PSA) in men. Consider a myeloma screen or tumour markers depending on the clinical picture.

Imaging
Imaging will depend on the likely cause of back pain and associated symptoms. Chest or abdominal causes may require contrast CT or ultrasound. Plain radiographs of the spine may reveal a compression fracture, but may appear normal despite the presence of a fracture, or significant degenerative change may compromise interpretation. CT of the spine may be indicated if there is a high clinical suspicion of a fracture, or if any of the features in Box 12.5 are present. Boxes 12.5 and 12.8 highlight the indications for CT and MRI of the spine.

Vertebral insufficiency fracture
Over 25% of post-menopausal women experience vertebral insufficiency fractures, with advanced age and osteoporosis being the greatest risk factors (25). Up to two-thirds will be asymptomatic, or have pain attributed to normal ageing or arthritis. In a similar manner to hip fractures, vertebral insufficiency fractures are indicative of increased frailty in an older adult, and are associated with a higher mortality rate than people without fractures (26). Vertebral fractures increase the risk of a further osteoporotic fracture fourfold (27).

Fractures occur when the vertebral body is unable to support the weight of the upper body. In severe osteoporosis, fractures may occur spontaneously or while sneezing, turning in bed, lifting an object or stepping out of the bath (28). In mild to moderate osteoporosis there is usually a history of a fall, or other trauma involving forced flexion. Most fractures occur at the thoracolumbar junction; T8–T12, L1 and L4 fractures are the commonest.

Diagnosis and classification

A vertebral insufficiency fracture can be diagnosed when there is over 20% loss of height in the anterior, middle or posterior column of the vertebral body, or a disruption of alignment of the anterior or posterior columns.

Radiographs should be taken of the whole spine as over 20% of vertebral fractures are multiple and may occur at different levels (2). Radiographs may not reliably distinguish between stable wedge fractures and potentially unstable fractures (29), and CT is increasingly used, particularly if any of the features in Box 12.5 are present. MRI should be organised urgently if there any features of neurological compromise (Box 12.8).

Several different quantitative classification systems can be utilised to describe vertebral fractures and plan management, for example, the Genant classification, which classifies fractures as wedge, biconcave or crush types (Figure 12.5) (31). The degree of vertebral height loss is also included to give a severity score of mild (grade 1, 20–25%), moderate (grade 2, 25–40%) and severe >40% (Figure 12.6).

Wedge compression fractures

These are the commonest fracture type. The anterior part of the vertebral body is crushed, resulting in loss of anterior height and a *wedge* deformity (Figure 12.4). As the middle and posterior columns are preserved, wedge fractures are usually stable and rarely associated with any neurological compromise. Examination may reveal a tender vertebral level, and the neurological examination is normal. Sequential vertebral wedge fractures are common and lead to a kyphotic deformity.

Biconcave fractures

These demonstrate a reduction in the mid-vertebral height but the anterior and posterior walls may remain intact.

Crush fractures

These demonstrate a reduction in the anterior and posterior vertebral height. As the posterior column is involved, there is the potential for neurological defects resulting from retropulsion of fragments into the spinal canal. They are the least common fracture type (32).

Management

Fractures complicated by neurological compromise or instability should be discussed urgently with a spinal surgeon.

In uncomplicated vertebral insufficiency fractures most patients improve slowly over 6–12 weeks as the fracture heals. Associated muscular pain may persist for some time after this. Early mobilisation should be encouraged, but patients may require a short period of bed rest initially. A back brace may be recommended, but this may be poorly tolerated in older patients due to increased pain.

Table 12.2 highlights important additional management points in any fragility fracture.

Surgical procedures such as percutaneous vertebroplasty or balloon kyphoplasty may be considered in stable fractures if the patient is failing to improve or cannot tolerate conservative management, if the pain is confirmed as originating from the fracture site (33).

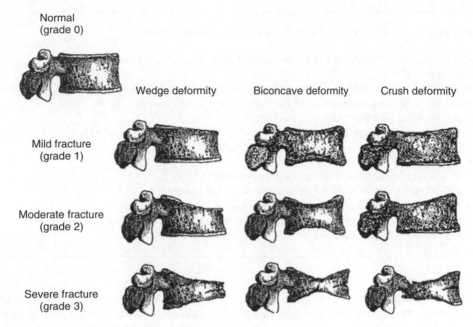

Figure 12.5 Schematic diagram of semiquantitative grading scale for vertebral fractures. Source: From Genant HK, Jergas M, Palermo L, Nevitt M, Valentin RS, Black D, et al. Comparison of semiquantitative visual and quantitative morphometric assessment of prevalent and incident vertebral fractures in osteoporosis The Study of Osteoporotic Fractures Research Group. *J Bone Miner Res*. 1996 Jul;11(7):984–96.(30) Reproduced with permission of John Wiley and Sons.

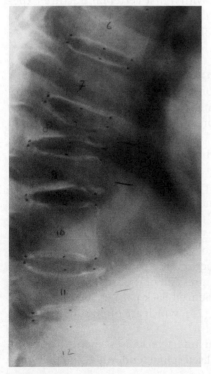

Figure 12.6 Lateral thoracic radiograph showing a grade 3 fracture of T8 and grade 2 fractures of T9 and T11 (41). Source: From Grigoryan M, Guermazi A, Roemer FW, Delmas PD, Genant HK. Recognising and reporting osteoporotic vertebral fractures. *Eur Spine J*. 2003 Oct;12 Suppl 2:S104–12. Reproduced with permission of Springer-Verlag.

Box 12.5 Indications for CT spine in acute back pain in the older patient.

- In the presence of polytrauma or where the mechanism would necessitate trauma imaging (Chapter 11)
- Suspected ruptured abdominal aortic aneurysm or other vascular emergency (Chapter 15)
- To identify fractures not seen on plain films where there is a high clinical suspicion
- In a suspected unstable fracture:
  - To assess fracture complexity and the state of the middle and posterior columns, and identify any encroachment of bone into the spinal canal
- In a potentially unstable fracture:
  - Increased interpedicular space on a anteriorposterior radiograph
  - Significant loss of vertebral height (e.g. over 40%; see Figure 12.5)
- Possible underlying malignancy causing a pathological fracture
- Suspected spinal cord compression where MRI is contraindicated or unavailable – CT scan may reveal spinal cord narrowing

---

Complications

Vertebral insufficiency fractures can lead to persistent back pain even after the fracture has healed. Reduced mobility results in associated problems such as deep vein thrombosis (DVT), constipation, pressure ulcers and deconditioning. Multiple wedge fractures lead to loss of body height, progressive thoracic kyphosis and lumbar lordosis. In severe cases, this may result in impaired respiratory function and a protuberant abdomen, causing early satiety and weight loss.

Vertebral insufficiency fractures may result in further fractures as adjacent vertebrae support the additional load. Up to 20% of patients with a first vertebral fracture experience a further vertebral fracture within 1 year (34).This may result in progressive instability and increase the possibility of later neurological compromise.

Spinal cord compression and cauda equina syndrome

Spinal cord compression and cauda equina syndrome make up a small proportion of cases of acute back pain presenting to the ED. Permanent neurological damage including paralysis and incontinence can be prevented or minimised by early diagnosis and treatment.

A low threshold of suspicion should be adopted in older adults, however, who are at higher risk of malignancy and who may present less typically. Delay in diagnosis is a frequent occurrence, and neurological deficits are often irreversible, leading to poor outcomes. Urgent MRI is required to confirm diagnosis (Box 12.8). Treatment, such as surgical decompression or external beam radiation therapy, needs to take place within 24 hours of diagnosis to prevent further neurological deterioration.

Metastatic malignancy accounts for the majority of cases: 4–6% of patients with cancer ultimately develop cord compression, which occurs due to pathological vertebral body collapse or direct tumour growth causing compression of the spinal cord or cauda equina (35). Eighty percent of patients have experienced back pain in the preceding 3 months prior to developing neurological symptoms (24), which are often subtle initially, leading to a delay in diagnosis.

Other causes include lumbar disc prolapse and infective causes such as epidural abscess or vertebral osteomyelitis. In the latter, localised spinal tenderness and pain may be absent, and white cell count may be normal, with a raised ESR (erythrocyte sedimentation rate) being more common (24). Epidural haematomas must be considered in patients taking anticoagulants.

History and examination

> **KEY POINT: Normal neurological examination does not exclude spinal cord compression. Severe pain is the first symptom in 95% of cases (36).**

Symptoms include the features in Box 12.6.

Box 12.6 Symptoms of spinal cord compression.

- Back pain
    Pain in the thoracic or cervical spine
    Severe, progressive lower spinal pain
    Spinal pain aggravated by straining
    Nocturnal spinal pain preventing sleep
- Weakness and altered sensation in the lower limbs
- Sphincter dysfunction: urinary retention or faecal incontinence
- Older patients may present with non-specific symptoms such as reduced mobility.

Examination findings may be normal initially. Above L1/L2, upper motor neuron signs (hyperreflexia, increased tone, upgoing plantar reflexes) may be present. There may be a clear sensory level or sensory signs may be absent or subtle. The spinal cord ends at L1/L2 and compression here will affect the cauda equina, containing the nerve roots of L1–L5 and S1–S5. Signs may include reduced tone, absent or reduced reflexes, downgoing plantars, altered sensation in the saddle area–groin, buttocks and back of thighs, and sphincter disturbance. Bedside bladder scanning and post-void residual volumes can be useful in identifying early urinary retention.

Management
Urgent intervention is required to prevent permanent disability. Box 12.7 summarises the key interventions required.

Box 12.7 Management of suspected malignant spinal cord compression (35).

- Arrange urgent MRI whole spine with contrast.
- Consult a neurosurgeon urgently, and a clinical/radiation oncologist in the case of suspected or known malignant disease.
- In patients with neurological defects, administer oral or intravenous dexamethasone.
- In the case of back pain with neurological signs, definitive treatment (radiotherapy or neurosurgery) should be undertaken within 24 hours of presentation.

Box 12.8 Indications for MRI in acute back pain.

Suspected spinal cord compression
Vertebral insufficiency fracture with neurological signs
Suspected osteomyelitis or discitis
Suspected malignancy e.g. primary bone neoplasm or multiple myeloma as a cause of pain.

Procedural sedation in the older patient

Procedural sedation involves administering sedative or dissociative agents with or without analgesic agents to facilitate painful procedures. Common procedures undertaken in older patients in the ED include manipulation of displaced distal radius and ankle fractures, reduction of dislocated hip prostheses or shoulder dislocations and occasionally DC cardioversion.

The advantages of procedural sedation in the ED include the following:
• The procedure is performed earlier, resulting in improved pain scores, less soft tissue damage in the case of fractures and dislocations, earlier mobilisation and better patient satisfaction.
• Potential avoidance of admission and the associated complications in the older patient.

Clinical guidelines and policies should be adhered to closely when performing procedural sedation in the ED. ACEP and CEM guidelines (37, 38) make the following recommendations:
• Ideally three healthcare professionals should be present: a 'sedation' clinician, who should be an experienced Emergency Physician (or anaesthetist) with advanced airway skills, someone to undertake the procedure, with a separate assistant if required, and a nurse or other qualified individual to record observations and drug dosages, seek additional equipment or personnel if required and monitor the patient for an extended period after the procedure is completed.
• Full monitoring and resuscitation facilities should be available including capnography, which allows the earlier detection of hypoventilation or apnoea.
• Pre-procedural fasting for any duration has not demonstrated a reduction in the risk of emesis or aspiration when administering procedural sedation. In the absence of fasting a decision to proceed should be based on the urgency of the procedure and the target depth of sedation with a careful assessment of aspiration risk (38).

Box 12.9 includes factors to consider when planning procedural sedation in the older patient.

Most side effects of sedative agents will be dose dependent, and may be avoided by using much smaller doses of sedative agents with slower titration in the older patient.

Choice of sedation agent will depend on characteristics of the patient and the required procedure, desired depth and duration of sedation and on the physician's experience. Table 12.3 highlights the commonest agents used, their advantages, and disadvantages. Seek local guidance for further information on dosages.

Other sedation agents utilised in different centres include nitric oxide, etomidate, ketofol (a mix of propofol and ketamine) and methohexital, among others.

Table 12.3 Frequently used sedative agents for procedural sedation in the emergency department.

Drug	Advantages	Disadvantages	Comments
Opioids e.g. fentanyl, morphine	Provides effective analgesia for painful procedures	Older patients are more susceptible to hypotension, CNS and respiratory depression	Used in combination with a sedative agent
Benzodiazepines e.g. midazolam	Physician and nursing staff familiarity. Well tolerated by patients. May be useful for longer procedures	Little or no analgesic effect. Respiratory and cardiovascular depression may occur, particularly if used with opioids. Duration of action may be prolonged in older patients. May cause or prolong delirium	Oxygen desaturation may be more frequent despite lower doses (39)
Propofol	Well tolerated, familiar drug Rapid onset and short duration of action	Increased risk of hypotension in older patients, particularly if hypovolaemic or cardiovascular compromise (28) Increased likelihood of apnoea or need for airway intervention	A study of propofol sedation in older and younger adults showed no significant increase in complications although lower doses were used. Overall there was an 8% risk of complications such as hypotension and oxygen desaturation in patients over 65 (40)
Ketamine	'Dissociative' sedation and analgesia Minimal cardiorespiratory inhibition Airway reflexes are usually maintained	May cause hypertension and tachycardia, or unpleasant emergence phenomena	Limited published data on use in older adults

CNS, central nervous system.

Box 12.9 Procedural sedation in the older patient.

- Arm–brain circulation time is prolonged, increasing the time taken for induction agents to take effect. Any sedative should be *more slowly titrated* than in the younger patient. *Significantly lower doses will be required*.
- Total body water is reduced in the older adult with a rise in total fat percentage. This leads to an increased volume of distribution for fat-soluble drugs such as propofol and benzodiazepines, prolonging drug clearance.
- Older patients are more likely to require a short period of bag-valve ventilation than younger patients during procedural sedation although this is rare. Note should be made of potential airway difficulties in the older patient (Figure 11.2, Chapter 11).
- Comorbidities and other medication may increase the risk of complications or adverse reactions.

KEY POINT: Procedural sedation is safe in the older adult but lower doses of sedative agents must be used. Mild sedation to general anaesthesia is a continuum, and it is not always possible to predict how individual patients will respond to sedative agents.

Take home messages

- Hip fracture is one not to miss: undertake further imaging if initial radiographs are unclear
- Do not give your patient HEADACHES (Table 12.1) by delaying surgery in fractured neck of femur: identify problems and treat them early
- Specialist orthogeriatrics care improves outcomes including mortality and length of stay and ideally all older patients with a hip fracture should have access to this
- Before diagnosing an isolated pubic ramus fracture, examine for posterior pelvic pain. A CT may demonstrate an occult posterior pelvic ring fracture
- Back pain is a concerning presentation in the older patient; note that it may not originate from the back
- Consider spinal cord compression in patients with severe progressive back pain. Once neurological signs are present, the outcome is poor
- Procedural sedation is safe in older patients, but lower doses and slower titration of sedative agents are required.

References

1 Johnell O, Kanis J. Epidemiology of osteoporotic fractures. *Osteoporos Int.* 2005;16 Suppl 2:S3–S7.
2 British Orthopaedic Association. The care of patients with fragility fracture. 2007.
3 Auron-Gomez M, Michota F. Medical management of hip fracture. *Clin Geriatr Med.* 2008;24(4): 701–719, ix.
4 Chatha HA, Ullah S, Cheema ZZ. Review article: magnetic resonance imaging and computed tomography in the diagnosis of occult proximal femur fractures. *J Orthop Surg (Hong Kong).* 2011;19(1):99–103.
5 The management of hip fracture in adults. National Institute for Health and Clinical Excellence (NICE) Guideline 2011.
6 Chesters A, Atkinson P. Fascia iliaca block for pain relief from proximal femoral fracture in the emergency department: a review of the literature. *Emerg Med J.* 2014 Oct;31(e1):e84–e87; doi:10.1136/emermed-2013 -203073.
7 Hip fracture. National Institute for Health and Care Excellence (NICE). Evidence Update 34. March 2013.
8 Elkhodair S, Mortazavi J, Chester A, Pereira M. Single fascia iliaca compartment block for pain relief in patients with fractured neck of femur in the emergency department: a pilot study. *Eur J Emerg Med.* 2011;18(6):340–343.
9 Fujihara Y, Fukunishi S, Nishio S, Miura J, Koyanagi S, Yoshiya S. Fascia iliaca compartment block: its efficacy in pain control for patients with proximal femoral fracture. *J Orthop Sci.* 2013;18(5): 793–797.
10 Singh SK, Gulyam Kuruba SM. The Loss of Resistance Nerve Blocks. ISRN Anesthesiol. 2011.
11 Burge R, Dawson-Hughes B, Solomon DH, Wong JB, King A, Tosteson A. Incidence and economic burden of osteoporosis-related fractures in the United States, 2005–2025. *J Bone Miner Res.* 2007;22(3):465–475.

12 Taillandier J, Langue F, Alemanni M, Taillandier-Heriche E. Mortality and functional outcomes of pelvic insufficiency fractures in older patients. *Joint Bone Spine*. 2003;70(4):287–289.

13 Scheyerer MJ, Osterhoff G, Wehrle S, Wanner GA, Simmen H-P, Werner CML. Detection of posterior pelvic injuries in fractures of the pubic rami. *Injury* 2012;43(8):1326–1329.

14 Krappinger D, Kammerlander C, Hak DJ, Blauth M. Low-energy osteoporotic pelvic fractures. *Arch Orthop Trauma Surg*. 2010;130(9):1167–1175.

15 Studer P, Suhm N, Zappe B, Bless N, Jakob M. Pubic rami fractures in the elderly – a neglected injury? *Swiss Med Wkly*. 2013;143:w13859.

16 Humphrey CA, Maceroli MA. Fragility fractures requiring special consideration: pelvic insufficiency fractures. *Clin Geriatr Med*. 2014;30(2):373–386.

17 Lau T, Leung F. Occult posterior pelvic ring fractures in elderly patients with osteoporotic pubic rami fractures. *J Orthop Surg (Hong Kong)* 2010;18(2):153–157.

18 Alnaib M, Waters S, Shanshal Y, Caplan N, Jones S, St Clair Gibson A, et al. Combined pubic rami and sacral osteoporotic fractures: a prospective study. *J Orthop Traumatol*. 2012;13(2):97–103.

19 Cummings SR, Kelsey JL, Nevitt MC, O'Dowd KJ. Epidemiology of osteoporosis and osteoporotic fractures. *Epidemiol Rev*. 1985;7:178–208.

20 Ring D, Jupiter JB. Treatment of osteoporotic distal radius fractures. *Osteoporos Int*. 2005;16 Suppl 2:S80–S84.

21 Nesbitt KS, Failla JM, Les C. Assessment of instability factors in adult distal radius fractures. *J Hand Surg Am*. 2004;29(6):1128–1138.

22 Blakeney WG. Stabilization and treatment of Colles' fractures in elderly patients. *Clin Interv Aging*. 2010;5:337–344.

23 Smith DW, Henry MH. Volar fixed-angle plating of the distal radius. *J Am Acad Orthop Surg*. 2005;13(1):28–36.

24 Broder J, Snarski JT. Back pain in the elderly. *Clin Geriatr Med*. 2007;23(2):271–289, v.

25 Melton LJ. Epidemiology of spinal osteoporosis. *Spine (Phila Pa 1976)*. 1997;22(24 Suppl):2S–11S.

26 Cauley JA, Thompson DE, Ensrud KC, Scott JC, Black D. Risk of mortality following clinical fractures. *Osteoporos Int*. 2000;11(7):556–561.

27 Chapman J, Bransford R. Geriatric spine fractures: an emerging healthcare crisis. *J Trauma*. 2007;62(6 Suppl):S61–S62.

28 Old JL, Calvert M. Vertebral compression fractures in the elderly. *Am Fam Physician*. 2004;69(1):111–116.

29 Ballock RT, Mackersie R, Abitbol JJ, Cervilla V, Resnick D, Garfin SR. Can burst fractures be predicted from plain radiographs? *J Bone Joint Surg Br*. 1992;74(1):147–150.

30 Genant HK, Jergas M, Palermo L, Nevitt M, Valentin RS, Black D, et al. Comparison of semi-quantitative visual and quantitative morphometric assessment of prevalent and incident vertebral fractures in osteoporosis The Study of Osteoporotic Fractures Research Group. *J Bone Miner Res*. 1996;11(7):984–996.

31 Genant H, Wu C, Van Kuijk C. Vertebral fracture assessment using a semiquantitative technique. *J Bone Min Res*. 1993;8:1137e48.

32 Alexandru D, So W. Evaluation and management of vertebral compression fractures. *Perm J*. 2012;16(4):46–51.

33 Percutaneous vertebroplasty and percutaneous balloon kyphoplasty for the treatment of osteoporotic vertebral fractures. National Institute for Health and Care Excellence (NICE) Guidelines. April 2013.

34 Lindsay R, Silverman SL, Cooper C, Hanley DA, Barton I, Broy SB, et al. Risk of new vertebral fracture in the year following a fracture. *JAMA*. 2001;285(3):320–323.

35 Diagnosis and management of adults at risk of and with metastatic spinal cord compression. National Institute for Health and Clinical Excellence Guidelines 2008. 2008.

36 Levack P, Graham J, Collie D, Grant R, Kidd J, Kunkler I, et al. Don't wait for a sensory level – listen to the symptoms: a prospective audit of the delays in diagnosis of malignant cord compression. *Clin Oncol (R Coll Radiol)* 2002;14(6):472–480.

37 Godwin SA, Burton JH, Gerardo CJ, Hatten BW, Mace SE, Silvers SM, et al. Clinical policy: procedural sedation and analgesia in the emergency department. *Ann Emerg Med*. 2014;63(2):247–58.e18.
38 Safe Sedation in Adults in the Emergency Department. Report and Recommendations by The Royal College of Anaesthetists and The College of Emergency Medicine Working Party on Sedation, Anaesthesia and Airway Management in the Emergency Department. November.
39 Yano H, Iishi H, Tatsuta M, Sakai N, Narahara H, Omori M. Oxygen desaturation during sedation for colonoscopy in elderly patients. *Hepatogastroenterology*. 1998;45(24):2138–2141.
40 Weaver CS, Terrell KM, Bassett R, Swiler W, Sandford B, Avery S, et al. ED procedural sedation of elderly patients: is it safe? *Am J Emerg Med*. 2011;29(5):541–544.
41 Grigoryan M, Guermazi A, Roemer FW, Delmas PD, Genant HK. Recognizing and reporting osteoporotic vertebral fractures. *Eur Spine J* 2003;12 Suppl 2:S104–S112.

CHAPTER 13
Skin trauma

Introduction

The ageing process causes changes in the structure and function of the skin, which make older adults more vulnerable to skin tears, lacerations and pressure injuries following falls or other trauma. Burns are more likely to be deeper and of a wider surface area, with markedly higher morbidity and mortality.

Any break in skin integrity, however minor, may lead to significant complications. The care of the older person's skin, both in health and following injury, should be seen as a priority.

Background

Figure 13.1 highlights the skin changes that occur with ageing.

Epidermal thinning results in reduced epidermal turnover and altered microcirculation, which delay healing. Lacerations are more likely following mild mechanical forces

Thinner subcutaneous tissue reduces protection against pressure injuries, fractures and hypothermia

Flattening of dermo–epidermal junction Shearing forces are likely to cause skin tears

Reduction in number of sweat glands leading to dry, itchy and fragile skin

Fragile vascular capillaries leading to ecchymosis and haematoma development following minor trauma

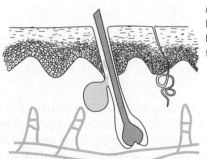

Figure 13.1 Age-related skin changes.

Dermal thinning results in a reduction in blood vessels, nerve endings and collagen, leading to reduced elasticity and strength of skin. There is also altered temperature control, reduced sensation and moisture retention. Burns are more likely to cause full dermal thickness injuries.

Geriatric Emergencies, First Edition.
Iona Murdoch, Sarah Turpin, Bree Johnston, Alasdair MacLullich and Eve Losman.
© 2015 John Wiley & Sons, Ltd. Published 2015 by John Wiley & Sons, Ltd.

In addition to the skin changes mentioned above, comorbid conditions and medications can lead to poor wound healing. The presence of localised oedema, poor circulation or neuropathy may result in the development of chronic wounds or ulceration.

History and examination

History taking should establish the mechanism and timing of the injury, along with a full assessment as per the guidance in Chapter 8. Document the presence of diabetes, anaemia, malignancy and cardiovascular disease as all these conditions may complicate wound healing. Medications implicated in delayed wound healing include corticosteroids, other immunosuppressive agents, non-steroidal anti-inflammatory drugs and anticoagulants. Note any history of chronic wounds or ulceration after previous injuries.

Assess pain and consider non-pharmacological methods of analgesia, such as dressings, elevation, and splinting, as well as analgesic medication (Chapter 3).

Box 13.1 highlights the important aspects to document when examining a skin wound in the older adult.

Box 13.1 Examination of skin trauma.
- Anatomical location and wound dimensions, degree of opposition of wound edges
- Presence of bleeding, haematoma and contamination
- Tissue viability in the wound edges or skin flap
- Type and amount of exudate
- Health of surrounding skin, presence of oedema, infection or bruising
- Signs of peripheral vascular disease, venous stasis and peripheral neuropathy
- Consider measuring ankle-brachial pressure index (ABPI) in lower limb injuries to detect arterial insufficiency
- Signs of systemic illness.

Tetanus status

Tetanus remains a rare condition, but the older patient is most at risk. The combination of waning immunity with ageing and delayed presentation or poor initial wound management contributes. Older women and those over 80 are at higher risk: men are more likely to have received vaccination as part of military service. Studies have demonstrated inadequate antibody titres in over 50% of older patients (1, 2). Immunisation history may be unreliable and extra precautions should be taken. Tetanus-prone injuries include a wound or burn sustained over 6 hours prior to treatment; puncture wounds; wounds with significant devitalised tissue including pressure ulcers; wounds in contact with soil or manure and evidence of sepsis.

Patients with tetanus-prone wounds who do not have a clear history of at least three tetanus vaccinations should be given tetanus immunoglobulin in addition to a tetanus vaccine (3). Consult local protocols in other circumstances.

Table 13.1 STAR skin tear classification system (5).

1a	A skin tear where the edges can be realigned to the normal anatomical position (without undue stretching) and the skin or skin flap colour is not pale, dusky or darkened
1b	The edges can be realigned to the normal anatomical position (without undue stretching) and the skin or skin flap colour is pale, dusky or darkened
2a	The edges cannot be realigned to the normal anatomical position and the skin or skin flap appears well perfused
2b	The edges cannot be realigned to the normal anatomical position and the skin or skin flap colour is pale, dusky or darkened
3	The skin flap is absent, and there is loss of skin

Specific injuries

Skin tears

Skin tears occur as a result of friction or sheering forces causing separation of skin layers. Partial thickness tears result from separation of the epidermis from the dermis and full thickness tears from the separation of the dermis from underlying subcutaneous tissue (4). Skin tears commonly occur on extremities, particularly on the dorsal aspect of the hand or forearm, the shin, as well as the back and buttocks. Skin tears can be classified according to the presence of skin loss or a skin flap. A suggested classification is detailed in Table 13.1.

Box 13.2 summarises the management of skin tears. Most skin tears will heal well with conservative treatment. When choosing a non-adherent dressing, it is important to maintain a moist wound environment while controlling the exudate. Some centres routinely use antibiotic ointment for wounds and burns, although the evidence base is limited (6). Routine oral antibiotics are not indicated unless there is significant contamination or the wound resulted from a human or animal bite.

Box 13.2 Management of skin tears.

- Control bleeding and clean the wound.
- Assess degree of tissue loss and skin or skin flap colour.
- Assess the surrounding skin condition, comorbidities and medication that may delay skin healing.
- Realign any skin or skin flap if possible and apply a non-adhesive dressing (e.g. hydrogel, silicone based, biocellulose). Mark instructions for removal on the dressing: dressings should be removed in the opposite direction of the skin flap. If there is no skin flap, gently clean and pat dry and apply a non-adhesive dressing. Hold in place with non-adherent products such as gauze, stockingette or tubular dressings. This will help absorb any excess exudate produced early in wound healing. Avoid the use of any adhesives that may cause tension.
- If skin or skin flap colour is pale, dusky or darkened arrange reassessment in 24–48 hours. Document any signs of improvement or deterioration such as increased pain, exudate, heat, oedema and malodour at each dressing change.
- Refer for surgical review if a skin tear is extensive or associated with a full thickness skin injury, significant bleeding or haematoma formation.

Scalp and face lacerations

Following infiltration of local anaesthesia, the base of the wound should be inspected and palpated for possible skull fracture or foreign material. If the galea aponeurosis layer (the tendon-like structure that covers the skull and inserts into the frontalis muscle of the forehead and into the occipitalis muscle posteriorly) is lacerated, this should be repaired with sutures. This will protect the underlying loose connective tissue from infection, prevent the frontalis muscle from contracting asymmetrically and also assist with haemorrhage control.

Primary closure of scalp lacerations can be achieved using staples, sutures, tissue glue or with a hair apposition technique. The particular method used will depend of the size, depth and location of the wound and the degree of tension the wound is under. Forehead lacerations can be closed with tissue glue, adhesive strips or sutures. Ensure tissue adhesive does not enter the wound, as it may form a barrier between the two wound edges and prevent healing.

Scalp and facial wounds may bleed heavily and a pressure dressing over the wound for 24 hours may limit haematoma formation and encourage haemostasis. Ensure a full head injury assessment takes place with referral for CT brain or admission for observation if required (Chapter 14).

Pre-tibial lacerations

The pre-tibial area has little protective soft tissue padding, and is particularly vulnerable to skin tears.

Management is similar to that of general skin tears as illustrated above. However, pre-tibial lacerations have a high likelihood of poor healing or necrosis due to poor blood supply. Skin necrosis is more likely with distally based flaps; with very thin flaps; where there is haematoma under the flap; or when the skin is replaced under tension. Suturing is likely to increase tension across a wound and will worsen necrosis. Adhesive tapes should only be used for simple linear lacerations or small, well-perfused skin flaps. Leave a space between adhesive strips to allow for the exudate to drain and accommodate for any wound swelling. Apply a non-adherent dressing and compression bandaging if there is no peripheral vascular disease. Arrange follow-up for dressing changes and monitoring of wound healing, through a specialist clinic or primary care facility depending on local resources (7).

Burns

Ten percent of burns occur in people aged over 65. Advancing age most closely correlates with mortality rates following a major burn, along with increased burn size, the presence of a full thickness burn, inhalation injury and female gender. The percentage total body surface area (TBSA) of a burn, the duration of stay as inpatient and the mortality related to a burn are all higher in the older patient. Despite many advances in burns treatment, patients aged 70 and older with burns over 20% TBSA have a mortality of 34% compared to 10% in patients aged 50–60 years. This rises to 84% mortality in 50% TBSA in those aged over 70 (8).

Table 13.2 Factors increasing the risk of burns in the older population.

Impaired visual and auditory perception	Inability to hear smoke alarm or observe that a stove remains on
Decreased manual dexterity	Increased risk of scalds when handling hot liquids
Peripheral neuropathy	Failure to appreciate that items remain hot
Reduced mobility	More likely to smoke indoors, increasing fire risk Reduced ability to escape from flames or smoke
Comorbidities, e.g. epilepsy, cardiac disorders	24% of burns result from a collapse, causing prolonged contact with a heat source (e.g. radiator or heater) or spillage of hot liquid (9)
Cognitive impairment, e.g. due to dementia, sedative medication, alcohol	Forgetting stove or fire is on Less recognition of danger Impaired reaction times and withdrawal from contact with heat source
Poverty	Small, cluttered accommodation increases fire risk Old-fashioned heaters or cooking appliances Lack of smoke or carbon monoxide alarms

Minor burns are usually managed in the community but problems with wound healing and infection are more common in the older patient, and secondary care advice should be sought early if necessary.

Background

The commonest burn injuries in the older adult are scalds, flame burns, and contact burns mostly occurring in the home environment. Cooking and bathing are the most common activities associated with burns. Table 13.2 demonstrates factors that increase the risk of burns in the older population.

Dermal atrophy and thinning of the subcutaneous fat in the older patient provide little protection against thermal insults and increase the surface area of burn and the likelihood of full thickness injury, compared to a younger patient exposed to the same heat source (Figure 13.1).

Initial assessment

Initial assessment should progress according to ATLS® principles (10): to include airway with cervical spine control, breathing, circulation, disability and exposure. Consider the safety of the treating medical team in the rare case of a chemical burn. See Box 13.3.

> **KEY POINT: As with all traumatic injuries in the older patient, consider whether another medical condition triggered the injury in the first place.**

History

This should include an exploration of the events leading to the injury to identify potential complications of the burn and to guide further investigation and management.

- Establish the type of burn (scald, flame, electrical, chemical).
- Inhalation injury and carbon monoxide poisoning are more likely if the fire was in an enclosed space, there was considerable time of exposure to fire and smoke, or if there was loss of consciousness. Burning plastics or furniture may cause cyanide poisoning.
- The burn may be as a result of a fall or collapse requiring investigation to identify the underlying cause. A syncopal episode due to an underlying cardiac arrhythmia may lead to prolonged contact with a hot radiator.
- Escaping from a fire may result in other injuries such as fractures.

Box 13.3 Initial assessment of an older patient presenting with burns.

Airway	Burns around the face and mouth, stridor, hoarseness, singed nasal hairs or dysphagia indicate potential airway compromise requiring immediate intervention. Give high-flow oxygen, position the patient in a position of comfort and obtain senior anaesthetic assistance, as it is likely that the airway will be challenging to control
Breathing	Products of combustion act as direct irritants to the lungs, leading to bronchospasm, inflammation and bronchorrhoea. Atelectasis and pneumonia may follow. Non-invasive or invasive ventilation may be required early. Arterial blood gases may demonstrate elevated carboxyhaemoglobin in carbon monoxide poisoning or hypoxia from cyanide poisoning or inhalation injury
Circulation	Establish intravenous access, preferably through non-burned tissue, taking routine bloods, coagulation, blood type and CK
	Circumferential burns to a limb or chest wall may impede peripheral circulation or ventilation some hours after a burn and fasciotomies or escharotomies may be required
	Hypotension due to hypovolaemia is not the usual initial physiological response to a burn. Exclude another source of hypotension such as chest, abdominal or pelvic trauma or other unrelated pathology
	Fluid requirements following major burns are increased in the older patient due to increased total body surface area of burns and reduced skin turgor causing increased oedema around the burn. Fluid overload risks pulmonary oedema and abdominal or limb compartment syndrome due to oedema, however. Be cautious using formulae for calculating fluid requirements in the older person due to other comorbidities. Early invasive monitoring with CVP (central venous pressure) and arterial lines or cardiac output monitoring may be helpful in guiding fluid management
Disability	Check and document GCS (Glasgow Coma Scale) and pupil size. Look carefully for signs of head injury
	In the obtunded patient, always consider carbon monoxide or cyanide poisoning
Exposure	Maintain core temperature above 36°C. Older patients can become hypothermic quickly, worsening the burn injury. Cover large burns with cling film, and use warming blankets if necessary

---

Past medical history and drug history are essential in identifying factors that may compromise wound healing. Social history is particularly important in identifying vulnerable older people in need of further social support, or possible elder abuse. Establish whether old, faulty, or poorly adapted equipment is in use, and whether this needs to be addressed before the patient can be discharged to their place of residence.

Table 13.3 Classification of burn depth.

Depth of burn	Layers of skin affected	Examination findings
Superficial	Epidermis is affected but the dermis is intact	Red and painful skin, similar to sunburn
Superficial dermal	Epidermis and upper layers of dermis	Painful pink skin with small blisters
Deep dermal	Epidermis, upper and deeper layers of dermis	Red, blotchy skin. Blisters may be present. Painful or painless
Full thickness	All skin layers through to subcutaneous tissues	Dry, white, brown on black skin. Leathery or waxy. Painless. Absent capillary refill

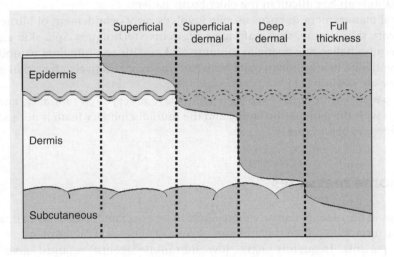

Figure 13.2 Burn depth. Source: From Enoch S, Roshan A, Shah M. Emergency and early management of burns and scalds. *BM J.* 2009 Jan 8;338:b1037. Reproduced with permission of BMJ Publishing Group Ltd.

Examination

Following the primary survey, examination should identify the TBSA of burned skin, utilising a Lund and Browder chart, and an estimate made of the burn thickness (Table 13.3; Figure 13.2).

It may be difficult to distinguish partial and full thickness burns immediately following an injury and a reassessment in 24–48 hours will be required.

Particular attention should be placed on general examination of the patient to identify skin integrity and cardiovascular status.

Management

Small burns should be cooled with tepid water pre-hospital, avoiding ice or very cold water, which can increase ischaemic damage to surrounding tissues. Cover with a non-adhesive dressing such as cling-film or paraffin-soaked gauze. Elevate if the burn involves a limb, and ensure tetanus prophylaxis.

Minor burns should be reassessed after 48 hours as until this time it is difficult to accurately assess the depth of a burn. The wound should be re-inspected and re-dressed every 3–5 days during healing to identify any early complications.

More significant burns may require referral to a burns unit. Criteria for referral may vary according to local policy, but usually include full thickness burns, burns greater than 3% TBSA, and burns to special areas such as face, genitalia or over joints. Since the older adult is more likely to have full thickness burns, inhalational injuries and complicating comorbidities, *discussion with a burns centre is advisable*.

Intravenous fluid is required for burns greater than 15% TBSA. Various formulas for calculating fluid requirements are available, such as the Parkland's formula; however, careful clinical assessment is required to avoid the complications of under- or over-estimation of fluid requirements. Managing pain control without causing delirium or over-sedation can be difficult in the older burns patient.

Surgical management of burns usually involves early debridement of burned tissue, and primary skin closure, skin grafting or alternative techniques. Split skin grafts may be technically challenging owing to thinning of skin with age. Impaired wound healing and susceptibility to infection in older burn patients may negatively affect skin graft take and donor site healing (11).

Older patients with burns over 50% TBSA have a very high mortality, and careful discussion with the patient, the family and the multidisciplinary team is necessary early on to agree on goals of care.

Take home messages

* Wounds in the older patient are more likely to be associated with delayed healing and chronic ulceration due to the presence of comorbidities and medications
* Older patients frequently have low immunity against tetanus: give tetanus immunoglobin and vaccinate in high-risk wounds
* Skin tears and pre-tibial lacerations may result in skin flaps. Adhesives, tape or sutures may compromise perfusion and result in necrotic tissue or wound breakdown. Always use a non-adherent dressing and ensure wound review is scheduled
* Burns are more likely to be of full thickness and of a greater surface area, and are associated with much higher mortality in the older patient.

References

1 Pepersack T, Turneer M, De Breucker S, Stubbe M, Beyer I. Tetanus immunization among geriatric hospitalized patients. *Eur J Clin Microbiol Infect Dis*. 2005;24(7):495–496.

2 Reid PM, Brown D, Coni N, Sama A, Waters M. Tetanus immunisation in the elderly population. *J Accid Emerg Med*. 1996;13(3):184–185.

3 Centers for Disease Control and Prevention (CDC). *Emergency Preparedness and Response: Tetanus Prevention*. http://www.bt.cdc.gov/disasters/disease/tetanus.asp [cited 2014 May 17].

4 LeBlanc K, Baranoski S. Skin tears: state of the science: consensus statements for the prevention, prediction, assessment, and treatment of skin tears©. *Adv Skin Wound Care*. 2011;24(9 Suppl):2–15.

5 Carville K, Lewin G, Newall N, Haslehurst P, Michael R, Santamaria P, et al. STAR: a consensus for skin tear classification. *Prim Intent*. 2007;15(1):18 – 28.

6 Barajas-Nava LA, López-Alcalde J, Roqué i Figuls M, Solà I, Bonfill Cosp X. Antibiotic prophylaxis for preventing burn wound infection Cochrane database. *Syst Rev*. 2013;6:CD008738.

7 Beldon P. Management options for patients with pretibial lacerations. *Nurs Stand*. 2008;22(32):53–54, 56, 58 passim.

8 American Burn Association. National Burn Repository Report of Data from 2002–2011. 2012, Chicago, IL

9 Hettiaratchy S, Dziewulski P. Introduction. What are the causes of burns? Who gets burnt? *BMJ*. 2004;328(7452):1366–1368.

10 American College of Surgeons Committee on Trauma. Advanced trauma life support program for doctors, 9th edn. 2012, Chicago, IL.

11 Keck M, Lumenta DB, Andel H, Kamolz LP, Frey M. Burn treatment in the elderly. *Burns*. 2009;35(8):1071–1079.

CHAPTER 14
Head injury

Introduction

Head injury is a common presentation to the emergency department in the older adult and may be isolated or occur in association with other traumatic injuries. There are 155,000 cases of head injury in the older adult annually in the United States, resulting in 12,000 deaths (1). More than two-thirds (81%) of head injuries in adults aged 65 and older are caused by falls, mostly from ground level (2). Ten percent of cases result from motor vehicle accidents, with the patient either as driver, passenger or pedestrian (3).

Traumatic brain injury results from both the initial focal injury to the brain, such as contusion or haemorrhage, and from the secondary insult due to poor cerebral circulation, hypoxia or oedema. Initial management of head injury is focused on preventing or limiting secondary brain injury.

Changes in the structure of the brain and skull with ageing (Figure 14.1) make intracerebral bleeding more common following a head injury. Comorbidities and medication such as anticoagulants and antiplatelet agents further increase the likelihood of complications and worsen prognosis.

Cerebral atrophy
Brain weight decreases by 10–20% by age 80 causing increased distance between the brain and the skull, resulting in:
- Greater movement of the brain in deceleration injuries
- Parasagittal bridging veins are stretched and more likely to rupture following injury
- A significant volume of blood can accumulate before symptoms are apparent

Cerebral blood flow is reduced by 20%, with impaired cerebrovascular autoregulation, increasing the risk of secondary brain injury

The dura becomes tightly adherent to the skull, so epidural haematomas are less common

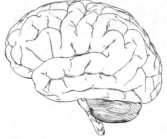

Figure 14.1 Structural changes in the ageing brain.

Geriatric Emergencies, First Edition.
Iona Murdoch, Sarah Turpin, Bree Johnston, Alasdair MacLullich and Eve Losman.
© 2015 John Wiley & Sons, Ltd. Published 2015 by John Wiley & Sons, Ltd.

Evidence for a head injury must be carefully sought when assessing a patient follow-ing a fall. Intracerebral bleeding may occur after a seemingly trivial injury and present with non-specific or delayed symptoms and signs. A low threshold for CT imaging should be adopted.

 KEY POINT: Remember that a head injury includes any injury to the face, nose or chin.

Initial assessment

The approach to an older patient with a traumatic injury should begin with a primary survey according to Advanced Trauma Life Support® (ATLS®) principles, covered in depth in Chapter 11. Serious head injuries may require urgent intervention.

Airway and cervical spine immobilisation
The airway should be rapidly assessed. Patients who have sustained a significant head injury may develop an obstructed or unprotected airway due to reduced consciousness. Basic airway opening manoeuvres and delivery of high flow oxygen are required. The patient may need airway adjuncts or endotracheal intubation following rapid sequence induction.

The neck should be triple immobilised (collar, blocks and tape; or other three-point system) if any of the factors in Box 14.1 are present. Immobilisation should be maintained until a cervical spine injury can be excluded. Imaging is usually required for this purpose in older patients in whom clinical examination can be insensitive. In patients with agitation or degenerative cervical spine disease, immobilisation may actually worsen outcome. Chapter 11 covers cervical spine injuries in more detail.

Box 14.1 Indications for cervical spine immobilisation in head injury (4).

- GCS <15 on initial assessment
- Neck pain or tenderness
- Focal neurological deficit
- Paraesthesia in the extremities
- Any other clinical suspicion of cervical spine injury – particularly if there is a *distracting* injury – defined as a condition thought by the clinician to be producing pain sufficient to distract the patient from a second (neck) injury – especially chest or upper limb injuries (5).

Breathing
Significant head injuries may cause a reduced conscious level with respiratory insuf-ficiency. Hypercapnoea causes vasodilatation of cerebral blood vessels, contributing to raised intracranial pressure (ICP) and secondary brain injury. Mechanical ventilation may be required to ensure adequate oxygenation.

Circulation with haemorrhage control

Cerebral blood flow decreases with age and an adequate mean arterial pressure is necessary to ensure cerebral perfusion. Prompt management of other injuries causing haemorrhage, including intravenous fluids, blood products or vasopressor support may be required to prevent secondary brain injury.

Disability

A brief neurological examination should take place during the primary survey and should include assessment of Glasgow Coma Scale (GCS), and pupillary size, equality and reactions. Ocular pathology such as glaucoma, cataract surgery and previous iritis may result in longstanding unequal pupils and may cause confusion when assessing the older patient.

Signs of critically raised ICP such as unequal pupils, hypertension or bradycardia necessitate immediate neurosurgical consultation and imaging. Temporary measures to reduce ICP include intravenous mannitol or hypertonic saline, mechanical ventilation and head elevation. Bedside INR measurement, if available, may indicate an urgent need for reversal of anticoagulants if there are signs consistent with intracerebral bleeding.

KEY POINT: In patients with dementia or a previous brain injury baseline mental and functional status should be established from family or carers. A change from baseline is always significant and should be investigated. Reduced conscious level is not a typical feature of dementia.

Exposure and environmental control

Inspect the patient for other life-threatening injuries. Hypothermia should be prevented with external warming devices.

History

Once the primary survey has been completed and any urgent issues arising from this addressed, a history of the head injury should be taken to guide examination and further investigation. Box 14.2 summarises the relevant aspects.

Box 14.2 Important questions in a head injury history.

- Timing and mechanism of injury
- Loss of consciousness or amnesia related to the injury
- Collateral history of events if available
- Symptoms such as headache, nausea and vomiting, blurred vision, diplopia, limb weakness, altered coordination or sensation and confusion
- Alcohol use
- Medication increasing bleeding risk such as anticoagulants and antiplatelet agents

---

- Medication that may have precipitated the injury such as antihypertensives, antidepressants and benzodiazepines (Table 8.1)
- Time of last oral intake, should airway interventions be required
- Past medical history and baseline cognitive and functional status
- Assessment of current cognition, for example using the 4AT score (Chapter 2).

Many head injuries are consequences of falls related to a syncopal event and these will require further work-up to elucidate the underlying cause (Chapter 8).

KEY POINT: A subdural haematoma may result from a trivial injury, or sudden deceleration, even where there is no direct impact to the head (6). Such injuries may not be remembered or reported.

Patients on anticoagulants such as warfarin are up to three times more likely to suffer from intracranial haemorrhage following head injury, with increasing likelihood as the INR rises above therapeutic levels (7). Patients receiving clopidogrel may have a higher prevalence of immediate traumatic intracranial haemorrhage compared with patients receiving warfarin (8). Antiplatelets as well as anticoagulants are associated with unfavourable outcome after head injury (9) and increased mortality following intracerebral haemorrhage (10–12). Dabigatran (a direct thrombin inhibitor) appears to be associated with a lower absolute risk of subdural haematoma than warfarin for patients with atrial fibrillation (13).

Excess use of alcohol increases the risk of serious head injury due to increased risk of falls and chronic liver disease resulting in coagulopathy. A low GCS should not be attributed to alcohol intoxification without first excluding other serious pathology.

Any head injury in an older adult should prompt consideration of elder abuse (Chapter 4).

Examination

Examination in the head-injured patient should include the points covered in Box 14.3.

Box 14.3 Examination of the head injury patient.

- Full external examination of scalp and face for signs of injury (Figure 14.2)
- Cervical spine examination
- Cranial nerve examination
- Peripheral neurological examination to include tone, power, reflexes and sensation
- Cerebellar examination to assess for ataxia, intention tremor, nystagmus and dysdiadochokinesis
- Secondary survey to evaluate for other injuries
- General examination to look for potential causes of a fall (Chapter 8)
- Gait assessment, when brain and cervical spine clearance is complete.

Eyes
Examine pupillary responses, visual acuity, visual fields and eye movements

Scalp
Inspect for a haematoma or laceration, and palpate for tenderness

Fundi
Look for papilloedema or retinal haemorrhages
Note any subconjunctival haemorrhages

Nose
Look for evidence of epistaxis or CSF (*cerebrospinal fluid*) rhinorrhoea

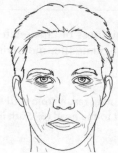

Ears
Examine the external ear and auditory canal. Look for CSF otorrhoea, haemotympanum or mastoid bruising

Figure 14.2 Examination of the head and face in the head injured patient.

Face
Look for facial lacerations or bruising. Palpate for tenderness over the facial bones. Check sensation and examine the cranial nerves

Cervical spine examination
Followed by imaging if required

Mouth
Check for missing teeth, mouth opening and mandibular tenderness

 KEY POINT: Abdominal, wrist and finger injuries are often missed in patients with a head injury.

Investigations

Initial investigations

Initial investigations should be guided by the severity of injury and informed by the primary survey, history and examination. As in all falls and injuries in the older adult, the head injury may have resulted from a medical problem such as arrhythmias, seizures, syncope or hypoglycaemia. Capillary blood glucose should be checked immediately in any patient with altered mental status. An ECG and routine blood tests (including coagulation studies if there is a history of anticoagulant use) will usually be required.

Computed tomography (CT) head

 KEY POINT: Most patients over the age of 65, and all those on anticoagulants, should undergo CT imaging following a head injury.

Patients with obvious signs of serious head injury such as reduced GCS, focal neurological deficit, post-traumatic seizures, vomiting or suspected open, depressed or basal skull fracture, or following a dangerous mechanism of injury, should undergo CT head urgently.

A dilemma may arise in the older patient who is GCS 15, and alert and orientated following a minor head injury. Physical examination has a low sensitivity for detecting intracranial injury in the older patient and as such a low threshold for imaging is necessary (14). In particular, any change in cognition, even if mild, should trigger imaging. The benefit of detecting an occult intracerebral haemorrhage far outweighs any possible risk of radiation exposure in the older patient. CT is a finite resource, however, and although in many centres all older adults will undergo CT following a head injury, in many this may not be feasible, and further risk stratification is necessary. Box 14.4 summarises the various guidelines for CT imaging in adults (4). Guidance may change, and up-to-date local guidelines should be consulted in all circumstances.

There is no specific guidance regarding patients with minor head injury on antiplatelet agents, but most consider these patients as having a coagulopathy and will arrange for CT imaging according to the above guidance.

The majority of abnormalities on CT imaging in the older patient are due to a subdural haematoma, which is discussed in more detail below. Epidural haematoma, traumatic subarachnoid haemorrhage, cerebral contusion or diffuse axonal injury are relatively less common in the older patient and usually result from higher impact trauma.

Box 14.4 Indications for CT head in mild head injury in older adults according to NICE, ACEP, CCHR, NOC and NEXUS II guidelines.

UK National Institute for Health and Care Excellence (NICE) Guidelines (4)
Perform CT head within 8 hours in
- All patients receiving anticoagulation with warfarin
- Patients aged over 65 with a history of loss of consciousness or amnesia
- Any history of bleeding or clotting disorders with a history of loss of consciousness or amnesia

American College of Emergency Physician (ACEP) Clinical Policy (15)
Perform CT head in
- All patients aged over 65
- Patients aged over 60 if there is loss of consciousness or post traumatic amnesia
- All patients taking anticoagulation (warfarin, fractionated or unfractionated heparin) or with documented coagulation disorder

The Canadian CT Head Rule (CCHR) (16)
Patients aged over 65 with a GCS 13–15 presenting with suspected head injury are at 'high risk' for an injury requiring neurosurgical intervention and head CT is necessary
Patients on anticoagulation were excluded from the contributory studies

New Orleans Criteria (NOC) (17)
In GCS 15 patients with a history of loss of consciousness in the setting of trauma, perform CT head if aged over 60
Patients with coagulopathy were underrepresented in this study

National Emergency X-Radiography Utilization Study (NEXUS)-II (18)
CT indicated if patient is aged over 65 or coagulopathic

Computed tomography (CT) cervical spine

The possibility of coexistent cervical spine injury should be carefully considered. ACEP guidelines (15) and UK College of Emergency Medicine guidelines (19) recommend concurrent CT imaging of the cervical spine for most older patients who are undergoing CT head. Plain radiographs can be inadequate or difficult to interpret due to degenerative changes, and may miss odontoid peg fractures (see Chapter 11).

Management

Management of head injury in the older patient will depend on findings gleaned from history, examination and imaging. Analgesia and cleaning and closure of any wound or lacerations will be required.

An intracranial bleed or other abnormality detected on CT imaging will require discussion with the local neurosurgical team. Endotracheal intubation and mechanical ventilation are necessary if the GCS is significantly reduced to ensure adequate oxygenation and normocarbia or to protect the airway during interhospital transfer. Measures to reduce ICP such as mannitol, hyperventilation and head elevation may be urgently indicated. Seizures should be treated promptly due to their deleterious effect on cerebral oxygen demand. If there are other injuries, balanced resuscitation is necessary to ensure an adequate blood pressure to perfuse the brain while limiting systemic bleeding. Blood glucose should be checked and controlled.

If neurological signs are present, but CT is normal, a repeat CT scan following a period of observation may be warranted. Magnetic resonance imaging (MRI) may reveal small subdural haemorrhages that are not visible on CT. Routine follow-up CT scans after a first negative scan have shown a low yield for detecting subsequent abnormalities (10), but repeat imaging is required if there is any change in neurological symptoms or signs.

Managing a head injured patient on anticoagulants

In a patient taking anticoagulants with a minor head injury, UK and US guidelines advise prompt CT imaging, regardless of INR – see Box 14.4.

Box 14.5 Anticoagulant reversal in the presence of life-threatening or serious bleeding (21,22).

In the presence of life-threatening or serious bleeding
Measure INR and take a blood sample for cross-matching
Administer 5 or 10 mg of vitamin K intravenously (maximum 1 mg/min)
Give prothrombin complex concentrate 25–50 units/kg*

---

*If unavailable, fresh frozen plasma 15 ml/kg is an alternative but is less effective and large volumes may cause fluid overload.

Prompt reversal of anticoagulation is required in patients taking warfarin who have signs of intracranial bleeding, and it improves mortality (20). All antiplatelets and anticoagulants should be stopped. Box 14.5 summarises current guidelines for anticoagulant reversal in the presence of life-threatening or serious bleeding.

New anticoagulants including direct thrombin inhibitors (e.g. dabigatran) and direct factor Xa inhibitors (e.g. rivaroxaban) do not have specific reversal agents. No routine laboratory tests are available that reliably measure the degree of anticoagulation. Although these drugs have a shorter half-life than warfarin, specialist advice from haematology should be sought as to how to manage bleeding in patients taking these medications. Prothrombin complex concentrate may be advocated.

Patients taking anticoagulants or antiplatelets with a normal CT head are at higher risk of delayed presentation of subdural haematoma. The role of routine admission for observation is unclear. European guidelines imply that anticoagulated patients with minor head injury should be admitted for 24 hours observation, followed by a second CT scan prior to discharge (23). A single centre prospective study supported this approach, with 5 of 87 (6%) patients having a delayed bleed identified on the second CT, four of whom had an INR greater than 3 (24), although only one bleed required neurosurgical intervention. A larger study observed that delayed intracerebral haemorrhage in patients on warfarin (4 in 687 patients) or clopidogrel (0 of 243 patients) was rare, and suggests that discharge from the emergency department, without reversal of anticoagulation or discontinuation of medication is reasonable if the patient or carer is aware of the indications to return (8). In the absence of clear guidance clinical judgement should be applied, with a low threshold to admit those with a supratherapeutic INR or higher impact injuries (25). In some patients the perceived risk of further falls weighed up against the risk of thromboembolic disease may prompt discontinuation of anticoagulation after careful consideration (see Chapter 19 for further discussion).

Discharging patients with head injuries

Patients with normal CT imaging may be considered for discharge to their usual place of residence provided they remain asymptomatic and can be observed by a family member or carer who is living with the patient. Consider an extended period of observation in patients who have other indications for admission (such as supratherapeutic anticoagulation; see above) or who live alone. A head injury advice sheet should be given outlining symptoms and signs indicating reassessment in the emergency department. Patients and their carers should be advised that a chronic subdural haematoma might present after a substantial interval of time after the initial head injury.

> KEY POINT: Older adults may develop a chronic subdural haematoma after a fall or head injury even though CT performed shortly afterwards may be normal, especially if they are on anticoagulants.

Subdural haematoma

Subdural haematoma is the commonest pathology detected in older patients following head injury, and increases in incidence with age. As the brain atrophies, bridging veins that lie between the cerebral cortex and the dural sinuses are more likely to tear causing bleeding. Due to the larger space between the brain and the skull a larger volume of blood can accumulate before clinical signs are evident (Figure 14.1).

Subdural haematomas can be classified into acute, subacute, chronic and acute on chronic. Risk factors include anticoagulation, antiplatelet medications, alcoholism, epilepsy and haemodialysis.

Acute subdural haematomas usually present within 72 hours of a head injury, and can occur following deceleration injuries or falls even when no impact to the head has occurred. Symptom onset is usually more rapid in patients taking anticoagulants. There can be a wide variation in presenting symptoms and signs in the older patient (Box 14.6), which will depend on the acuity and extent of bleeding. The patient may be entirely asymptomatic.

KEY POINT: The absence of neurological signs does not exclude the possibility of a chronic subdural haematoma.

Box 14.6 Symptoms and signs of subdural haematoma (26).

Headache
Drowsiness
Nausea or vomiting
New or worsening cognitive impairment
Behavioural or personality changes
Hemiparesis
Dysphasia
Reduced conscious level
Seizures.

Chronic subdural haematoma occurs due to slower bleeding over a period of time or following organisation of an acute subdural haematoma and can present more insidiously. It may be detected as an incidental finding following brain imaging for another indication. In up to half of cases there is no recollected head injury or fall (27).

CT imaging in subdural haematoma demonstrates a crescentic collection of blood and may be associated with midline shift. A hyperdense collection of blood will appear white on CT scanning and suggests an acute bleed (Figure 14.3), whereas a hypodense collection will be dark and implies a chronic subdural haematoma. Chronic subdural haematomas can be complicated by a new acute bleed, and CT will demonstrate blood of mixed densities.

Management decisions are usually made after discussion with the local neurosurgical team and will depend on the patient's neurological signs, extent of the bleeding on imaging and comorbidities.

Asymptomatic patients or those who are neurologically stable with a small bleed and no midline shift may be observed. One-third of patients undergo surgical treatment, such as craniotomy (removal and replacement of a section of skull) or craniostomy (drilling a hole through the skull) to evacuate the haematoma. The choice of surgical management will depend on patient comorbidities and the anticipated difficulty of clot evacuation (28). Observational studies suggest that corticosteroids may have a role in conservative management of subdural haematoma, and potentially as an adjunct to surgery (29). Typically, older people have had poorer functional outcomes than their

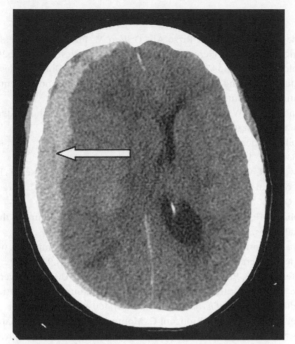

Crescentic right side high attenuation subdural collection (arrow),
suggesting acute subdural haematoma. There is substantial mass
effect and oedema with effacement of the ventricle and midline shift

Figure 14.3 Acute subdural haematoma. CT demonstrating crescentic right sided high attenuation subdural collection (arrow), with midline shift. From Teale EA, Iliffe S, Young JB. Subdural haematoma in the elderly. BMJ. 2014 Jan 11;348(mar11_11):g1682. Reproduced with permission of BMJ Publishing Group Ltd.

younger counterparts following a traumatic brain injury (30). However, age should not be a sole determinant in treatment decisions (31). Multidisciplinary rehabilitation is required following any traumatic brain injury.

In cases of a severe bleed with suspected poor prognosis, significant comorbidities or advanced frailty, neurosurgery may not be appropriate. Older patients with a subdural haematoma presenting with a GCS less than 8 have a mortality rate approaching 100%.

Careful discussion should take place between the proxy decision maker, family and relevant specialties. If the decision is made not to undergo surgery, supportive treatment is usually provided alongside palliation of symptoms. See Chapter 3 for further information.

Take home messages

- Significant intracerebral injury can occur from seemingly minor trauma in the older patient
- CT imaging should be strongly considered in all adults over 65 years
- Exclude concurrent cervical spine injury, which may present with minimal symptoms
- Delayed presentation of intracerebral bleeding commonly occurs with ageing, and caution should be taken when discharging patients from hospital.

References

1 Richmond R, Aldaghlas TA, Burke C, Rizzo AG, Griffen M, Pullarkat R. Age: is it all in the head? Factors influencing mortality in elderly patients with head injuries. *J Trauma*. 2011;71(1):E8–E11.

2 Faul M, Xu L, Wald M, Coronado V. Traumatic brain injury in the United States: emergency department visits, hospitalizations, and deaths. Centers for Disease Control and Prevention, National Center for Injury Prevention and Control; 2010. Atlanta, GA; 2010.

3 Langlois J, Rutland-Brown W, Thomas K. Traumatic brain injury in the United States: emergency department visits, hospitalizations, and deaths. Atlanta, GA; 2004.

4 Hodgkinson S, Pollit V, Sharpin C, Lecky F. Early management of head injury: summary of updated NICE guidance. *BMJ*. 2014;348(jan22_2):g104.

5 Hoffman JR, Mower WR, Wolfson AB, Todd KH, Zucker MI. Validity of a set of clinical criteria to rule out injury to the cervical spine in patients with blunt trauma. National Emergency X-Radiography Utilization Study Group. *N Engl J Med* 2000;343(2):94–99.

6 Flanagan SR, Hibbard MR, Riordan B, Gordon WA. Traumatic brain injury in the elderly: diagnostic and treatment challenges. *Clin Geriatr Med*. 2006;22(2):449–468, x.

7 Claudia C, Claudia R, Agostino O, Simone M, Stefano G. Minor head injury in warfarinized patients: indicators of risk for intracranial hemorrhage. *J Trauma*. 2011;70(4):906–909.

8 Nishijima DK, Offerman SR, Ballard DW, Vinson DR, Chettipally UK, Rauchwerger AS, et al. Immediate and delayed traumatic intracranial hemorrhage in patients with head trauma and preinjury warfarin or clopidogrel use. *Ann Emerg Med*. 2012;59(6):460–468.e1–7.

9 Fabbri A, Servadei F, Marchesini G, Bronzoni C, Montesi D, Arietta L. Antiplatelet therapy and the outcome of subjects with intracranial injury: the Italian SIMEU study. *Crit Care*. 2013;17(2):R53.

10 Mak CHK, Wong SKH, Wong GK, Ng S, Wang KKW, Lam PK, et al. Traumatic brain injury in the elderly: is it as bad as we think? *Curr Transl Geriatr Exp Gerontol Rep*. 2012;1(3):171–178.

11 Ohm C, Mina A, Howells G, Bair H, Bendick P. Effects of antiplatelet agents on outcomes for elderly patients with traumatic intracranial hemorrhage. *J Trauma*. 2005;58(3):518–522.

12 Wong DK, Lurie F, Wong LL. The effects of clopidogrel on elderly traumatic brain injured patients. *J Trauma*. 2008;65(6):1303–1308.

13 Hart RG, Diener H-C, Yang S, Connolly SJ, Wallentin L, Reilly PA, et al. Intracranial hemorrhage in atrial fibrillation patients during anticoagulation with warfarin or dabigatran: the RE-LY trial. *Stroke*. 2012;43(6):1511–1517.

14 Mack LR, Chan SB, Silva JC, Hogan TM. The use of head computed tomography in elderly patients sustaining minor head trauma. *J Emerg Med*. 2003;24(2):157–162.

15 Jagoda AS, Bazarian JJ, Bruns JJ, Cantrill S V, Gean AD, Howard PK, et al. Clinical policy: neuroimaging and decisionmaking in adult mild traumatic brain injury in the acute setting. *Ann Emerg Med*. 2008;52(6):714–748.

16 Stiell IG, Wells GA, Vandemheen K, Clement C, Lesiuk H, Laupacis A, et al. The Canadian CT head rule for patients with minor head injury. *Lancet*. 2001;357(9266):1391–1396.

17 Haydel MJ, Preston CA, Mills TJ, Luber S, Blaudeau E, DeBlieux PM. Indications for computed tomography in patients with minor head injury. *N Engl J Med*. 2000;343(2):100–105.

18 Mower WR, Hoffman JR, Herbert M, Wolfson AB, Pollack C V, Zucker MI. Developing a decision instrument to guide computed tomographic imaging of blunt head injury patients. *J Trauma*. 2005;59(4):954–959.

19 Guideline on the management of alert, adult patients with potential cervical spine injury in the emergency department. College of Emergency Medicine, UK. 2010.

20 Ivascu FA, Howells GA, Junn FS, Bair HA, Bendick PJ, Janczyk RJ. Rapid warfarin reversal in anticoagulated patients with traumatic intracranial hemorrhage reduces hemorrhage progression and mortality. *J Trauma*. 2005;59(5):1131–1137; discussion 1137–1139.

21 British National Formulary Website. http://www.bnf.org [cited 2014 Apr 17].

22 Cushman M, Lim W, Zakai NA. Clinical Practice Guide on Anticoagulant Dosing and Management of Anticoagulant-Associated Bleeding Complications in Adults. American Society of Hematology. 2011.

23 Vos PE, Alekseenko Y, Battistin L, Ehler E, Gerstenbrand F, Muresanu DF, et al. Mild traumatic brain injury. *Eur J Neurol*. 2012;19(2):191–198.

24 Menditto VG, Lucci M, Polonara S, Pomponio G, Gabrielli A. Management of minor head injury in patients receiving oral anticoagulant therapy: a prospective study of a 24-hour observation protocol. *Ann Emerg Med*. 2012;59(6):451–455.

25 Barbosa RR, Jawa R, Watters JM, Knight JC, Kerwin AJ, Winston ES, et al. Evaluation and management of mild traumatic brain injury: an Eastern Association for the Surgery of Trauma practice management guideline. *J Trauma Acute Care Surg*. 2012;73(5 Suppl 4):S307–S314.

26 Teale EA, Iliffe S, Young JB. Subdural haematoma in the elderly. *BMJ*. 2014;348(mar11_11):g1682.

27 Adhiyaman V, Asghar M, Ganeshram KN, Bhowmick BK. Chronic subdural haematoma in the elderly. *Postgrad Med J*. 2002;78(916):71–75.

28 Ducruet AF, Grobelny BT, Zacharia BE, Hickman ZL, DeRosa PL, Anderson K, et al. The surgical management of chronic subdural hematoma. *Neurosurg Rev*. 2012;35(2):155–169; discussion 169.

29 Berghauser Pont LME, Dirven CMF, Dippel DWJ, Verweij BH, Dammers R. The role of corticosteroids in the management of chronic subdural hematoma: a systematic review. *Eur J Neurol*. 2012;19(11):1397–1403.

30 Mosenthal AC, Lavery RF, Addis M, Kaul S, Ross S, Marburger R, et al. Isolated traumatic brain injury: age is an independent predictor of mortality and early outcome. *J Trauma*. 2002;52(5):907–911.

31 McIntyre A, Mehta S, Janzen S, Aubut J, Teasell RW. A meta-analysis of functional outcome among older adults with traumatic brain injury. *NeuroRehabilitation*. 2013;32(2):409–414.

CHAPTER 15

Abdominal emergencies

Introduction

Abdominal pain is the fourth commonest presentation to the Emergency Department in the older adult. It is a worrisome symptom, associated with a mortality rate of 5–10% (1). Abdominal pain may be minimal or even absent in the older patient despite the presence of serious intra-abdominal pathology. Vomiting, change in bowel habit, gastrointestinal bleeding, urinary symptoms or non-specific presentations such as delirium or immobility may predominate.

Identifying the cause of abdominal symptoms can be difficult due to the frequency of atypical presentations, comorbid conditions and sometimes limited history due to cognitive impairment. The wide range of potential differentials leads to misdiagnosis occurring in up to 30% of cases (2). The older patient may initially appear well with normal vital signs despite serious underlying pathology. Early abdominal CT is often helpful in reaching a diagnosis (3), but caution must be taken when using IV contrast in dehydrated patients (Chapter 2). Many older people will have radiological evidence of gallstones or diverticular disease without these necessarily being the cause of their symptoms. Early, effective analgesia is vitally important in managing the older person with abdominal pain (Chapter 3). Gastrointestinal bleeding increases in incidence with age, partly due to the more widespread use of anti-platelet agents in the older person. Prompt resuscitation and early endoscopy are required in the older patient due to the increased mortality risk. Up to 30% of older adults admitted with abdominal pain undergo surgery (4). The mortality rate for emergency abdominal surgery in older adults is 15–34%, predominantly due to complications arising from coexisting disease (5).

Background

Age-related changes in the gastrointestinal system are shown in Figure 15.1. Biliary disease is the responsible for 20–30% of cases of abdominal pain in the older patient, followed by bowel obstruction, peptic ulcer disease (PUD), diverticulitis and appendicitis. In 20% of cases, no diagnosis is made by the time of discharge.

Geriatric Emergencies, First Edition.
Iona Murdoch, Sarah Turpin, Bree Johnston, Alasdair MacLullich and Eve Losman.
© 2015 John Wiley & Sons, Ltd. Published 2015 by John Wiley & Sons, Ltd.

Decreased gastric emptying, atrophy of gastric mucosa and rise in carriage of *Helicobacter pylori* increases the likelihood of peptic ulcer disease, gastritis and reflux. Acid production may increase.

Immobility significantly prolongs colonic transit time, increasing risk of constipation or post-operative ileus.

Slower colonic transit with increased water re-absorption results in harder faeces, exacerbating constipation and causing faecal impaction and formation of diverticulae.

Increasing laxity of gastro-oesophageal sphincter may lead to hiatus herniae and reflux symptoms.

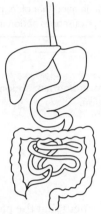

Figure 15.1 Age-related change in the gastrointestinal system.

Two-thirds of older adults have incidental colonic diverticulae that may or may not develop complications.

Changes in bile salt composition and decreased responsiveness to cholecystokinin with depressed gallbladder motility predispose the older patient to gallstone formation. Approximately 20% of 70 year olds and 40% of 80 year olds will have gallstones.

Atherosclerosis, atrial fibrillation, hypertension, and peripheral artery disease increase the risk of vascular causes of abdominal pain in the older adult such as mesenteric ischaemia and abdominal aortic aneurysm.

Initial assessment

An older patient presenting with abdominal pain should be assessed promptly (Box 15.1) to exclude life-threatening causes such as acute myocardial infarction or ruptured abdominal aortic aneurysm (AAA).

Box 15.1 Initial assessment in the older patient with abdominal pain.

Airway	Assess patency and provide high flow oxygen initially
Breathing	Measure oxygen saturations, and observe the pattern of breathing. Tachypnoea is a sensitive sign for serious illness. Peritonitis may cause rapid shallow breathing in part due to pain and as a compensatory mechanism for a metabolic acidosis
Circulation	Record heart rate and blood pressure, and note the presence of cool peripheries and prolonged capillary refill time indicating circulatory compromise. If there are signs of shock, insert two large bore intravenous cannulae, take urgent blood tests and give an initial bolus of intravenous fluid. Request urgent blood products if a ruptured abdominal aortic aneurysm or gastrointestinal bleeding are suspected. Tachycardia may occur in response to pain but should be assumed to be due to serious pathology until proven otherwise. Tachycardia may be absent due to beta-blocker therapy, reduced catecholamine response to hypovolaemia in the older adult, or cardiac conduction abnormalities. 'Normal' blood pressure may reflect significant hypotension if a patient is usually hypertensive

| Disability | Record level of consciousness. Assess pain severity and provide analgesia such as small doses of intravenous opioids repeated as necessary |
| Exposure | Examine the abdomen for signs of peritonitis or a pulsatile mass. Consider undertaking a bedside ultrasound to identify abdominal free fluid or an aortic aneurysm. Measure temperature; however bear in mind that older patients may be normothermic or hypothermic in the presence of serious abdominal pathology |

KEY POINT: Perform an urgent electrocardiogram: abdominal pain can be the only presenting symptom of acute myocardial infarction.

History

Once it is clear from the initial assessment that the patient is stable, a pain history should take place, incorporating the mnemonic SOCRATES (Table 15.1). Altered pain perception in the older adult and cognitive impairment may affect the ability to report and describe pain (Chapter 3).

Past surgical history should include past operations, their indications and any complications. Past medical history should include risk factors for vascular causes including cardiovascular disease, smoking, atrial fibrillation, or peripheral vascular disease. Diabetes may be associated with atypical presentations. Medications such as non-steroidal anti-inflammatories, anti-platelet agents, SSRI (selective serotonin reuptake inhibitors) antidepressants, and steroids may increase the risk of peptic ulceration and gastrointestinal bleeding. Anticoagulants may require urgent reversal where there is evidence of bleeding or surgery is required.

Examination

In addition to an abdominal examination, a cardiorespiratory examination is important to assess circulatory status and detect medical causes of abdominal pain such as pneumonia or congestive cardiac failure. Signs of chronic liver disease should be sought. The presence of atrial fibrillation should prompt consideration of mesenteric ischaemia. Postural blood pressure is useful if gastrointestinal bleeding is suspected.

Inspection
Initial inspection may reveal abdominal distension or previous surgical scars. There may be a visible hernia or mass. Rarely, bruising in the flanks may be visible in necrotic pancreatitis or ruptured AAA.

Palpation
Focal tenderness may point towards a particular aetiology, and guarding and rigidity indicates localised peritoneal irritation. However, this may be much less marked or even

Table 15.1 Points to cover in an abdominal pain history.

Site	Figure 15.2 illustrates sites of abdominal pain and potential underlying causes. The older patient is less likely to identify a precise area of pain. Back pain may originate from retroperitoneal structures such as the aorta and kidneys
Onset	Sudden onset of pain may indicate a ruptured viscus or ruptured aortic aneurysm. However, even abdominal catastrophes such as a perforated peptic ulcer may be associated with insidious onset of symptoms
Character	Establish whether pain is dull and aching indicating visceral pathology or sharp and localised indicating peritoneal irritation
Radiation	Radiation to the back may be characteristic of pancreatitis, peptic ulceration or aortic aneurysm. Ureteric calculi typically cause flank pain radiating to the groin. Diaphragmatic irritation may cause pain referred to the shoulder
Associated symptoms	Establish any additional features: • General symptoms such as anorexia, fever, night sweats, reduced mobility and altered mental state. • Collapse or pre-syncope which is suspicious for ruptured AAA • Vomiting, haematemesis and jaundice. • Urinary symptoms (dysuria, frequency and haematuria) and approximate urine output. • Bowel movements, passage of stool and flatus, diarrhoea, rectal bleeding or melaena. Other important subacute symptoms include weight loss, dysphagia, early satiety, fatigue and change in bowel habit, which may point to abdominal pain as a result of an underlying malignancy
Timing	A history of recurrent pain episodes should prompt consideration of mesenteric ischaemia, biliary disease, ureteric colic or malignancy. Persistent or worsening pain is usually more concerning than pain that has improved spontaneously
Alleviating and aggravating factors	Pain with movement, coughing or deep breathing may indicate peritoneal irritation. Pain after eating may reflect peptic ulcer disease, biliary disease or mesenteric ischemia
Severity	Pain in the older adult is often reported as less severe for any given pathology. Mild pain should not dissuade the clinician from considering a serious underlying cause

absent in the older patient due to reduced abdominal wall musculature and muscle fatigue. One study demonstrated that only 21% of older adults with perforated peptic ulcers presented with rigidity and guarding (6). Abdominal pain that does not worsen with palpation is typical of mesenteric ischaemia. Feel for a pulsatile mass and check the femoral and distal limb pulses, which may be absent in ruptured AAA. Take care to examine the inguinal regions and scrotum, for herniae, masses and skin changes. Figure 15.2 illustrates different sites of abdominal pain and their potential causes.

Percussion

A dull percussion note may reveal urinary retention, organomegaly or a solid malignancy. Hyperresonant percussion may reflect dilated bowel loops due to obstruction. There may be evidence of ascites in advanced malignancy or liver or congestive cardiac failure.

Auscultation
High-pitched bowel sounds may be audible in small bowel obstruction. Absent bowel sounds is a concerning sign, potentially indicating ileus due to peritonitis or severe intra-abdominal infection or inflammation.

Rectal examination
Rectal examination should be performed in most patients and may reveal melaena, rectal bleeding, faecal impaction, rectal masses or prostatic enlargement.

Epigastric
Pancreatitis
Peptic ulcer disease
Gastritis
Myocardial Infarction
Cholecystitis

Right-sided
Cholecystitis
Pyelonephritis
Pneumonia
Hepatic congestion
Renal colic
Appendicitis
Renal calculi
Caecal tumour
Right-sided diverticulitis

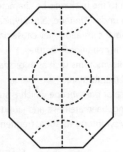

Figure 15.2 Potential causes and sites of abdominal pain in the older person.

Suprapubic
Acute urinary retention
Incarcerated inguinal hernia
Gynaecological malignancy
Urinary tract infection

Left sided
Pneumonia
Peptic ulcer disease
AAA
Diverticulitis
Renal calculi
Colon cancer

Non-specific or central
Mesenteric ischaemia
Small bowel obstruction
AAA
Malignancy
Extra-abdominal or medical causes
(Table 15.3)

Investigations

An urgent **blood gas**, venous or arterial, may demonstrate acid–base derangement and/or an elevated lactate, which would increase concern for perforation, bowel infarction, intra-abdominal sepsis or vascular catastrophe.

Full blood count may reveal a leucocytosis but frequently conditions such as cholecystitis and appendicitis are not associated with raised or left-shifted white cells in the older patient (7). Amylase should always be checked in older patients with abdominal pain. It is frequently raised in mesenteric ischaemia or perforated peptic ulcer and pancreatitis and lipase is more specific for pancreatic inflammation. Liver function tests are often normal in acute cholecystitis, unlike in younger patients (8).

KEY POINT: Thirty percentages of older adults with a surgical abdomen do not present with either a fever or leucocytosis.

Microscopic haematuria on urine dipstick testing may signal potential ureteric colic but can also result from urethral irritation due to AAA, appendicitis or diverticulitis.

Plain radiographs may identify perforation or dilated bowel loops due to bowel obstruction. Sensitivity, however, is low and films may be normal in 40–50% of confirmed perforations.

Formal or bedside ultrasound may assist in the diagnosis of cholecystitis, biliary obstruction, appendicitis and AAA. In the latter case, ultrasound will not be able to identify whether an aneurysm is leaking, but in the setting of an unstable patient, this signals the need for immediate transfer to the operating theatre.

Abdominal CT is sensitive for diagnosing perforation, AAA, diverticulitis, pancreatitis and occult malignancy. In one study of patients aged 65 years and older with abdominal pain CT imaging lead to a change in diagnosis in 45% of cases (9). See Chapter 2 for a discussion on the risks of contrast agents in the older patient. Non-contrast CT may be a useful compromise in some circumstances.

> **KEY POINT: Plain abdominal radiographs are of limited utility in the evaluation of acute abdominal pain in the older patient. Have a low threshold for urgent CT imaging but consider also the risk of contrast-induced acute kidney injury.**

Specific causes of abdominal pain in the older adult

Abdominal aortic aneurysm (AAA)

AAAs are present in 5–9% of those over 65 years (10) and are four to five times more common in men than in women. They are most often infrarenal and may extend into the iliac vessels. Rupture of an AAA has an overall mortality rate of approximately 80% (11), with around 30–50% of patients dying pre-hospital (12). Early diagnosis and intervention to control bleeding, such as cross-clamping of the aorta or endovascular balloon placement, is required. The diagnosis, however, is often delayed or missed as AAA may mimic more benign conditions such as ureteric colic, musculoskeletal back pain or diverticulitis.

> **KEY POINT: AAA is common and should be strongly considered in all patients over 60 with back or abdominal pain.**

Box 15.2 Emergency management of suspected ruptured AAA.

Provide high flow oxygen

Insert two large bore cannulae and send blood for cross-match

Request at least 10 units of red cells, fresh frozen plasma and platelets. Reverse anticoagulants (see Chapter 11)

Give fluid and blood products, targeting a lower systolic blood pressure to limit bleeding and clot disruption (termed **permissive hypotension**)

Inform the theatre team, anaesthetist and vascular surgeon

Provide analgesia and an antiemetic e.g. intravenous opioid

The classical presentation of a ruptured AAA includes hypotension, sudden severe abdominal or back pain, and a pulsatile abdominal mass, although this triad is present in only 25–50% of individuals (13). Tamponade of bleeding in the left retroperitoneal cavity can result in normal initial vital signs. Atypical presentations include symptoms of lumbar root compression, testicular pain and gastrointestinal bleeding in the event of an aorto-enteric fistula. Microscopic haematuria may be present in up to 87% cases of ruptured AAA, due to irritation of the ureter by the aneurysm (6).

The primary goal in ruptured AAA is control of bleeding by aortic cross-clamping or endovascular balloon occlusion; without this, resuscitation efforts are futile. If the patient is stable, CT with close monitoring will confirm the diagnosis of a ruptured AAA and identify the aortic anatomy involved to guide operative or endovascular approach. Box 15.2 summarises the initial emergency management.

Open surgical treatment of ruptured AAAs is associated with a 30–50% mortality rate (12, 14). Age and haemodynamic stability on presentation are among the most important risk factors for immediate post-operative death (15). Surviving surgery is the first step in an often lengthy critical care admission followed by rehabilitation. Up to 40% of patients will not undergo operative management because of the perceived high peri-operative mortality and poor prognosis (12). Decisions as to whether to treat the oldest old with ruptured AAA are clinically and ethically challenging and require the involvement of senior clinicians.

Biliary disease

Gallstones affect 15% of men and 24% of women by the age of 70 (16). Gallstones are frequently asymptomatic, but complications such as biliary colic, cholecystitis, cholangitis and pancreatitis occur when they obstruct the neck of the gallbladder or the common bile duct. Complications of gallstones are more common in the older population. They account for 20–30% of abdominal pain presentations to the ED and are the commonest reason for abdominal surgery in the older adult.

Biliary colic causes pain, nausea and vomiting, usually triggered by eating, and settles over a few hours with analgesia. Prompt elective cholecystectomy should be considered to prevent more serious complications and hospital admissions.

Cholecystitis is characterised by right upper quadrant tenderness, pyrexia and raised leucocytes and inflammatory markers. However, raised inflammatory markers, abnormal liver function tests and fever are absent in more than half of cases in older patients. Anorexia, nausea and vomiting may predominate in the absence of pain.

Diagnosis can be confirmed on ultrasound, which demonstrates a thickened gallbladder wall in the presence of biliary calculi. Older patients have an increased likelihood of acalculous cholecystitis, however, which is not appreciated as readily on ultrasound and is associated with a higher mortality (17). If ultrasound findings are non-diagnostic, a hepatobiliary (HIDA) scan or abdominal CT may confirm cholecystitis.

Initial management of cholecystitis includes intravenous fluids, analgesia and broad-spectrum antibiotics. Early definitive cholecystectomy is often considered ideal in the older patient with good functional status, resulting in decreased hospital length of stay (18). Non-operative management is associated with a 38% gallstone-related readmission rate over the subsequent 2 years (16). Percutaneous drainage of the gallbladder (percutaneous cholecystotomy) may be an option in the frail older patient.

Biliary obstruction occurs when a gallstone becomes lodged in the cystic duct or common bile duct. Stools become pale and the urine dark. Ascending cholangitis may develop, classically resulting in Charcot's triad: jaundice, abdominal pain, and fever. Patients may become systemically septic and require fluid resuscitation and intravenous antibiotics. Urgent endoscopic retrograde cholangiopancreatography (ERCP) is required to remove the obstructing stone and allow drainage of infected bile.

Biliary obstruction may also be due to malignancy in the pancreas or gallbladder. Clues to this may be preceding weight loss or chronic pain. Further imaging such as magnetic resonance cholangiopancreatography (MRCP) and/or endoscopic ultrasound can provide further delineation of the underlying cause and can additionally detect bile duct stones with higher sensitivity and specificity than standard ultrasound.

Other serious complications of gallstones include gangrenous cholecystitis leading to gallbladder perforation or empyema of the gallbladder. In addition, gallstone ileus, the migration of a biliary calculus into the small bowel, accounts for up to 25% of small bowel obstructions in those aged over 65 years (19).

Pancreatitis

Pancreatitis is the most common non-surgical cause of abdominal pain in the older adult (20), usually as a result of gallstones (65–70%). Mortality rates are much higher in older patients at 20–25% (21), with older age an independent risk factor for organ failure or death. Older patients with severe pancreatitis should be managed in a high dependency environment.

Diagnosis of pancreatitis requires two of the following three characteristics: abdominal pain, elevated pancreatic enzymes (usually three to five times the upper limit of normal) or imaging demonstrating pancreatic inflammation. The classical presentation is of upper abdominal pain radiating to the back, but it may present as isolated back or chest pain. Nausea and vomiting occur frequently.

Lipase is the biochemical assay of choice, as it is equal in sensitivity to amylase but has a higher specificity and longer duration of elevation. Amylase may be raised because of other abdominal or extra-abdominal pathology.

Box 15.3 Bedside index for severity in acute pancreatitis score (22).

Blood urea rise	>25 mg/dL or >8.9 mmol/L
Impaired mental status	Disorientation, lethargy, somnolence, coma or stupor
Systemic inflammatory response syndrome	≥2 of: • Temperature >38°C (100.4°F) or < 36°C (96.8°F) • Heart rate > 90 • Respiratory rate > 20 or $PaCO_2$ < 32 mmHg • WBC > 12,000/mm³ and 4,000/mm³
Age over 60 years	
Pleural effusion	As detected on imaging

Patients with a BISAP score >0 have an increasing risk of mortality, especially with a score of 3 or more. A score of 5 has a mortality rate of 22%.

CT, ultrasound or MRI may reveal pancreatic inflammation confirming the diagnosis. ERCP is used as a diagnostic and therapeutic procedure if gallstones are suspected as the cause, for example where common bile duct dilatation is visible on imaging.

Various scoring systems are available for assessing severity and risk stratifying acute pancreatitis, each with advantages and disadvantages. The key aim is early recognition of shock and multi-organ failure. The bedside index for severity in acute pancreatitis (BISAP) score (Box 15.3) has been identified as a useful tool in early pancreatitis that is appropriate for use in the ED (22, 23).

Peptic ulcer disease

Symptoms and signs of peptic ulcer disease (PUD) are often absent: 30% of patients older than 60 years with peptic ulceration have no abdominal pain (24). Vague symptoms may include anorexia, reflux, dyspepsia, nausea, weight loss, and symptoms of anaemia. Perforation or gastrointestinal haemorrhage may be the first presentation. Risk factors for PUD include non-steroidal anti-inflammatory drugs and infection with *Helicobacter pylori* of which intestinal carriage increases with age.

Perforation typically presents with acute severe epigastric pain, often radiating to the shoulder, signs of peritonitis and absent bowel sounds. However severe pain and abdominal rigidity is absent in up to 50% and 80%, respectively (25). 'Silent' perforation is more common in older patients with diabetes or those who take steroids.

Free air under the diaphragm on chest radiograph may be absent in 40% of patients with a perforation (25). Blood tests may reveal raised leucocytes and amylase. Bedside ultrasound may identify intra-peritoneal free air or fluid. CT may be required to confirm the diagnosis. Ensure adequate resuscitation is carried out whilst simultaneously preparing for operative intervention. The mortality rate rises to 30% in the geriatric population (6).

Gastrointestinal haemorrhage

The incidence of gastrointestinal (GI) bleeding rises in adults aged 60 and above. The widespread use of anti-platelet agents increases the incidence of bleeding and impacts on its outcome.

The basic principles of diagnosis and management of GI bleeding are the same in older and younger patients. However, older patients have higher rates of hospitalisation, re-bleeding, requirement for surgical intervention, blood transfusion and death (26, 27). Patients who have been started on dual anti-platelet therapy due to recent acute coronary syndrome or angioplasty with acute GI bleeding present a particular challenge (Chapter 5).

Gastrointestinal bleeding may occur from the upper or lower tract. Upper GI bleeding usually presents with haematemesis or melaena, with lower GI bleeding presenting with fresh blood rectally or darker red blood mixed with stool. However, brisk upper GI bleeding may result in fresh blood per rectum, and caecal bleeding may cause melaena. Older patients may not specifically report rectal bleeding or melaena and may present with symptoms related to anaemia or hypovolaemia.

Upper GI bleeding is most commonly due to peptic ulcer disease but other pathologies include oesophagitis, oesophageal or gastric varices, Mallory-Weiss tear or malignancy. Syncope, light headedness or postural hypotension may be presenting features in the absence of overt bleeding. Antecedent symptoms such as dyspepsia or abdominal pain in cases of peptic ulceration are less common in older people. The extent of bleeding may be underestimated because of the absence of tachycardia due to reasons mentioned earlier. Comorbidities such as cardiac failure, ischaemic heart disease, liver failure, renal failure and malignancy greatly increase mortality. Scoring systems such as the Rockall and Blatchford score identify the contribution of older age and/or comorbidities to mortality and re-bleeding risk (28).

> **KEY POINT: Always inspect the nose and throat to exclude bleeding from the upper respiratory tract mimicking upper GI bleeding.**

Haemodynamic compromise necessitates resuscitation with balanced blood products (red cells, platelets and fresh frozen plasma) and reversal of anticoagulation, in line with local protocols. Similar to the trauma or ruptured AAA scenario, targeting a lower systolic blood pressure (**permissive hypotension**) may limit bleeding and clot disruption whilst awaiting endoscopy. Most patients receive a bolus of intravenous proton pump inhibitor (PPI). Prompt interventional endoscopy, for example with clipping of bleeding vessels or epinephrine injection, is life saving and well tolerated in older patients (27). However, patients with delirium or dementia may lack the capacity to consent and find the procedure itself confusing and frightening. Careful liaison and communication with the practitioners doing the procedure is required to determine the optimal approach. Intravenous PPI infusions reduce re-bleeding after interventional endoscopic procedures. Variceal bleeding is an indication for vasopressin or somatostatin analogues, which reduce portal hypertension. If *H. Pylori* is identified as a contributing factor to peptic ulceration, eradication with antibiotics and PPI is necessary with confirmation of clearance.

Lower GI bleeding is most commonly due to complications of diverticular disease, followed by angiodysplasia, haemorrhoids, mesenteric ischaemia, colitis and malignancy. Options for investigation and/or treatment include sigmoidoscopy or colonoscopy, CT imaging or angiography. Fresh rectal blood may also result from brisk upper GI bleeding. This may be suggested by a raised blood urea to creatinine ratio or aspiration of blood stained nasogastric fluid and requires investigation with upper GI endoscopy.

Small bowel obstruction

Bowel obstruction presents with abdominal distension, colicky pain, nausea and vomiting. Older patients often have a protuberant abdomen due to kyphoscoliosis and reduced abdominal wall musculature and it is useful to ask whether their abdomen appears more distended. Establish when their bowels last opened and if they are passing flatus. Examine the abdomen carefully, including the groins and scrotum to look for herniae.

Small bowel obstruction is most commonly caused by adhesions following previous abdominal surgery (50–74%), obstructed herniae (15%), and malignancy (15%). Gallstone ileus is more common in the older person, in one study causing up to 20% of small bowel obstructions (19).

Plain radiography may demonstrate distended bowel loops, air fluid level, or collapsed bowel distal to obstruction but it is limited by a sensitivity of just 66% and specificity of

57% (29). CT usually identifies the site, degree and cause of bowel obstruction, with an improved sensitivity of 92% and specificity of 93% (30).

 KEY POINT: Look carefully for an incarcerated hernia, which may be missed on initial examination.

30–50% of small bowel obstructions will resolve with conservative treatment, which includes nasogastric decompression, analgesia, intravenous fluids and bowel rest. Adequate hydration and maintenance of electrolyte balance are essential. Morbidity and mortality in older adults with small bowel obstruction is approximately 26% (6): high dependency care will be required with careful monitoring of urine output and vital signs. Deterioration may indicate strangulation or bowel ischemia requiring immediate surgical intervention.

Large bowel obstruction

Large bowel obstruction is less common than small bowel obstruction and occurs mostly due to malignancy (60%), volvulus (10–15%), or diverticulitis. Volvulus, a twist of the bowel along its own mesentery, may occur in the sigmoid colon (70–80% of cases) or caecum (Figure 15.3). Risk factors for volvulus include chronic distension, previous abdominal surgery and adhesions, laxative use and medication, which reduces bowel motility (Box 15.4).

Presentation of large bowel obstruction is similar to small bowel obstruction but onset may be more gradual. Half of patients will have no vomiting and 20% will have diarrhoea (17). Vomiting is more likely to be faeculant in view of the more distal obstruction. A background history of symptoms suggestive of malignancy such as weight loss or iron deficiency anaemia may be present. Delayed diagnosis due to subtlety of symptoms leads to a mortality rate approaching 40% (17).

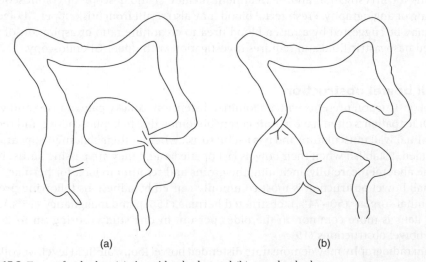

(a)   (b)

Figure 15.3 Types of volvulus: (a) sigmoid volvulus and (b) caecal volvulus.

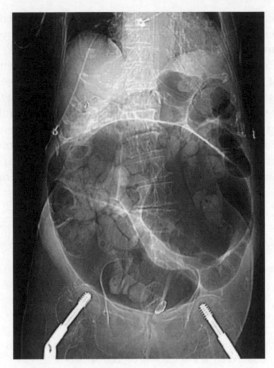

Figure 15.4 'Coffee bean sign' in an older patient with sigmoid volvulus. Source: From Ladizinski B, Amjad H, Rukhman E, Sankey C. The coffee bean sign and sigmoid volvulus in an elderly adult. *J Am Geriatr Soc.* 2013 Oct;61(10):1843–4. Reproduced with permission from John Wiley & Sons.

Plain radiographs may reveal a dilated colon, identified by incomplete haustral lines. Sigmoid volvulus may reveal the classic 'coffee bean sign' on plain radiograph (Figure 15.4). CT should be undertaken promptly to identify the site and cause of obstruction and any associated complications.

Sigmoid volvulus may be decompressed via sigmoidoscopy and placement of a rectal tube. If unsuccessful urgent surgical intervention is required as delay will lead to rapid bowel ischaemia. Laparotomy will be required in other cases of large bowel obstruction due to the risk of imminent perforation.

Non-mechanical causes of bowel obstruction

Functional disturbances in intestinal motility are thought to be due to a disruption of the enteric nervous system that governs peristalsis, owing to a number of possible factors (Box 15.4). Any part of the gastrointestinal tract can be affected, but most commonly dysfunction of the small bowel and colon, termed **ileus** and **acute colonic pseudo-obstruction** (or Ogilvie's syndrome), respectively. These are more common in the older patient because of medication, critical illness and comorbidities (Box 15.4).

> **KEY POINT:** The critical aspect in the management of acute colonic pseudo-obstruction is exclusion of mechanical obstruction.

Presenting symptoms are similar to mechanical bowel obstruction with cramping abdominal pain, vomiting and abdominal distension, but as the bowel is atonic, bowel sounds will be reduced.

Investigations should be focused on identifying an underlying cause and ruling out a mechanical cause of obstruction.

Plain radiographs may demonstrate distended loops of small bowel. Massive colonic dilatation is usually visible in Ogilvie's syndrome and also involves the rectum, helping to distinguish from more proximal causes of obstruction where the rectum will usually be collapsed. However, the distinction between mechanical and functional obstruction cannot be made with plain radiography alone. CT, barium enema and/or colonoscopy are usually required to exclude a mechanical obstruction due to tumour or stricture.

Box 15.4 Causes of non-mechanical bowel obstruction and constipation (31).

Critical illness e.g. sepsis, acute kidney injury, multi-organ failure and trauma

Prolonged immobility, hospitalisation

Pancreatitis or other intra-abdominal infection or inflammation

Post-operative, following abdominal or non-abdominal surgery

Medication e.g. opioids, anticholinergics, tricyclic antidepressants, anti-Parkinson medication, phenothiazines, iron, calcium channel blockers and benzodiazepines

Electrolyte disturbances such as hypokalaemia, hypomagnesaemia, hyponatraemia, hyperglycaemia and hypercalcaemia, also hypothyroidism

Neurological disorders e.g. Parkinsonism, dementia, multiple sclerosis and spinal cord syndromes

---

Management of acute non-mechanical bowel obstruction is based on treating the underlying cause, stopping causative medications and ensuring adequate hydration and electrolyte balance. Nasogastric decompression and bowel rest are required. In acute colonic pseudo-obstruction, colonoscopy itself is successful in decompressing the bowel in 80% of cases, but recurrence occurs in 22%(32). Pharmacologic decompression can be achieved with the use of intravenous neostigmine, but there are several contraindications and potential complications (33). Prolonged colonic distension, particularly over 5 days duration, can result in mural ischemia and perforation and a need for urgent laparotomy (33). Daily physical and radiological examination is important to identify emerging complications early. Poor outcome is usually related to underlying comorbidities.

Constipation and faecal impaction

Constipation becomes more common due to age-related change (Figure 15.1) or secondary to other factors, such as medication, dehydration or biochemical disturbances (Box 15.4). Anorectal diseases such as anal fissure, strictures and haemorrhoids may contribute. Constipation can be defined in a number of ways such as decreased stool frequency, increased hardness of stool, straining or sensation of incomplete evacuation.

Symptoms associated with constipation include abdominal pain, inability to pass stool, distension, rectal bleeding, faecal impaction and overflow diarrhoea.

> **KEY POINT: In a patient with 'constipation' who has severe abdominal pain or abnormal vital signs, abdominal CT may be required to exclude a more serious diagnosis such as obstruction, perforation or ischaemia.**

Faecal impaction occurs when a compacted mass of faeces fills the distal colon or rectum. It may lead to absolute constipation with signs of mechanical bowel obstruction or cause overflow diarrhoea: the passage of liquid stool around the impaction. Older people with cognitive impairment have an increased risk of faecal impaction because of decreased awareness of the need to defecate, reduced mobility and reduced thirst sensation. If untreated, faecal impaction can be life threatening. It can cause the intra-luminal pressure within the colon to increase, potentially resulting in pressure necrosis of the bowel wall leading to ulceration and perforation.

Rectal examination may reveal hard impacted stool but faecal impaction may also occur more proximally in the colon and the rectum may be empty. Plain radiography may identify the site of impaction, but CT may be required to exclude an alternative mechanical cause of large bowel obstruction. Faecal impaction commonly results in acute urinary retention, and this should always be excluded as a complication.

The treatment of a faecal impaction requires enemas and suppositories to soften the stool and stimulate the bowel. If impaction is relieved in the ED and the underlying cause has been addressed, the patient may be discharged with a laxative regime to prevent recurrence. In some circumstances, however, manual evacuation of faeces, occasionally under sedation or anaesthesia, may be required. This can be hazardous and is best performed by the surgical team. In the event of bowel necrosis or perforation, urgent laparotomy is indicated.

Mesenteric ischaemia

Acute mesenteric ischaemia is a relatively rare cause of abdominal pain, accounting for <1% of presentations, but mostly occurs in the older patient because of the increased incidence of hypertension, peripheral arterial disease, atherosclerosis and atrial fibrillation (8). Mesenteric ischaemia often presents insidiously resulting in diagnostic delay and has a mortality rate of over 50% (34).

Mesenteric ischaemia occurs due to four different pathological processes that can be associated with varying clinical presentations (Table 15.2). The superior mesenteric artery (SMA) is the commonest site where emboli lodge, owing to the oblique angle as the SMA emerges from the aorta, and it is also the commonest site of severe atherosclerosis predisposing to thrombus formation (35).

Initial symptoms include diffuse abdominal pain, with nausea, vomiting and diarrhoea and minimal initial findings on abdominal examination. As ischaemia progresses to infarction signs of peritonism develop, and rectal bleeding may be apparent.

Blood tests may or may not reveal a metabolic acidosis, raised lactate, inflammatory markers, white cell count, liver function tests or amylase.

Table 15.2 Causes of mesenteric ischaemia (35).

Cause	Clinical features
Superior mesenteric artery embolus (50%)	Caused by an obstructing embolus, usually cardiac in origin. Associated with atrial fibrillation, acute myocardial infarction with mural thrombus, or endocarditis. Symptoms may be sudden in onset
Superior mesenteric artery thrombosis (25%)	Progressive atherosclerosis of mesenteric vessels may lead to a chronic history of pain after eating ('intestinal angina'). Development of collateral vessels may cause a more gradual presentation of ischaemia and infarction in the event of an acute occluding thrombus, which may delay diagnosis and worsen mortality
Mesenteric venous thrombosis (8%)	Mesenteric vein thrombosis is associated with a hypercoagulable state or concomitant intra-abdominal inflammation or sepsis. 50% of patients have a personal or family history of venous thromboembolism (36). Onset is usually gradual
Non-occlusive mesenteric ischaemia (17%)	Intestinal hypoperfusion occurs due to sepsis, severe dehydration, or congestive heart failure, particularly in patients receiving critical care support for multi-organ failure. Vasopressin and catecholamines, in addition to beta-blockers, digoxin and ACE inhibitors may compromise mesenteric blood flow

Plain radiographs may reveal dilated or thickened bowel loops. Abdominal CT may demonstrate bowel wall oedema or haemorrhage but may miss arterial thrombi. CT angiography is the investigation of choice, with a sensitivity of 93% and a specificity of 100% (37).

 KEY POINT: If pain appears to be out of proportion to examination findings, consider mesenteric ischaemia.

If the diagnosis is made early, treatment modalities such as intra-arterial thrombolytics, vasodilators, endovascular techniques or anticoagulation (in the case of mesenteric venous thrombosis) may be considered. In cases where peritonitis is present, exploratory laparotomy is usually required to assess bowel viability and perform mesenteric arterial revascularisation, such as embolectomy or mesenteric vessel bypass, followed by bowel resection if required. Delayed anastomosis or stoma formation after a second look at bowel viability after 24–48 hours is often required (38). Supportive treatment in intensive care with broad-spectrum antibiotics and fluid resuscitation should be instigated. Owing to the high mortality rate associated with emergency surgery, a palliative, non-operative approach may be more appropriate in certain cases (Chapter 3).

Appendicitis

Appendicitis accounts for 5% of all cases of acute abdomen in the older patient and is the third most common reason for abdominal surgery in the older population. It is often considered a condition affecting the young but 10% of appendicitis occurs in those aged over 60. Less than a third have the classical presentation of leucocytosis, fever and right lower abdominal pain (4). Half of patients demonstrate no guarding or rebound tenderness and up to a quarter have no right lower quadrant tenderness at all (39). Non-specific symptoms such as urinary frequency, abdominal distension, diarrhoea or systemic sepsis may confuse the clinical picture and delay definitive diagnosis. CT is not 100% sensitive, and diagnostic laparoscopy should be considered earlier in older patients in whom appendicitis is suspected rather than watchful waiting (17). Up to 70% of older adults have a perforated appendix at the time of operation with associated complications and higher mortality (40). This number is decreasing with increased utilisation of early CT in undifferentiated abdominal pain. Antibiotics and intravenous fluids should be given promptly before surgery.

Diverticular disease

Diverticulae are narrow mucosal outpouchings of the colon mucosa associated with aging and a low fibre diet, most often affecting the sigmoid colon. Diverticulosis occurs in two-thirds of older persons, 10–30% of whom develop symptomatic disease (41). Complications are more common in the older patient and may include diverticulitis, diverticular abscess, bowel obstruction, perforation or fistula formation (8). Diverticular disease is the most common cause of rectal bleeding in the older population (see above).

The presentation of diverticulitis is classically with left lower quadrant cramping abdominal pain, fever, leucocytosis and change in bowel habit. Rectal bleeding may be present and occasionally brisk. As with appendicitis, proximity of the bladder or ureter to the site of inflammation may lead to pyuria or haematuria, leading to the erroneous diagnosis of urinary tract infection. Acute diverticulitis may also develop on the right side of the colon although this is less common. Contrast CT is useful in identifying diverticulitis and other complications of diverticular disease; however, CT may appear normal early in the disease process. Other differential diagnoses to consider are colitis due to *Clostridium difficile*, inflammatory bowel disease or mesenteric ischaemia.

Mild symptoms may be managed with oral antibiotics in the community with close follow up. More severe cases will require admission for broad-spectrum intravenous antibiotics and fluids, with careful monitoring and re-examination to detect any complications. Perforation will require urgent laparotomy with colonic resection. Diverticular abscess may be amenable to CT guided drainage. A total of 25% of patients will have a recurrence of diverticulitis following an initial episode (42).

Genitourinary causes

> KEY POINT: Be wary of diagnosing more benign conditions such as gastroenteritis or UTI in the older patient without first excluding serious alternative pathology.

Urinary tract causes account for 5–10% of abdominal pain in the older adult (6). Urinary tract infections may be associated with lower abdominal pain or flank pain. UTIs are frequently over diagnosed in the older person due to high rates of asymptomatic bacteriuria (Chapter 7), and a serious alternative cause should be excluded before abdominal pain is ascribed to a UTI.

Acute urinary retention should always be considered as a cause of acute abdominal pain, as it is so easily identified and treated. This is particularly the case in those who

Table 15.3 Other causes of abdominal pain.

Cardiac causes	Acute myocardial infarction, most commonly of the inferior wall, pericarditis, congestive cardiac failure with hepatic congestion or aortic dissection
Respiratory causes	Pneumonia and pulmonary embolus may present with upper abdominal pain
Intra-abdominal malignancy	May present as bowel, biliary or urinary obstruction or with isolated pain
Gastrointestinal infection and inflammation	Gastroenteritis, gastritis, oesophagitis and gastroeosophageal reflux disease
Neuropathic causes	Nerve root compression or herpes zoster infection
Gynaecological or urological causes	Ovarian torsion, gynaecological malignancy, epididymoorchitis and prostatitis
Abdominal wall	Rectal sheath haematomas, especially in anti-coagulated patients. Abdominal muscle strain or Spigelian hernia
Medical causes	Hepatitis, diabetic ketoacidosis, hyperosmolar hyperglycaemic state, adrenal insufficiency, acute intermittent porphyria and hypercalcaemia
Medication	Metformin, antibiotics and digoxin can cause abdominal cramps, nausea, diarrhoea and vomiting

are unable to communicate reduced or absent urine output. A bladder scan or bedside ultrasound will confirm a distended bladder found on examination. Causes include medications such as anticholinergics, tricyclic antidepressants and antihistamines; alcohol; constipation; clot retention due to haematuria; prostatic enlargement or neurological conditions such as cauda equina syndrome.

Urinary tract stones occur in 4–5% of older patients with abdominal pain. They may be identified on non-contrast CT, which will also rule out an AAA, the most important diagnosis to exclude when considering renal colic.

Non-surgical or extra-abdominal causes of abdominal pain

History and examination may point to a non-surgical or extra-abdominal cause of abdominal pain, such as those given in Table 15.3.

Non-specific abdominal pain

20% of patients will have no diagnosis ascribed to their abdominal pain after assessment and imaging. The causes in Table 15.3 should be carefully considered and excluded if relevant. If symptoms have resolved and vital signs and investigations are reassuring, it is sensible to observe patients for a few hours to ensure that there are no further episodes of pain, check they are managing food and fluid and perform a repeat examination. If the patient is discharged home, it is important to inform the primary care physician of their attendance and advise the patient to return should any symptoms redevelop. Up to 10% of patients presenting with transient non-specific abdominal pain will have an abdominal malignancy diagnosed in the year following their attendance (43, 44), and it is wise to schedule routine follow up with a primary care physician following discharge.

Take home messages

- Rapid initial assessment should exclude immediately life-threatening causes of abdominal pain such as acute myocardial infarction, ruptured aortic aneurysm and aortic dissection
- Diagnostic accuracy in acute abdominal pain decreases with increasing age. History, examination findings and blood results may be misleading. Early CT imaging should be considered when the diagnosis remains unclear
- Biliary disease is the commonest cause of abdominal pain in the older adult. However, care should be taken not to presume that pain is due to biliary colic or cholecystitis just because the patient is known to have gallstones: the same applies for diverticular disease
- Avoid diagnosing benign conditions such as urinary tract infection, gastroenteritis, ureteric colic, gastro-oesophageal reflux or constipation without excluding more serious pathology. Consider the worst possible diagnosis first.

References

1 Marco CA, Schoenfeld CN, Keyl PM, Menkes ED, Doehring MC. Abdominal pain in geriatric emergency patients: variables associated with adverse outcomes. *Acad Emerg Med*. 1998;5(12):1163–8.
2 Kizer KW, Vassar MJ. Emergency department diagnosis of abdominal disorders in the elderly. *Am J Emerg Med*. 1998;16(4):357–362.
3 Hustey FM, Meldon SW, Banet GA, Gerson LW, Blanda M, Lewis LM. The use of abdominal computed tomography in older ED patients with acute abdominal pain. *Am J Emerg Med*. 2005;23(3): 259–265.
4 Yeh EL, McNamara RM. Abdominal pain. *Clin Geriatr Med*. 2007;23(2):255–270.
5 Lyon C, Clark D. Diagnosis of acute abdominal pain in older patients. *Am Fam Physician*. 2006; 74(9):1537–1544.
6 Ragsdale L, Southerland L. Acute abdominal pain in the older adult. *Emerg Med Clin North Am*. 2011;29(2):429–448.
7 Potts F, Vukov L. Utility of fever and leukocytosis in acute surgical abdomens in octogenarians. *J Gerontol A Biol Sci Med Sci*. 1999;54:M55–M58.
8 Chang C-C, Wang S-S. Acute abdominal pain in the elderly. *Int J Gerontol*. 2007;1(2):77–82.
9 Esses D, Birnbaum A, Bijur P, Shah S, Gleyzer A, Gallagher E. Ability of CT to alter decision making in elderly patients with acute abdominal pain. *Am J Emerg Med*. 2004;22(4):270–272.
10 Ho M-P, Chou A-H, Cheung W-K. Ruptured abdominal aortic aneurysm in an elderly man. *J Am Geriatr Soc*. 2013;61(12):2261–2262.
11 Biancari F, Venermo M. Open repair of ruptured abdominal aortic aneurysm in patients aged 80 years and older. *Br J Surg*. 2011;98(12):1713–1718.
12 Reimerink JJ, van der Laan MJ, Koelemay MJ, Balm R, Legemate DA. Systematic review and meta-analysis of population-based mortality from ruptured abdominal aortic aneurysm. *Br J Surg*. 2013;100(11):1405–1413.
13 Banerjee A. Atypical manifestations of ruptured abdominal aortic aneurysms. *Postgrad Med J*. 1993;69(807):6–11.
14 Mani K, Lees T, Beiles B, Jensen LP, Venermo M, Simo G, et al. Treatment of abdominal aortic aneurysm in nine countries 2005–2009: a vascunet report. *Eur J Vasc Endovasc Surg*. 2011;42(5): 598–607.

15 Biancari F, Mazziotti MA, Paone R, Laukontaus S, Venermo M, Lepäntalo M. Outcome after open repair of ruptured abdominal aortic aneurysm in patients >80 years old: a systematic review and meta-analysis. *World J Surg. Springer-Verlag.* 2011;35(7):1662–1670.

16 Riall TS, Zhang D, Townsend CM, Kuo Y-F, Goodwin JS. Failure to perform cholecystectomy for acute cholecystitis in elderly patients is associated with increased morbidity, mortality, and cost. *J Am Coll Surg Elsevier.* 2010;210(5):668, 679.

17 Martinez JP, Mattu A. Abdominal pain in the elderly. *Emerg Med Clin North Am.* 2006;24(2):371–388.

18 Gurusamy KS, Samraj K. Early versus delayed laparoscopic cholecystectomy for acute cholecystitis. *Cochrane database Syst Rev.* 2006 Oct 18;(4):CD005440.

19 Kirchmayr W, Mühlmann G, Zitt M, Bodner J, Weiss H, Klaus A. Gallstone ileus: rare and still controversial. *ANZ J Surg.* 2005;75(4):234–238.

20 Martin SP, Ulrich CD. Pancreatic disease in the elderly. *Clin Geriatr Med.* 1999;15(3):579–605.

21 Ross SO, Forsmark CE. Pancreatic and biliary disorders in the elderly. *Gastroenterol Clin North Am.* 2001;30(2):531–545.

22 Wu BU, Johannes RS, Sun X, Tabak Y, Conwell DL, Banks PA. The early prediction of mortality in acute pancreatitis: a large population-based study. *Gut.* 2008;57(12):1698–1703.

23 Papachristou GI, Muddana V, Yadav D, O'Connell M, Sanders MK, Slivka A, et al. Comparison of BISAP, Ranson's, APACHE-II, and CTSI scores in predicting organ failure, complications, and mortality in acute pancreatitis. *Am J Gastroenterol.* 2010;105(2):435–441; quiz 442.

24 Hilton D, Iman N, Burke GJ, Moore A, O'Mara G, Signorini D, et al. Absence of abdominal pain in older persons with endoscopic ulcers: a prospective study. *Am J Gastroenterol.* 2001;96(2):380–384.

25 Fenyö G. Acute abdominal disease in the elderly: experience from two series in Stockholm. *Am J Surg.* 1982;143(6):751–754.

26 Farrell JJ, Friedman LS. Gastrointestinal bleeding in older people. *Gastroenterol Clin North Am.* 2000;29(1):1–36.

27 Yachimski PS, Friedman LS. Gastrointestinal bleeding in the elderly. *Nat Clin Pract Gastroenterol Hepatol.* 2008;5(2):80–93.

28 Wang C-Y, Qin J, Wang J, Sun C-Y, Cao T, Zhu D-D. Rockall score in predicting outcomes of elderly patients with acute upper gastrointestinal bleeding. *World J Gastroenterol.* 2013;19(22):3466–3472.

29 Maglinte DD, Balthazar EJ, Kelvin FM, Megibow AJ. The role of radiology in the diagnosis of small-bowel obstruction. *AJR Am J Roentgenol.* 1997;168(5):1171–1180.

30 Mallo RD, Salem L, Lalani T, Flum DR. Computed tomography diagnosis of ischemia and complete obstruction in small bowel obstruction: a systematic review. *J Gastrointest Surg.* 2005;9(5):690–694.

31 Jain A, Vargas HD. Advances and challenges in the management of acute colonic pseudo-obstruction (ogilvie syndrome). *Clin Colon Rectal Surg.* 2012;25(1):37–45.

32 Vanek VW, Al-Salti M. Acute pseudo-obstruction of the colon (Ogilvie's syndrome). An analysis of 400 cases. *Dis Colon Rectum.* 1986;29(3):203–210.

33 Saunders MD, Kimmey MB. Systematic review: acute colonic pseudo-obstruction. *Aliment Pharmacol Ther.* 2005;22(10):917–925.

34 Sise MJ. Acute mesenteric ischemia. *Surg Clin North Am.* 2014;94(1):165–181.

35 Ozden N, Gurses B. Mesenteric ischemia in the elderly. *Clin Geriatr Med.* 2007;23(4):871–887, vii–viii.

36 Rhee RY, Gloviczki P, Mendonca CT, Petterson TM, Serry RD, Sarr MG, et al. Mesenteric venous thrombosis: still a lethal disease in the 1990s. *J Vasc Surg.* 1994;20(5):688–697.

37 Aschoff AJ, Stuber G, Becker BW, Hoffmann MHK, Schmitz BL, Schelzig H, et al. Evaluation of acute mesenteric ischemia: accuracy of biphasic mesenteric multi-detector CT angiography. *Abdom Imaging.* 2009;34(3):345–357.

38 Acosta S, Björck M. Modern treatment of acute mesenteric ischaemia. *Br J Surg.* 2014;101(1): e100–e108.

39 Storm-Dickerson TL, Horattas MC. What have we learned over the past 20 years about appendicitis in the elderly? *Am J Surg.* 2003;185(3):198–201.

40 Sheu B-F, Chiu T-F, Chen J-C, Tung M-S, Chang M-W, Young Y-R. Risk factors associated with perforated appendicitis in elderly patients presenting with signs and symptoms of acute appendicitis. *ANZ J Surg.* 2007;77(8):662–666.

41 Farrell RJ, Farrell JJ, Morrin MM. Diverticular disease in the elderly. *Gastroenterol Clin North Am.* 2001;30(2):475–496.

42 Issa N, Dreznik Z, Dueck DS, Arish A, Ram E, Kraus M, et al. Emergency surgery for complicated acute diverticulitis. *Colorectal Dis.* 2009;11(2):198–202.

43 Laurell H, Hansson LE, Gunnarsson U. Why do surgeons miss malignancies in patients with acute abdominal pain? *Anticancer Res.* 2006;26(5B):3675–3678.

44 Sanson TG, O'Keefe KP. Evaluation of abdominal pain in the elderly. *Emerg Med Clin North Am.* 1996;14(3):615–627.

CHAPTER 16

Diabetic and environmental emergencies

Part 1: Diabetic emergencies

Introduction

Ageing is associated with decreased glucose tolerance, due to insulin resistance and decreasing pancreatic beta-cell function. Impaired glucose tolerance may manifest itself as type 2 diabetes mellitus or raised blood glucose in the presence of physiological distress such as infection or infarction. The prevalence of type 2 diabetes mellitus peaks in persons aged between 65 and 74 years, and approximately 20% of people aged over 65 years are affected (1, 2). Up to 40% of patients with type 2 diabetes are undiagnosed. Type 1 diabetes is most commonly a disease of the young but can present at any age, and increasing numbers of type 1 diabetics are surviving into old age with the associated challenges. This section addresses type 2 diabetes in older patients only.

In addition to diabetic emergencies such as hypoglycaemia, hyperglycaemic hyperosmolar syndrome (HHS) and diabetic ketoacidosis (DKA), older adults with diabetes have an increased risk of other serious acute conditions. Accelerated atherosclerosis increases the risk of myocardial infarction, cerebrovascular disease and peripheral vascular disease. Risk of infection and systemic sepsis is higher. Frailty and functional decline is more common, and diabetics are at increased risk of falling and sustaining hip fractures. Presenting symptoms and signs are even more likely to be atypical in older diabetic patients.

Box 16.1 History taking in older adults with diabetes.

Duration and type of diabetes

Associated complications (e.g. vascular, neuropathy and retinopathy)

Previous diabetic emergencies

Treatment regimen and ability to manage this independently

If on insulin, establish whether the patient is insulin dependent (insulin required to prevent ketosis) or on insulin for improved glycaemic control

Usual blood glucose measurements, frequency of hypoglycaemic episodes, the presence or absence of hypoglycaemic symptoms and whether these necessitated external help

---

Geriatric Emergencies, First Edition.
Iona Murdoch, Sarah Turpin, Bree Johnston, Alasdair MacLullich and Eve Losman.
© 2015 John Wiley & Sons, Ltd. Published 2015 by John Wiley & Sons, Ltd.

Older diabetic patients are at increased risk of in hospital mortality and prolonged length of stay (3), whether their presenting complaint is directly related to their diabetes or not. An adequate diabetic history is important to ensure that patients receive appropriate treatment and monitoring during their admission (Box 16.1). Diabetic medication may need adjustment. Deranged glycaemic control may result from acute illness, reduced adherence to treatment secondary to dementia or delirium, change in diabetic regimen, diet, alcohol or drugs such as steroids and beta-blockers. Sulphonylureas or long-acting insulin may cause persistent hypoglycaemia, particularly in the presence of acute kidney injury or sepsis. Metformin may cause lactic acidosis and should usually be withheld in acute illness. There is some evidence that hyperglycaemia *may* be associated with poor outcome in acute stroke, acute MI and sepsis but tight glycaemic control with an insulin sliding scale may expose the patient to an unnecessary risk of serious hypoglycaemia.

Hypoglycaemia

Incidence of hypoglycaemia rises with age and duration of diabetes (4). Around 20% of hospital inpatients with diabetes will experience a blood glucose <4 mmol/L during their admission, increasing mortality and length of stay (5). Reduced glucagon secretion, poor nutritional intake and effects of comorbidities such as renal failure or concurrent infection increase the likelihood of hypoglycaemia. Frail older persons, on sulphonylureas or insulin, with polypharmacy and frequent hospitalisations are at a highest risk for drug-associated hypoglycaemia (6). Other contributory causes, which may result in hypoglycaemia in the non-diabetic, include alcohol, liver failure, sepsis or adrenal insufficiency.

Presentation of hypoglycaemia includes *autonomic features* such as sweating, tachycardia, pallor; *neuroglycopaenic symptoms* such as irritability, agitation, confusion or seizures and *general symptoms* such as headache and nausea. Hypoglycaemia may mimic or precipitate acute stroke or myocardial infarction. Recognition of hypoglycaemia may be delayed due to reduced autonomic response in older adults, impaired awareness of hypoglycaemia with duration of diabetes and pre-existing cognitive impairment. Hypoglycaemia is more likely to be severe in the older patient; often requiring treatment from a second person (5). Older adults who have chronic poor glycaemic control may experience symptoms of hypoglycaemia with a blood glucose above 4.0 mmol/L.

KEY POINT: **Always check blood glucose in any older person presenting with falls, altered mental state or collapse.**

A blood glucose <4 mmol/L should be treated immediately, as summarised in Figure 16.1. Patients who are very drowsy, agitated or having seizures will require rapid administration of intravenous glucose. If possible a laboratory blood glucose measurement should be taken to confirm hypoglycaemia, especially if an alternative endocrine cause is considered.

Glucagon mobilises glycogen from the liver and will be less effective in older patients with chronically malnourishment, alcohol dependence or those taking sulphonylureas.

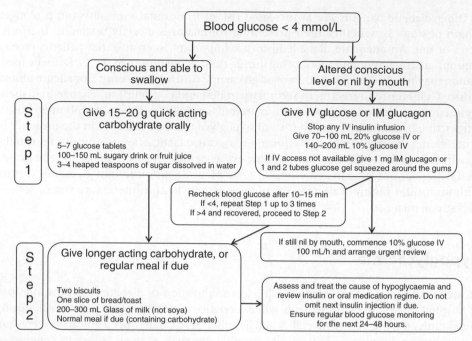

Figure 16.1 Management of hypoglycaemia (5).

Once the episode of hypoglycaemia has been adequately treated, the underlying cause should be considered and the patient's diabetic regime reviewed. A less stringent long-term glycaemic target may be appropriate in the older population, reducing the potential for hypoglycaemia. If the hypoglycaemia was due to sulfonylurea or long-acting insulin therapy, then the risk of hypoglycaemia may persist for up to 24–36 hours following the last dose, especially if there is concurrent renal impairment, and admission for monitoring is necessary.

 KEY POINT: Avoid 50% glucose IV in the older patient where peripheral veins are more vulnerable to extravasation injury. Rebound hyperglycaemia is less common with smaller doses of 10–20% glucose (5).

If the cause for hypoglycaemia has been fully corrected, the patient may be discharged after a period of observation. Ensure that the patient or carer monitors their blood glucose closely over the following 24–48 hours, understands the management of hypoglycaemia and arrange follow up with the primary care physician or diabetes specialist nurse.

Hyperglycaemic hyperosmolar syndrome

Hyperglycaemic emergencies include DKA and HHS. HHS may be the first presentation of type 2 diabetes and is more common in the older patient. Delayed presentation may occur due to reduced thirst sensation, cognitive impairment and reduced access to and intake of fluids, particularly in patients with reduced mobility.

HHS is characterised by increased osmolality, severe hyperglycaemia, dehydration, mild acidosis and absent or minimal ketosis (2). Mortality is higher in HHS than in DKA, due to comorbid illnesses precipitating or resulting from HHS such as infection or organ failure (7). Dehydration places patients at risk of thrombotic complications such as myocardial infarction, stroke or peripheral arterial thrombosis. Age is an independent predictor of mortality (8).

In contrast to DKA, which develops over hours, patients with HHS become progressively dehydrated over a period of days, amounting to fluid deficits of several litres. As a result, electrolyte disturbances may be more severe and require careful and slow correction to avoid cerebral oedema, osmotic demyelination syndrome or seizures.

Diagnosis

Transient hyperglycaemia occurs commonly in the diabetic patient, but diagnosis of HHS requires sustained hyperglycaemia with associated dehydration (Box 16.2).

Box 16.2 Diagnostic criteria in HHS (9).

- Marked hyperglycaemia (blood glucose 30 mmol/L or more) without significant hyperketon-aemia (ketones <3 mmol/L) or acidosis (pH > 7.3, bicarbonate >15 mmol/L)
- Osmolality over 320 mosmol/kg (measured or calculated as $2Na^+$ + urea + glucose)
- Hypovolaemia

Management

Management of HHS is centred on four principles as in Box 16.3.

Box 16.3 Treatment priorities in HHS.

1 Treat the underlying cause e.g. broad-spectrum antibiotics for suspected sepsis
2 Replace fluid and electrolyte losses cautiously
3 Normalise blood glucose
4 Prevent complications such as arterial or venous thrombosis and cerebral oedema

---

Local guidelines should be consulted and expert advice from the diabetic team sought. Total fluid losses in HHS are typically between 100 and 220 mL/kg (10). Rehydration with isotonic fluid usually results in a fall in blood glucose without a requirement for insulin. The aim should be to replace approximately 50% of estimated fluid loss within the first 12 hours and the remainder in the following 12 hours, although caution must be exercised in patients with heart failure. Monitor fluid balance and urine output carefully. Low dose (0.05 units/kg/h) insulin infusion should only be commenced if blood glucose fails to fall despite IV fluids or there is significant ketosis (9). Measure glucose, electrolytes and osmolality regularly to ensure rate of correction is gradual. Reduction in blood glucose should not exceed 5 mmol/h and sodium

10 mmol/24 hours. Total body potassium is usually low, and potassium replacement may be required, but be wary of coexistent acute kidney injury with the potential for hyperkalaemia. Prophylactic anticoagulation e.g. low-molecular-weight heparin should be given in the absence of other contraindications.

Part 2: Temperature homeostasis

Introduction

Older people are less able to control body temperature due to changes in skin and muscle mass, altered autonomic nervous system function and behavioural and cognitive factors (Figure 16.2). They are particularly sensitive to extremes of environmental temperature. In temperate climates, hypothermia is a more common occurrence but a spectrum of heat illnesses, from heat stress to heat stroke, may occur with exposure to high environmental temperatures.

Cold exposure due to poverty, climate, inadequate clothing or heating systems.

Lack of fans or air conditioning in hot conditions.

Reduced heat production from lower metabolic rate.

Less subcutaneous fat and muscle mass resulting in reduced insulation. Reduced shivering due to lower muscle mass.

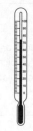

Figure 16.2 Factors leading to altered thermoregulation in the older adult.

Alcohol, sedative drugs and cognitive impairment alter temperature perception, thirst and reduce shivering.

Poor mobility or falls risk may lead to prolonged exposure to cold or hot conditions.

Reduced number and function of sweat glands limiting ability to reduce core temperature

Reduced autonomic nervous system activity resulting in reduced shivering, sweating and vasoconstriction or vasodilatation.

Antihypertensives and other medication may limit vasoactive responses to temperature.

Infection may precipitate or complicate hypothermia or hyperthermia.

Hypothermia

Hypothermia may follow a fall or a period of immobility in a cold environment.

Definition

Hypothermia is defined as an involuntary drop in core body temperature to <35°C. It can be categorised into mild (<35°C), moderate (<32°C) and severe (<30°C). Hypothermia may be due to inadequate heat conservation due to excessive cold, termed *primary hypothermia*, or due to another disease process such as sepsis, hypothyroidism or adrenal insufficiency, termed *secondary hypothermia*.

Background

The initial response of the body when exposed to cold is to maintain a normal core temperature by means of active movement and involuntary shivering, in addition to seeking external heat sources and applying clothing. Figure 16.2 illustrates the factors that may compromise the ability of an older person to respond appropriately to cold.

> KEY POINT: In moderate to severe hypothermia, oral or tympanic temperature management may be inaccurate and underestimate severity. Core temperature should be measured using a low-reading rectal thermometer, oesophageal or bladder probe.

Initial assessment

Assess airway, breathing and circulation and attach monitoring and high flow oxygen.

Airway and breathing

Hypothermia may lead to reduced conscious level and respiratory depression, requiring airway interventions and ventilatory support.

Circulation

Hypothermia eventually results in myocardial suppression, bradycardia and hypotension. Atrial fibrillation (AF) with a reduced ventricular rate is a common presenting arrhythmia. Ventricular fibrillation (VF) and asystolic cardiac arrest may occur. Continuous cardiac monitoring is required.

Disability

Neurological signs such as confusion, ataxia, seizures, focal neurological deficits and speech disturbances may be present.

Hypothermia leads to impaired coagulation, increased risk of pancreatitis, renal failure and eventual multi-organ failure. Critical care admission may be required.

History and examination

If available, a history of exposure to cold and other precipitating factors should be established. In moderate to severe hypothermia, conscious level is usually depressed and a collateral history is essential.

Examine for contributing or consequential medical conditions such as pneumonia or other infections and assess for any injuries that may have occurred as a result of falls or immobility.

> KEY POINT: Hypothermia is a marker of poor prognosis in sepsis.

Investigations
Blood tests
Routine bloods plus creatine kinase, thyroid function tests, blood glucose, amylase and lipase, and venous or arterial blood gases should be taken. Blood and urine cultures should be taken if sepsis is suspected.

ECG
An ECG may demonstrate the classical changes of hypothermia, including prolonged PR interval, J waves or AF.

Management
Management of hypothermia depends on the severity and level of respiratory and cardiac depression, as well as the likely aetiology.

Consider broad-spectrum antibiotics to cover for infection and treat any precipitating cause.

If there are no immediately life-threatening complications, re-warming should occur gradually, at 0.5–1°C per hour. Rapid re-warming may lead to hypotension, cerebral and pulmonary oedema or trigger arrhythmias. Re-warming may also cause an *afterdrop*: a further drop in core temperature due to cool blood returning from the peripheries.

Passive re-warming
In a patient with mild hyperthermia, stable circulation and who is shivering, dry clothes and warm blankets reduce conductive losses and allow re-warming.

Active external re-warming
Hot air blankets reduce conductive heat losses and provide a heat source and are indicated for mild to moderate hypothermia.

Active internal re-warming
Simple internal re-warming includes warm IV fluids (at 43°C), and warm, humidified oxygen. In severe hypothermia, invasive warming methods such as bladder, peritoneal or pleural cavity irrigation with warm fluid may be required. Extracorporeal membrane oxygenation (ECMO) or cardiopulmonary bypass should be considered for patients with hypothermia and cardiac instability or cardiac arrest who do not respond to the above-mentioned methods, but resources for this may not be available.

> KEY POINT: Moving or transferring a severely hypothermic patient or performing procedures may trigger arrhythmias, particularly VF.

Cardiac arrest
As core temperature decreases, sinus bradycardia may lead to AF, VF and asystole. Bradycardia and AF tend to spontaneously improve with rising temperature without the need for cardiac pacing or other treatments. In the event of cardiac arrest, commence

CPR and advanced life support. A few adjustments to the life support algorithm should be adopted as shown in Box 16.4 (11).

Box 16.4 Adjustments to advanced life support in severe hypothermia.

- Look for signs of life and at the ECG trace for up to 1 min before determining that there is no cardiac output and starting CPR.
- Do not give adrenaline or other cardiac arrest drugs until the core temperature is over 30°C. Double the time interval between drug doses until the temperature reaches 35°C, when the normal ALS protocol can resume.
- In the case of a shockable rhythm (VF or VT), a maximum of three shocks can be given if the temperature remains below 30°C: further attempts should be delayed until the temperature rises above this threshold.

Hyperthermia and heat illness

Hyperthermia occurs when the body gains heat energy quicker than it is able to cool. Hyperthermia may be caused by heat from the environment or due to endogenous heat production (Box 16.5). People aged over 60 years are the worst affected by extreme heat, with those living in institutions, confined to bed or living alone having the highest rates of morbidity and mortality (12, 13).

Box 16.5 Differential diagnosis of hyperthermia.

Environmental hyperthermia
Sepsis
Central nervous system infection
Drug toxicity or withdrawal
Serotonin syndrome
Neuroleptic malignant syndrome
Malignant hyperthermia
Endocrine disorders e.g. thyroid storm or phaeochromocytoma

A history of exposure to heat, for example after a collapse in direct sunlight during the summer months or very high environmental temperatures during a heat wave, will usually help to distinguish exogenous from endogenous causes of hyperthermia. In the older patient, there is more likely to be an underlying trigger for the initial exposure, such as sepsis or medication side effects. Risk factors for heat illness in the older adult include lack of acclimatisation, dehydration, obesity, alcohol and cardiovascular disease. Drugs such as antihypertensives, beta-blockers and calcium channel blockers, diuretics, anticholinergics and antipsychotics may cause dehydration or lead to an inability to compensate for heat-related vasodilatation.

Hyperthermia can be classified according to a spectrum of severity, from minor heat stress, to heat exhaustion and then heat stroke with multi-organ failure (Box 16.6).

Box 16.6 Classification of heat illness (14, 15).

Heat stress: Muscle cramps, tachycardia and malaise due to elevated core temperature (37–39°C). Sweating, thirst and vasodilatation are preserved, with normal mental status.

Heat exhaustion: Sodium and water loss leads to syncope, weakness, vomiting, dizziness and headache. The patient complains of feeling hot and appears flushed and sweaty with a core temperature <40°C. Mild confusion and irritability may occur, but CNS function is otherwise intact. Heat exhaustion may progress to heat stroke.

Heat stroke: Non-exertional heat stroke is a systemic inflammatory response with loss of all thermoregulatory control. Core temperature rises to above 40.6°C accompanied by mental state change. The skin is hot and dry with the absence of sweating. Multi-organ failure may include rhabdomyolysis and acute kidney injury, respiratory failure and acute respiratory distress syndrome (ARDS), seizures and coma, arrhythmias and hypotension, coagulopathy and liver failure. Mortality is high. Exertional heat stroke occurs in association with exercise.

Management

Management of heat illness will depend on severity.

In the case of heat stress, remove clothing, provide cool oral rehydration solution, spray or sponge tepid water onto the skin and apply a bedside fan.

In heat exhaustion or heat stroke, assess airway, breathing and circulation. Obtain experienced help. Undress the patient, apply ice packs over the axillae, groins and neck and give cool intravenous fluid. Check venous or arterial blood gases, electrolytes, renal and liver function and creatine kinase. In the presence of neurological signs and symptoms, cool rapidly to 39°C and then stop active cooling to avoid hypothermia (11). Large volumes of IV fluid may be required but may cause pulmonary or cerebral oedema, especially in the older patient. Monitor ECG, blood pressure, electrolytes and acid–base, blood glucose and conscious level in a high dependency environment.

Take home messages

- Diabetes is very common in the older adult and is an important risk factor for most other geriatric emergencies. Diabetes is often undiagnosed and may present in the context of an acute hospital admission. Deranged glycaemic control may be the first indication of an infection or other acute illness
- Symptoms of hypoglycaemia in the older patient may be atypical and blood glucose should be checked in all cases of acute illness. Remember that 'Four is the floor': treat blood glucose <4 mmol/L. Give 10% or 20% dextrose rather than 50% dextrose.
- HHS develops more gradually than DKA and is associated with significant dehydration and electrolyte disturbances. Complications include infection and thrombosis. Rehydration with intravenous fluid should occur before use of insulin is considered

- Older patients are prone to disorders of thermoregulation due to extreme environmental conditions, medical conditions or medication
- In general, normalising temperature should be done rapidly if there are features of altered mental status or cardiovascular instability, but more slowly if there are no life-threatening sequelae, due to the risks of precipitating hypotension, pulmonary or cerebral oedema or arrhythmias.

References

1 Morley JE. Diabetes and aging: epidemiologic overview. *Clin Geriatr Med*. 2008;24(3):395–405.

2 Lee A. Management of elderly diabetic patients in the subacute care setting. *Clin Geriatr Med*. 2000; 16(4):833–852.

3 NHS Information Centre, National Diabetes Inpatient Audit 2012. Health and Social Care Information Centre. http://www.hscic.gov.uk/catalogue/PUB10506.

4 Leese GP, Wang J, Broomhall J, Kelly P, Marsden A, Morrison W, et al. Frequency of severe hypo-glycemia requiring emergency treatment in type 1 and type 2 diabetes: a population-based study of health service resource use. *Diabetes Care*. 2003;26(4):1176–1780.

5 Joint British Diabetes Societies Inpatient Care Group. The Hospital Management of Hypoglycaemia in Adults with Diabetes Mellitus. Joint British Diabetes Society Guideline. 2010. www.diabetes.org.uk /About_us/what-we-say/Improving-diabetes-healthcare/The-hospital-management-of -hypoglycaemia-in-adults-with-Diabetes-Mellitus/ (accessed online 6 Jun 2014).

6 Shorr RI. Incidence and risk factors for serious hypoglycemia in older persons using insulin or sul-fonylureas. *Arch Intern Med* 1997;157(15):1681.

7 Nugent BW. Hyperosmolar hyperglycemic state. *Emerg Med Clin North Am*. 2005;23(3):629–648.

8 MacIsaac RJ, Lee LY, McNeil KJ, Tsalamandris C, Jerums G. Influence of age on the presentation and outcome of acidotic and hyperosmolar diabetic emergencies. *Intern Med J*. 2002;32(8):379–385.

9 The management of the hyperosmolar hyperglycaemic state (HHS) in adults with diabetes. Joint British Diabetes Societies Guideline. 2012.

10 Kitabchi AE, Umpierrez GE, Miles JM, Fisher JN. Hyperglycemic crises in adult patients with diabetes. *Diabetes Care*. 2009;32(7):1335–1343.

11 Cardiac Arrest in Special Circumstances, Chapter 12 Advanced Life Support, Resuscitation Council (UK). 2010.

12 Kenny GP, Yardley J, Brown C, Sigal RJ, Jay O. Heat stress in older individuals and patients with common chronic diseases. *CMAJ*. 2010;182(10):1053–1060.

13 Bouchama A, Knochel JP. Heat stroke. *N Engl J Med*. 2002;346(25):1978–1988.

14 Heat Stress in the Elderly. Centers for Disease Control and Prevention. http://www.bt.cdc.gov/ disasters/extremeheat/elderlyheat.asp [cited 2014 May 15].

15 Wilson L, Black D, Veitch C. Heatwaves and the elderly – the role of the GP in reducing morbidity. *Aust Fam Physician*. 2011;40(8):637–640.

CHAPTER 17

Acute kidney injury and metabolic emergencies

Although specific management of metabolic disturbances and acute kidney injury in the older adult does not differ hugely from the younger patient, these conditions are increasingly common, and often co-exist with other acute and chronic illnesses, complicating management. Metabolic disturbances may present with non-specific symptoms and signs and can be easily missed if blood tests are not undertaken. The workup and treatment of all metabolic disturbances in older patients should be modified according to the patient's other comorbidities, prognosis and goals of care.

Acute kidney injury

Acute kidney injury (AKI) commonly complicates acute illness in older adults, occurring in 15% of adult hospital admissions. Patients over the age of 70 have a 3.5-fold increase in AKI (1), with advancing age an independent risk factor. AKI is associated with significant morbidity and mortality, with impaired recovery of renal function in older adults (2). As AKI is a biochemical diagnosis, often with no symptoms and signs, a high degree of vigilance is required.

Decrease in the number of functional nephrons.

Reduced tubular conservation of sodium and water during periods of dehydration, increasing the risk of volume depletion.

Decreased capacity for the excretion of drugs and drug metabolites.

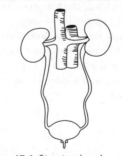

Figure 17.1 Structural and functional changes in the aging kidney reducing renal reserve (3).

Autoregulation of renal blood flow is less effective leading to lack of glomerular filtration rate preservation in dehydration states.

Ageing of systemic vessels results in decreased renal blood flow and a rise in renal vascular resistance. There is a variable reduction in glomerular filtration rate with age.

Geriatric Emergencies, First Edition.
Iona Murdoch, Sarah Turpin, Bree Johnston, Alasdair MacLullich and Eve Losman.
© 2015 John Wiley & Sons, Ltd. Published 2015 by John Wiley & Sons, Ltd.

Definition

AKI is typically identified by an increase in serum creatinine levels or a reduction in urine output. A number of different criteria for diagnosis and staging of AKI are in use such as the RIFLE, AKIN or KDIGO definitions (4–6). Box 17.1 outlines the criteria suggested by the National Institute for Health and Care Excellence (NICE) (and based on the above definitions) for the detection of AKI.

Box 17.1 Standard criteria for the detection of acute kidney injury in adults (7).

- A rise in serum creatinine of 26 mmol/L (0.3 mg/dL) or greater within 48 h *or*
- 50% or greater rise in serum creatinine within the past 7 days *or*
- A fall in urine output to <0.5 mL/kg/h for more than 6 h

These criteria have limitations in the older patient. In many cases, previous blood results may not be available for comparison, and decreased muscle mass with ageing

Table 17.1 History and examination in pre-renal, renal and post-renal causes of acute kidney injury (1).

	Causes	History	Examination
Pre-renal *Decreased renal perfusion*	Fluid loss or redistribution	Vomiting, diarrhoea, haemorrhage, diuretics, osmotic diuresis due to hyperglycaemia and sepsis	Signs of volume depletion
	Decreased cardiac output	Heart failure, arrhythmias and valve disease	Evidence of cardiac failure
	Impaired renal autoregulation	Medications: non-steroidal anti-inflammatories, angiotensin-converting enzyme inhibitors and angiotensin receptor blockers	
Renal *Intrinsic renal damage*	Acute tubular necrosis	Sepsis, prolonged volume depletion, recent administration of radio-contrast material, chemotherapy and rhabdomyolysis	Signs of sepsis or source of infection
	Vascular	Recent angiography causing cholesterol embolisation	
	Glomerulonephritis	Possible history of autoimmune disease or vasculitis	
	Acute interstitial nephritis	Infection, new medication e.g. antibiotics or non-steroidal anti-inflammatories	
Post-renal *Obstructive*	Upper urinary tract	Renal and ureteric stones, pelvic malignancy and retroperitoneal disease	Renal angle tenderness and pelvic masses
	Lower urinary tract	Prostatic cancer or hypertrophy, prolonged urinary retention, bladder stones and urethral strictures	Acute urinary retention, enlarged prostate on rectal examination

may lead to seemingly reassuring creatinine levels. Fifty percentage of renal function may be lost before serum creatinine rises, delaying recognition of AKI (8).

Background
Structural and functional changes occur in the ageing kidney, in part due to hypertension and other comorbidities as well as the ageing process itself (Figure 17.1). These changes increase susceptibility to AKI due to the combination of a precipitating illness with comorbid conditions, nephrotoxic medications, contrast agents and urinary obstruction due to prostatic enlargement.

Initial assessment
Assess airway, breathing and circulation. Record vital signs and examine to determine the patient's volume status – fluid resuscitation may be required immediately. Exclude life-threatening complications of AKI as illustrated in Box 17.2 and involve critical care early if necessary.

History and examination
AKI can be classified according to its cause: pre-renal (33% of cases in older adults), renal (58% of cases) or post-renal (9% of cases) (9). Table 17.1 highlights these causes and points to note on history and examination.

The history should establish any risk factors for AKI, such as recent medication change, recent illness with associated dehydration, reduced fluid intake (e.g. due to delirium), radiological imaging, surgical procedures and other comorbidities such as hypertension and diabetes. Older patients are often unaware that they have chronic kidney disease, even if this has been identified previously.

Investigations
Blood tests
Urgent *urea, creatinine and electrolytes* as well as a *venous or arterial blood gas* will indicate the severity of acute kidney injury and demonstrate any serious complications such as metabolic acidosis or hyperkalaemia (Box 17.2).

Other investigations will depend on the likely cause.

Bedside bladder scanning
This can be performed rapidly at the bedside to exclude urinary retention.

Urinary tract ultrasound
Urinary tract ultrasound should be considered in patients with a possible obstructive cause and may demonstrate hydronephrosis or ureteric dilatation. Small kidneys on ultrasound may indicate pre-existing chronic kidney disease, although reduced renal mass may be due to ageing alone.

Urinalysis
Urine dipstick may reveal blood or protein suggestive of a renal cause. Urine should be sent for microscopy to look for casts suggestive of acute tubular necrosis or glomerulonephritis. White blood cells in the urine may suggest interstitial nephritis

Table 17.2 Treatment of AKI depending on cause.

Cause	Treatment strategy
Pre-renal	Volume repletion with intravenous crystalloid Stop diuretics and antihypertensive medication Optimise cardiac output and oxygenation
Renal	Stop nephrotoxic medication Avoid or delay radiographic contrast use Consider specific treatment e.g. steroids for glomerulonephritis
Post-renal	Catheterisation Nephrostomy or ureteric stenting if higher obstruction is present

in the absence of other signs of infection. Renal biopsy may be indicated to confirm diagnosis.

Urinary electrolytes

Urinary electrolytes may help in identifying pre-renal causes of AKI, where renal tubules retain sodium and water, resulting in low urinary sodium and osmolality. This may be less useful in the older patient due to reduced sodium-conservation ability and diuretic use.

Management

General management of AKI should involve careful monitoring of vital signs, fluid balance and treatment of the underlying cause. Blood pressure and oxygenation should be optimised. Careful medication review is required to stop or suspend nephrotoxic drugs or drugs causing dehydration. Doses of several other drugs need to be adjusted in AKI, or alternative drugs with no or fewer renally excreted metabolites selected: consult a pharmacist or other specialist.

Repeated creatinine and electrolytes are necessary to assess progress and detect complications. In more serious cases, catheterisation with careful monitoring of urine output, high dependency care and/or invasive monitoring may be required.

Specific management of AKI will depend on the likely aetiology, as given in Table 17.2.

> **KEY POINT:** In older patients with mild AKI with a clear cause, no urinary retention on bladder scanning, and in whom there are signs of improvement with treatment, avoid catherisation if possible to reduce the risk of introducing infection.

Complications

> **KEY POINT:** Where AKI progresses despite initial treatment, seek specialist help.

Box 17.2 Common acute complications of AKI.

- Pulmonary oedema and fluid overload due to oliguria
- Hyperkalaemia
- Uraemia
- Metabolic acidosis
- Hypocalcaemia
- Toxicity from accumulation of renally excreted drugs or drug metabolites (e.g. morphine-6-glucuronide)

Hyperkalaemia will require cardiac monitoring, intravenous calcium administration and insulin–dextrose infusion. Sodium bicarbonate may be administered in the case of severe metabolic acidosis with cardiac compromise. Signs and symptoms of uraemia include weakness, vomiting, altered mental status, seizures and pericarditis. Urgent renal replacement therapy (RRT) such as haemodialysis or haemofiltration may be required if these complications are refractory to initial treatment. The decision to undertake RRT may be difficult. For older patients with advanced frailty, reduced cardiovascular reserve, increased bleeding risk or competing comorbidities, acute RRT may be a burdensome treatment with a poor chance of recovery. Studies to date have not identified age alone as a risk factor for hospital mortality (10); however, an individualised approach should be taken to decision making. See Chapter 3 for further discussion on critical care in the older patient.

Prevention of acute kidney injury

The risk of AKI is high in all hospitalised older patients and should be at the forefront of the mind of all clinicians working in acute care. Maintaining hydration, adequate blood pressure, oxygenation and stopping or reducing nephrotoxic drugs in high risk patients can all help to reduce the risk of AKI.

Early recognition and vigorous management is critical to prevent progression to more serious AKI associated with reduced chance of renal recovery and increased mortality. AKI can develop over a short time period, for example 2–3 days, without any symptoms or changes in vital signs. A high degree of vigilance is required.

Older adults in the community should be advised to stop taking potentially nephro-toxic drugs such as angiotensin-converting enzyme inhibitors (or seek urgent advice with respect to this) in the event of acute illness or gastrointestinal disturbance. Older patients should be warned of the risks of over-the-counter non-steroidal anti-inflammatories. Rehydration with intravenous fluid where possible should occur before administration of contrast agents in unwell hospitalised patients.

Hyponatraemia

Hyponatraemia, defined as a blood sodium level of <135mmol/L, is the most common electrolyte abnormality in the older patient. The cause may be immediately obvious or complex and multi-factorial. Older patients have a decreased ability to maintain fluid and electrolyte balance in acute illness. The commonest causes of hyponatraemia are loss of sodium and water from the gastrointestinal system and diuretic therapy, constituting

65% of cases presenting to the Emergency Department (11). Severe hyponatraemia in geriatric patients has significant morbidity and mortality, and expert advice should be sought regarding specific management.

Definition
Mild hyponatraemia (130–134 mmol/L)
Mild hyponatraemia may be asymptomatic or may cause anorexia, cramps, nausea, vomiting and headache.

Moderate hyponatraemia (125–129 mmol/L)
Moderate hyponatraemia may cause disorientation, delirium, weakness and lethargy. More severe symptoms usually occur when the drop in sodium is acute.

Severe hyponatraemia (<125 mmol/L)
The symptoms of severe hyponatraemia may be similar to those of moderate hyponatraemia. When a severe drop in sodium occurs acutely, seizures, coma and respiratory arrest may occur.

Background
For links to further resources in understanding osmolality and sodium homeostasis, please see the end of the chapter.

Sodium is a key contributor to *plasma tonicity (or effective osmolality)* and a low sodium will result in hypotonicity (hypotonic hyponatraemia). Exceptions to this occur in hyperglycaemia, or following infusion of osmotic diuretics such as mannitol. Hyperlipidaemia or hyperparaproteinaemia may result in a pseudohyponatraemia.

Most simply, two key features to determine the cause of hypotonic hyponatraemia are *volume status* and *urinary sodium* levels.

CAUTION: Hyponatraemia may be multi-factorial. Assessing volume status in the older patient may be difficult in the presence of other comorbidities. Interpretation of urinary electrolytes and osmolality may be less reliable in older patients. Figure 17.2 is intended as an aid to understanding, but expert advice should be sought in more difficult cases.

In hypovolaemic hyponatraemia, there is evidence of volume depletion (Box 17.3). Sodium loss may be renal, resulting in raised urinary sodium, or extra renal such as from the GI tract. Hypervolaemic hyponatraemia is caused by water (and sodium) retention in conditions such as congestive cardiac failure, nephrotic syndrome and liver cirrhosis. Acute or chronic renal failure may cause hypervolaemic hyponatraemia with urinary sodium loss.

In euvolaemic hyponatraemia, there is no evidence of volume overload or depletion. In primary polydipsia or infusion of hypotonic fluids, urine sodium and osmolality will be low. A urine osmolality >100 mOsml/L, with a urinary sodium over 20 mmol/L (in patients not taking diuretics), indicates inappropriate conservation of water by the kidneys, leading to impaired urinary dilution. This is termed the syndrome of inappropriate antidiuresis (SIAD). Causes include pulmonary pathology, malignancy, central nervous system disorders, and drugs, including some anticonvulsants, antidepressants, and opioids. However, SIAD is greatly overdiagnosed in older patients and may lead to

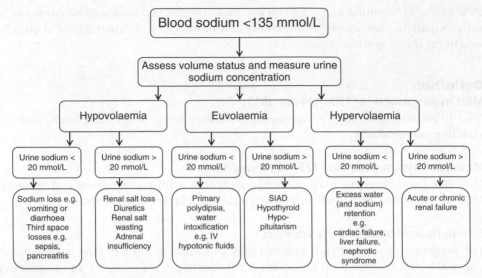

Figure 17.2 A summary of causes of hyponatraemia (12).

inappropriate fluid restriction and adverse outcomes. SIAD is a diagnosis of exclusion and certain criteria must be met including euvolaemia, low plasma osmolality <260 mOsml/L, urine osmolality >200 mOsml/L and urine sodium >20 mmol/L, and the absence of hypothyroidism, adrenal insufficiency, renal, hepatic or cardiac failure or diuretic use (13).

History and Examination

The signs and symptoms of hyponatraemia depend on both the serum sodium level and the rate of decline. Gradual changes in sodium levels will often be asymptomatic due to central nervous system compensation. It is important to try to establish whether the fall in sodium is acute (<24–48 hours) or chronic (>48 hours), by noting symptom onset or comparing old blood results. Rapid correction of chronic hyponatraemia may cause *osmotic demyelination syndrome*, which is associated with long-term neurodisability or death. History may help guide assessment of volume status and provide clues as to the cause of hyponatraemia: such as vomiting and diarrhoea, infusion of hypotonic intravenous fluids or use of diuretics.

Physical examination should assess for complications of hyponatraemia (such as delirium and altered conscious level) and causes, including an assessment of volume status as given in Box 17.3. The patient can be considered to be euvolaemic if there is no hypotension and no peripheral oedema. However, chronic extracellular fluid excess may make determining volume status more difficult in older adults.

Box 17.3 Assessing fluid status.

Hypervolaemia: peripheral oedema, distended neck veins, wheeze, bibasal crackles, third heart sound and weight gain

Hypovolaemia: dry mucus membranes, dry axillae, reduced skin turgor, postural hypotension, tachycardia and weight loss

Investigations

When a low sodium level is identified, the following tests may be useful (Table 17.3):

Table 17.3 Investigations in hyponatraemia.

Investigation	Comments
Blood glucose	A cause of hyponatraemia with raised plasma osmolality
Urea and creatinine	Acute and chronic kidney injury
Plasma and urine electrolytes and osmolality	Interpretation of urinary electrolytes and osmolality may be difficult in older patients due to impaired tubular sodium retention or diuretic use (Figure 17.1)
Thyroid function tests	Exclude hypothyroidism
Inflammatory markers, full blood count	Infection causing hypovolaemic hyponatraemia or SIAD
Bone profile, tumour markers	Malignancy causing SIAD
CXR	Pulmonary cause of SIAD
CT head scan	Intra-cerebral cause of SIAD

Management

The principles of managing hyponatraemia include

- Rapid correction of sodium in case of life-threatening or neurological emergency with hypertonic saline.
  CAUTION: obtain urgent senior and specialist advice in these circumstances
- Treating the underlying cause e.g. pneumonia causing SIAD, stopping diuretics or other responsible medication.
- Slow correction of sodium in minimally or asymptomatic patients with chronic hyponatraemia (maximum 10 mmol/24 hours); rapid correction in these cases can lead to osmotic demyelination syndrome.

Patients with hypovolaemic hyponatraemia should be fluid resuscitated with normal saline. Both in hyponatraemia and hypernatraemia, tools such as the Adrogue formula (14), may assist with the calculation of total body water excess or deficit that may guide the rate of fluid replacement and predict the change in sodium levels after a certain volume of saline solution.

Treatment of confirmed SIAD is initially fluid restriction, although this may be poorly tolerated and is often ineffective (13). Medication such as demeclocycline, which induces nephrogenic diabetes insipidus, or vasopressin receptor antagonists, which act by increasing free water excretion, may be indicated.

Hypervolaemic patients with cardiac failure, renal failure or nephrotic syndrome should be fluid restricted initially. Diuretic therapy or vasopressin receptor antagonists may be required.

In hyponatraemic patients, sodium levels should be regularly checked to ensure that the rate of correction is not too rapid.

Hypernatraemia

Hypernatraemia (serum sodium >145 mmol/L) is characterised by a deficit of total body water relative to total body sodium and resulting cellular dehydration. It is common in the frail older patient with immobility or cognitive impairment, with reduced water intake due to impaired thirst response or lack of access to water. It may also result from net water loss, such as in diarrhoea; vomiting; fever; osmotic diuresis due to hyperglycaemia; or diuretic therapy. Other rare causes include diabetes insipidus or iatrogenic sodium excess such as due to hypertonic saline or sodium bicarbonate.

The history may elucidate the most likely cause and give an idea as to the speed of onset. Symptoms of hypernatraemia include thirst, lethargy and weakness. Examination will reveal signs of hypovolaemia as illustrated in Box 17.3. Severe hypernatraemia (>160 mmol/L) is associated with coma, seizures or other neurological signs. Significant dehydration may result in complications such as venous thrombosis and intracerebral bleeding caused by stretching of vessels with reduction in brain size (3).

Blood tests may reveal additional evidence of dehydration such as raised urea and creatinine, high albumin, raised haemoglobin and haematocrit. Despite the high serum sodium, patients often have a total body sodium deficit in addition to the larger water deficit.

Management consists of addressing the underlying cause and correcting the hypernatraemia. The enteral route should be used for rehydration if possible, but intravenous fluid is usually required. Normal 0.9% saline should be given if the patient is initially hypovolaemic (3).

Once the patient is normovolaemic, hypotonic fluid such as 0.45% saline or 5% dextrose may be required; however, the sodium concentration should not be reduced faster than 1 mmol/h, as there is increased risk of cerebral oedema, particularly if the initial hypernatraemia was subacute or chronic.

Hypercalcaemia

Hypercalcaemia requiring emergency treatment in the older adult is usually due to malignancy, most commonly breast, prostate, lung cancers and myeloma. Hypercalcaemia in malignancy may result from direct bone invasion or secretion of parathyroid hormone-related protein (PTHrP) by a solid tumour. Other causes include primary hyperparathyroidism, medications such as thiazide diuretics or calcium carbonate/vitamin D supplements; immobility; hyperthyroidism and granulomatous disease such as sarcoidosis and tuberculosis. Reduced renal clearance of calcium and a rise in intestinal absorption of calcium with ageing increase the likelihood of symptomatic hypercalcaemia (3).

History and examination

The symptoms of hyperglycaemia can be remembered as 'stones, groans, bones and moans' indicating the frequency of renal stones, constipation, bone pain and delirium as presenting symptoms. There is usually a history of thirst and polyuria, and the patient will appear dehydrated.

Stones
Renal stones commonly develop in hypercalcaemia. Hypercalcaemia also causes a nephrogenic diabetes insipidus-like syndrome, impairing the ability of the kidney to concentrate urine. This causes a polyuria that can result in severe dehydration. AKI may result from both of these processes.

Groans
The patient may experience abdominal pain, nausea and vomiting due to constipation, pancreatitis or peptic ulcer disease.

Bones
Malignancy and hyperparathyroidism may cause bone pain.

Moans
Common symptoms include delirium, anxiety, depression or fatigue.

Symptoms and signs of malignancy or granulomatous disease should be sought. These may include weight loss, night sweats, cough, haemoptysis, masses, bony tenderness or lymphadenopathy.

Management
Mild
Calcium levels <3.0 mmol/L (<12 mg/dL) are often asymptomatic and usually do not require urgent treatment.

Moderate
Calcium levels >3.0 mmol/L (>12 mg/dL) may be symptomatic and usually require urgent treatment.

Severe
Calcium levels >3.5 mmol/L (>14 mg/dL) require urgent treatment.

If calcium levels have risen slowly, symptoms may be less marked. Patients with severe hypercalcaemia, or those who have changes in mental status, require urgent treatment and admission. The treatment priority in the ED is rehydration. Management is highlighted in Box 17.4.

Older adults with cardiac dysfunction may develop pulmonary oedema following large volume fluid resuscitation. Central venous pressure monitoring may be helpful. Loop diuretics may need to be given if signs of fluid overload develop but are no longer recommended as part of routine management of hypercalcaemia as they are not effective in reducing serum calcium levels (15). Specialist advice should be sought if it appears that second-line treatments, such as glucocorticoids, calcitonin or calcimimetics, may be required (16).

Box 17.4 Emergency management of hypercalcaemia (16).

- Severe hypercalcaemia may cause circulatory collapse due to dehydration, dysrhythmias and coma: assess airway, breathing and circulation before proceeding.
- Send blood for urea and electrolytes, calcium, albumin, phosphate and a PTH level. If PTH is elevated, this suggests primary hyperparathyroidism.
- Calculate corrected calcium levels.

    Corrected calcium (mmol/L) = total calcium + 0.02 × (40−albumin)

    Calcium levels should always be corrected for albumin as 40% of calcium is protein bound. Low serum albumin levels may give falsely low calcium levels, leading to false reassurance.
- Rehydrate with intravenous fluids; 4−6 L over the first 24 hours is usually required. Aim for a urine output of 100−150 mL/h.
- Once rehydrated give IV bisphosphonates e.g. pamidronate or alendronate. Monitor calcium levels daily; bisphosphates take 2−4 days to take effect.
- In severe, symptomatic hypercalcaemia, subcutaneous calcitonin may provide a small, temporary reduction in calcium levels over the first 48 hours before bisphosphonates take effect (17).
- Investigate for underlying malignancy.

Take home messages

- Renal ageing, coupled with medication and comorbidities, elevates the risk of AKI in older adults. AKI may occur both on initial presentation and arise during hospital admission. A high degree of vigilance is required, and AKI should always be treated vigorously. Where AKI progresses despite initial treatment, seek specialist help
- The management of AKI involves treating any precipitating causes and ensuring high-quality supportive care, including maintaining adequate blood pressure and oxygenation
- Electrolyte disturbances are associated with delirium, increased falls and fracture risk and higher morbidity and mortality. Acute disturbances present with more signs and symptoms than chronic changes, in which central nervous system compensation may occur
- Acute severe hyponatraemia associated with reduced conscious level or seizures requires urgent treatment with hypertonic saline to prevent worsening cerebral oedema. Overly rapid correction of chronic hyponatraemia, however, is associated with osmotic demyelination syndrome
- Always check the calcium in any older patient with delirium or other non-specific symptoms.

Recommended resources

http://www.learnphysiology.org An introductory tutorial on fluid compartments, sodium and osmolality

http://www.anaesthesiamcq.com/FluidBook/index.php An online textbook on fluid physiology

References

1 Abdel-Kader K, Palevsky PM. Acute kidney injury in the elderly. *Clin Geriatr Med*. 2009;25(3): 331–358.

2 Schmitt R, Coca S, Kanbay M, Tinetti ME, Cantley LG, Parikh CR. Recovery of kidney function after acute kidney injury in the elderly: a systematic review and meta-analysis. *Am J Kidney Dis*. 2008; 52(2):262–271.

3 AlZahrani A, Sinnert R, Gernsheimer J. Acute kidney injury, sodium disorders, and hypercalcemia in the aging kidney: diagnostic and therapeutic management strategies in emergency medicine. *Clin Geriatr Med*. 2013;29(1):275–319.

4 Kellum JA, Lameire N. Diagnosis, evaluation, and management of acute kidney injury: a KDIGO summary (part 1). *Crit Care*. 2013;17(1):204.

5 Ftouh S, Thomas M. Acute kidney injury: summary of NICE guidance. *BMJ*. 2013;347(aug28_2): f4930.

6 Ricci Z, Cruz D, Ronco C. The RIFLE criteria and mortality in acute kidney injury: a systematic review. *Kidney Int*. 2008;73(5):538–546.

7 Acute Kidney Injury. National Institute for Health and Care Excellence (NICE) clinical guideline 169. 2013.

8 Chronopoulos A, Rosner MH, Cruz DN, Ronco C. Acute kidney injury in elderly intensive care patients: a review. *Intensive Care Med*. 2010;36(9):1454–1464.

9 Cheung CM, Ponnusamy A, Anderton JG. Management of acute renal failure in the elderly patient: a clinician's guide. *Drugs Aging*. 2008;25(6):455–476.

10 Rosner MH. Acute kidney injury in the elderly. *Clin Geriatr Med*. 2013;29(3):565–578.

11 Lee C, Guo H, Chen J. Hyponatremia in the emergency department. *Am J Emerg Med*. 2000; (18):264–268.

12 Assadi F. Hyponatremia: a problem-solving approach to clinical cases. *J Nephrol*. 2012;25(4): 473–480.

13 Lehrich RW, Ortiz-Melo DI, Patel MB, Greenberg A. Role of vaptans in the management of hyponatremia. *Am J Kidney Dis*. 2013;62(2):364–376.

14 Adrogué HJ, Madias NE. Hypernatremia. *N Engl J Med*. 2000;342(20):1493–1499.

15 LeGrand SB, Leskuski D, Zama I. Narrative review: furosemide for hypercalcemia: an unproven yet common practice. *Ann Intern Med*. 2008;149(4):259–263.

16 Acute Hypercalcaemia: Emergency Endocrine Guidance. Society for Endocrinology (UK). 2013.

17 Wisneski LA. Salmon calcitonin in the acute management of hypercalcemia. *Calcif Tissue Int*. 1990;46 (Suppl):S26–S30.

CHAPTER 18

Delirium

Introduction

Delirium affects at least 10% of older patients in the ED and up to 30% of older medical inpatients. As well as being very common, it is associated with multiple adverse outcomes. Delirium is greatly under detected in the ED and in acute wards (1, 2), and care is often suboptimal.

This chapter focuses on the assessment and management of acute delirium in older patients, both on initial presentation to the ED and on the ward. Other causes of behavioural disturbance in the older patient will be considered in the section titled Differential Diagnosis'. This chapter also aims to provide general guidance on the use of legislation to safely manage delirious patients who lack capacity regarding their healthcare decisions, although exact laws vary depending on location.

Definition

Box 18.1 Clinical features of delirium.

Disturbance in attention, level of arousal and other aspects of mental status.

Acute onset and fluctuating course.

Psychosis (hallucinations and delusions) occurs in 30–50%.

There may or may not be clear precipitants on review of the history, physical and laboratory findings.

KEY POINT: Delirium is distinct from dementia, although they often co-exist.

Delirium can be hyperactive, hypoactive or mixed and can present very differently in individual patients (Figure 18.1).

Background

Delirium in older patients is linked with poor outcomes. Delirious patients are twice as likely to die, have longer hospital admissions and are more likely to develop dementia or require institutional care on discharge. Failure to detect delirium in the ED is associated with increased mortality and is an independent predictor of increased hospital stay (3–6).

Geriatric Emergencies, First Edition.
Iona Murdoch, Sarah Turpin, Bree Johnston, Alasdair MacLullich and Eve Losman.
© 2015 John Wiley & Sons, Ltd. Published 2015 by John Wiley & Sons, Ltd.

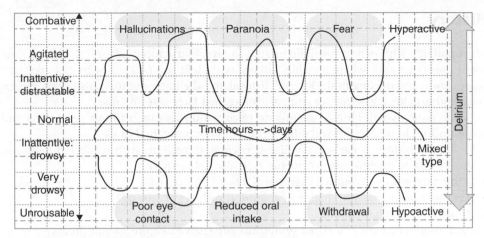

Figure 18.1 A graphical depiction of the different types of delirium.

Many patients who experience an episode of delirium never return to their cognitive baseline. In addition, a significant proportion of patients can recall the experience of acute delirium, and 70–80% of these patients experience significant distress as a result of these recollections (7, 8).

Box 18.2 Terminology in delirium.

Many formal and informal terms for delirium exist. These include 'acute confusional state' 'septic encephalopathy', 'ICU psychosis', 'knocked-off', and 'obtunded'.

It is best to use the standard term 'delirium' rather than these other synonyms, so as to aid communication and facilitate consistent management.

 KEY POINT: Patients with dementia are much more likely to develop delirium (9).

 KEY POINT: Most older patients with delirium also have dementia. Delirium in older patients without current dementia is associated with an eightfold risk of future dementia (10).

Risk factors for delirium
- Increasing age
- Male sex
- Multiple comorbidities
- Pre-existing dementia
- Previous episode of delirium
- History of stroke or other neurological disorder
- Depression
- Current or past alcohol abuse
- Chronic hepatic or renal impairment

History

Most patients with delirium will be unable to give a structured history. However, time spent observing and, where possible, talking with delirious patients is an essential part of assessment to document the level of arousal and the nature of their disturbed mental state and provide a baseline for comparison against later assessments.

Some patients will be able to provide information relating to their symptoms and presentation; however, this will differ depending on individual cases.

Collateral history as early as possible is *essential* in patients with suspected delirium. It should aim to establish the following: (see also Table 18.1).
- Is the patient more confused than normal?
- Has there been an acute change in cognition or level of arousal?
- Do the symptoms fluctuate?
- Have there been any associated symptoms suggestive of a precipitant illness?
- Have there been any changes in medication?
- Have the symptoms been present for hours/days/weeks or months?
- Was there evidence of background cognitive impairment before this acute change?

Almost any medical condition or drug can lead to delirium. In addition, physiological disturbance from medical conditions can directly lead to delirium. Box 18.3 contains a list of precipitants to consider early in the assessment.

Box 18.3 Precipitants of delirium (1, 2, 11, 12).

Drugs	Other precipitants
Confirmed association: • Anti-cholinergics • Opioids • Benzodiazepines, Z-drugs • Dihydropiridines (e.g. nifedipine) • Antihistamines Possible association: • H$_2$ agonists • Tricyclic antidepressants • Antiparkinson medications • Steroids • Diuretics • NSAIDs	• Infection: UTI/pneumonia/biliary sepsis/cellulitis/diverticulitis • Drug withdrawal (e.g. antidepressants, benzodiazepines and alcohol) • Hypoxia and hypercapnia • Cardiac: acute coronary syndromes/heart failure • Trauma: head injury/hip fracture • Primary CNS disorders: stroke/subdural haemorrhage/tumour/non-convulsive status epilepticus/encephalitis/meningitis • Metabolic: electrolyte disturbance/hypoglycaemia/dehydration • Acute kidney injury • Pain which is unrecognised or undertreated • Acute physiological stress e.g. surgery, pancreatitis • Change in environment e.g. new surroundings, sleep deprivation, restraint • Urinary retention • Urinary catheterisation • Constipation

Table 18.1 Taking an informant history for a patient with delirium.

Question	Reason you are checking	Why it is important
Have they had any recent illnesses, accidents or falls or complained of any particular problems?	Searching for precipitant: e.g. infection/head injury	Identifying and treating potential precipitating causes
Have had contact with the health services (e.g. primary care physician)? If so, why?	Searching for precipitant: e.g. new medication, inter-current illness	Primary care physicians can provide useful collateral information
Have their bowels and bladder been working normally?	Searching for precipitant: e.g. constipation, retention and UTI	Identifying and treating potential precipitating causes. E.g. constipation and urinary retention commonly co-exist
Have they been eating and drinking normally?	Searching for precipitant: e.g. dehydration Identifying possible consequence: e.g. reduced oral intake secondary to delirium	Reduced oral intake and dehydration can be a cause and a consequence of delirium. Nutritional status should be actively checked
Is there any change in their sleeping pattern?	Searching for precipitant/establishing diagnosis: sleep disturbance can precipitate delirium and also indicate delirium	Optimising sleep hygiene and establishing a routine can help treat delirium and reduce its chance of recurring
Do they have a walking aid?	Searching for precipitants: e.g. immobility Identifying possible consequences: falls	Immobility can precipitate or worsen delirium and patients should be encouraged to mobilise safely; delirious patients are at increased risk of falling and this needs to be considered when planning their care
Do they have hearing or visual aids?	Searching for precipitants: e.g. sensory impairment	Sensory impairment can precipitate or worsen delirium; ensuring patients can see and hear can improve recovery from delirium
What medicines are they on?	Searching for precipitant: e.g. medication. Ensuring important medications are not omitted	Intercurrent illness or increasing age may affect drug metabolism leading to adverse effects
Have their medicines been changed?	Searching for precipitant: e.g. new medication	Starting or stopping medications suddenly can precipitate delirium
Do they manage their own pills?	Searching for precipitant: e.g. medication error Establishing cognitive baseline	This may increase the risk of a medication error; it is also a helpful introduction question to discussing the patient's normal cognitive abilities
Have they had any memory problems in the past?	Establishing cognitive baseline	Patients with dementia are at increased risk of delirium and need to be regularly screened when in hospital

Table 18.1 (*continued*)

Question	Reason you are checking	Why it is important
Do they seem more confused, upset, agitated or drowsy than normal?	Establishing diagnosis: recent change in cognition	Differentiates delirium from dementia
Has this happened before? If so, what happened?	Identifying potential tendency to delirium	Patients with prior delirium are at increased risk of developing it again and need regular screening
Do they sometimes seem OK and other times become confused?	Establishing diagnosis: fluctuation	Differentiates delirium from dementia
Any sign of them hearing or seeing things that are not real?	Establishing diagnosis: Identifying hallucinations	Hallucinations are a common symptom of delirium and can be very distressing
Were they like this last week? How about the week before that? (and so on)	Establishing diagnosis: timescale (typically hours-days-weeks rather than months-years)	Differentiates delirium from dementia
Have they been distressed, e.g. by not understanding what is happening to them?	Managing symptoms: detecting distress	Distress is very common in delirium but is greatly underestimated
Have they shown any signs of having hallucinations, or suspicious beliefs?	Managing symptoms: detecting psychosis	Psychosis is common in delirium and is an important cause of distress. It is often undetected

Differential diagnosis

Delirium is generally readily distinguished from other mental disorders because of its acute onset and fluctuating course. However, a clear informant history is not always available. The following conditions should be considered in the differential diagnosis.
• Dementia (fluctuations can occur, especially in dementia with Lewy bodies)
• Brainstem stroke ('locked-in' syndrome)
• Autoimmune encephalitis (can resemble delirium but often has longer course)
• Post-ictal state
• Psychiatric diagnoses: agitated depression, mania, schizophrenia, acute stress disorder

Examination

Physical examination: general

Many patients with delirium are acutely unwell and the initial examination should be directed at detecting acute life-threatening illness, physiological disturbance or drug intoxication. Use a systematic ABCDE approach to ensure that serious underlying illness is not overlooked. Document level of arousal using an objective and commonly used technique such as the AVPU score (Box 18.4). Check capillary blood glucose. Look for evidence of opioid toxicity, alcohol withdrawal or other acute drug-related precipitants.

After life-threatening illness has been excluded, patients with delirium then require a thorough and systematic physical examination of all body systems with specific assessment for urinary retention, constipation and faecal impaction, neurological assessment including speech and an active search for infections such as pneumonia.

Box 18.4 The AVPU score.

ALERT: The patient is awake
VERBAL: The patient responds to verbal stimulation
PAIN: The patient responds to painful stimulation
UNRESPONSIVE: The patient is completely unresponsive

KEY POINT: Unless an older person's level of arousal and cognition is objectively assessed and documented, there is no baseline for comparison throughout the hospital stay.

Specific areas of focus on examination

A thorough systemic examination must take place to actively search for precipitants of delirium (Figure 18.2).

Assessing for and documenting delirium

A formal assessment for delirium should be completed in all older acute patients and documented in the patient's case notes. A recently validated rapid method for identifying delirium is the 4AT (see www.the4AT.com for further information and download). A copy of this test is provided in Chapter 2.

Investigations

Initial investigations

All patients with delirium should have a comprehensive set of laboratory tests including:
- Full blood count, urea and electrolytes (including calcium), liver function tests, glucose, C-reactive protein, thyroid function tests, B12 and folate.
- Urine culture.
- Chest radiograph.
- ECG.

Further investigations
Arterial blood gases

Arterial blood gases should be considered if there are signs suggestive of respiratory failure: hypoxia and hypercapnia may cause delirium.

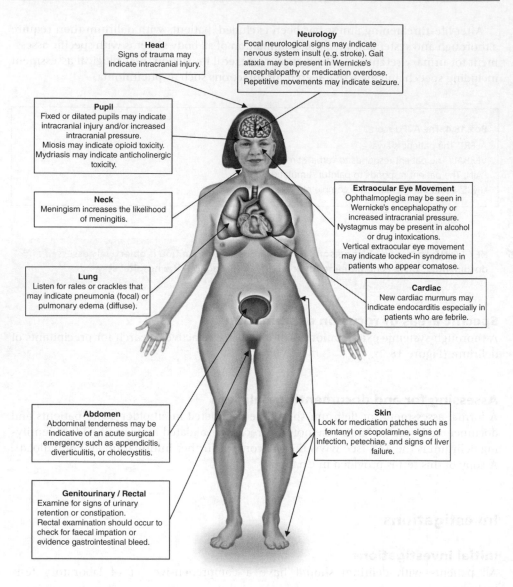

Head
Signs of trauma may indicate intracranial injury.

Neurology
Focal neurological signs may indicate nervous system insult (e.g. stroke). Gait ataxia may be present in Wernicke's encephalopathy or medication overdose. Repetitive movements may indicate seizure.

Pupil
Fixed or dilated pupils may indicate intracranial injury and/or increased intracranial pressure.
Miosis may indicate opioid toxicity. Mydriasis may indicate anticholinergic toxicity.

Neck
Meningism increases the likelihood of meningitis.

Extraocular Eye Movement
Ophthalmoplegia may be seen in Wernicke's encephalopathy or increased intracranial pressure. Nystagmus may be present in alcohol or drug intoxications.
Vertical extraocular eye movement may indicate locked-in syndrome in patients who appear comatose.

Lung
Listen for rales or crackles that may indicate pneumonia (focal) or pulmonary edema (diffuse).

Cardiac
New cardiac murmurs may indicate endocarditis especially in patients who are febrile.

Abdomen
Abdominal tenderness may be indicative of an acute surgical emergency such as appendicitis, diverticulitis, or cholecystitis.

Skin
Look for medication patches such as fentanyl or scopolamine, signs of infection, petechiae, and signs of liver failure.

Genitourinary / Rectal
Examine for signs of urinary retention or constipation.
Rectal examination should occur to check for faecal impation or evidence gastrointestinal bleed.

Figure 18.2 Areas of focus when examining a delirious patient. Source: From Han JH, Wilber ST. Altered mental status in older patients in the emergency department. *Clin Geriatr Med*. 2013 Feb;29(1):101–36. Reproduced with permission of Elsevier.

Venous lactate

Venous lactate should be measured if there are concerns about sepsis or other potential causes of metabolic derangement.

Troponin

Troponin should be considered if there are symptoms suggesting cardiac pathology, signs of cardiac failure or ECG abnormalities.

CT head

There is considerable geographical and practitioner variability in the routine use of CT scanning in patients initially presenting with delirium. However, the evidence suggests that routine use of CT head scanning in delirious patients is not helpful (13). Unnecessary scanning can be harmful because of the potentially disorienting effects of moving a delirious patient to different locations. Some guidelines recommend that CT head is indicated in the initial workup of delirious patients if the patient has:

- focal neurological signs
- delirium developing after head injury
- delirium developing after a fall
- a prescription for anticoagulants
- evidence of raised intracranial pressure

CT head should also be considered in the event of prolonged delirium (5 days or more) with no alternative precipitating causes found.

Lumbar puncture

This is not routinely helpful in patients with delirium unless there is a suspicion that the underlying cause is meningitis or encephalitis (13). Therefore, it is only indicated (after CT head if appropriate) in

- patients with signs of meningism
- patients with a severe headache and fever

Electroencephalogram (EEG)

This test is frequently abnormal in delirium, but in practice it is not part of the routine assessment of delirious patients (13). It is usually ordered following an assessment by a specialist. EEG can be useful in helping to

- differentiate delirium from dementia
- differentiate delirium from non-convulsive status epilepticus and temporal lobe epilepsy
- identify those patients in whom the delirium is due to a focal intracranial lesion, rather than a global abnormality

Management

General management

The key principles in delirium management are as follows:

- Identify and treat the precipitating causes (usually there is more than one precipitant)
- Optimise conditions for recovery
- Prevent and manage complications
- Reduce distress in patients
- Communicate with carers
- Prevent of delirium in high risk patients

Identifying and treating precipitating causes

The key first step is to look for and treat acute life-threatening causes. These can include both disease processes such as pneumonia, and the physiological consequences of these disease processes, such as hypoxia and low blood pressure. The next step is to carefully define all the remediable precipitating causes and to treat these comprehensively. Combinations of precipitants are common. For example, a patient might have a UTI that then leads to delirium, which is then further complicated by dehydration (drinking less, increased sweating) and then acute kidney injury. Thus, treat *all the causes*.

Optimise conditions for recovery

Alongside treating specific precipitating causes, it is crucial to optimise conditions such that the injured brain is able to recover. This means ensuring adequate oxygenation, providing hydration and nutrition, early mobilisation, reducing or stopping potentially deliriogenic drugs (even if these are long-term), detecting and managing any pain or other discomfort (e.g. dry mouth), providing ongoing psychological intervention including frequent explanations and reassurance, avoiding constipation and ensuring any sensory impairments are addressed where possible.

Preventing and managing complications

Delirium has many potential complications, including
- Aspiration pneumonia from reduced level of arousal and associated unsafe swallow
- Inadequate/inconsistent drug treatment because of lack of compliance with oral or parenteral routes of administration
- Dehydration because the patient is unable to drink enough or because of difficulties in administering parenteral fluids
- Malnourishment
- Immobility leading to deconditioning and pressure sores
- Prolonged hospital stay leading to functional decline
- Difficult rehabilitation leading to increased risk of new institutionalisation

   Addressing these complications requires ongoing proactive systematic assessment and a multi-disciplinary approach.

Managing distress

To manage distress in delirious patients, it needs first to be identified: check proactively for any potentially distressing symptoms such as hallucinations. Some patients will not volunteer these symptoms unless asked directly.

   Ask: 'How are you feeling today?' 'Are you in pain?' 'Are you concerned about anything?' 'Are you seeing anything strange around the bed?'

   The management of distress in delirium can be divided into non-pharmacological (Table 18.2) and pharmacological (Table 18.3); in general, non-pharmacological techniques should be attempted first and if these techniques are unsuccessful, pharmacological management should be considered in addition to ongoing supportive care.

Non-pharmacological management

Table 18.2 outlines potential non-pharmacological methods to assist in the management of a delirious patient.

Pharmacological management

Management of distressed or dangerously agitated patients

Current guidelines advocate the use of anti-psychotic medication in patients in whom non-pharmacological strategies have been unsuccessful and who are highly distressed

Table 18.2 Non-pharmacological management of a patient with delirium.

Behavioural adaptations	Environmental adaptations	Address specific causes of distress
Calm non-confrontational manner	Single room	Urinary retention
Reassurance	Well lit area	Pain
Reorientation	Clear signs indicating day,	Thirst/dry mouth
Distraction	time, season and place	Hunger
One-to-one nursing	Familiar objects	Feeling too cold or too warm
		Specific fears (e.g. 'I'm locked up'; 'My husband doesn't know where I am')
		Not understanding what is happening
		Hallucinations
		Delusions

Table 18.3 Pharmacological adjuncts to the management of delirium.

Drug	Normal starting dose in older patients	Cautions
Haloperidol	0.5–1.0 mg daily	Extra-pyramidal side effects Long QTc Avoid in patients with LBD or PD
Olanzapine	2.5–5 mg daily	Extra-pyramidal side effects (possibly less than haloperidol) Long QTc Avoid in patients with LBD or PD
Risperidone	0.25–0.5 mg once daily	Extra-pyramidal side effects (possibly less than haloperidol) Long QTc Avoid in patients with LBD or PD
Lorazepam (Note: Use generally reserved for patients in whom antipsychotics are contraindicated or where there is alcohol or benzodiazepine withdrawal)	0.5 mg PRN 4 h	Benzodiazepines can worsen and prolong delirium Paradoxical excitation Respiratory depression Falls risk Acceptable for use in patients with LBD or PD

LBD Lewy body dementia
PD Parkinson's disease

(especially when the delirium involves psychotic features) or who are considered a significant risk to themselves or others. Medication should be started as a single agent at the lowest clinically appropriate dose and titrated according to symptoms. There is a very limited evidence base to support drug treatment.

Some pharmacological therapies currently used in the treatment of delirium are shown in Table 18.3.

Communication with carers

Delirium is associated with high levels of carer stress. Because delirium is under-detected, carers are frequently left with no explanation from a healthcare professional as to why their loved one has had a profound change in their mental functioning. Carers often think that their relative has developed dementia or another mental disorder because public awareness of delirium is low. It is thus very important not only to make the diagnosis formally and communicate this with the whole team but also to provide clear and consistent information to carers. This process can greatly be assisted by use of written materials, e.g. the 'Think Delirium' leaflet available from Healthcare Improvement Scotland (14).

Specific management considerations in older patients

It is often the case that there are multiple precipitating causes for delirium in older patients, and therefore, a systematic approach to investigating and examining delirious patients is important to ensure that simple causes are not overlooked.

Age-related changes in drug metabolism mean that older patients require much lower doses of anti-psychotic medication; this is particularly true in patients with pre-existing dementia.

Dementia is present in around two-thirds of older patients with delirium, and this has often not been previously detected. Informant history can help identify possible background dementia. Cognitive tests during or just after a delirious episode are unhelpful in detecting dementia because of the acute effects of delirium on cognitive function. Patients in whom dementia is suspected but who lack a formal diagnosis of dementia should be considered for referral for further assessment, typically through their general practitioner or through older adult psychiatry services.

Legislation and delirious patients

The following section considers general circumstances in which relevant healthcare legislation needs to be considered with regard to the management of delirious patients.

Legislation, documentation and guidelines in the United Kingdom to be aware of include:

- Mental Capacity Act (MCA) (2005)
- Adults with Incapacity (AWI) (Scotland) Act 2000
- Common Law
- Power of Attorney
- Mental Health Act (MHA) 1983 as amended by Mental Health Act (MHA) 2007
- Mental Health (Care and Treatment) (Scotland) Act 2003
- Deprivation of Liberty Safeguards (DOLS).

Legislation may change: always seek local, up-to-date information when dealing with these issues.

Capacity

Decision-making capacity is a key issue when managing delirious patients. Often, patients lack capacity regarding health and welfare decisions, and in this situation, local law must be consulted to ensure appropriate documentation and proper adherence to legislation.

Capacity is complex; legislation and guidance exists in the United Kingdom to assist healthcare professionals in assessing and treating patients who lack capacity. For detailed guidance on assessing capacity, best interest decisions and advance directives in older patients see Chapter 3.

> **KEY POINT: Capacity is not a blanket term – it relates to specific decisions and can change with time.**

Medical treatments and other healthcare interventions

Medical treatments can be administered within the confines of the Mental Capacity Act / Adults with Incapacity Act as long as they are felt to be in the patient's best interests, in keeping with previously expressed wishes of the patient and the least restrictive option. In an emergency, intramuscular injections can be given to a patient who is resisting treatment under the MCA or common law. However, repeated administration of medication under restraint should prompt a careful review of the ongoing use of the MCA or AWI. In Scotland, repeated restraint and medication administration should prompt consideration of the use of the Mental Health Act (if treating a mental disorder e.g. administering anti-psychotic) or welfare guardianship (if treating a physical disorder e.g. administering insulin). This requires full psychiatric assessment. In England and Wales, the MCA can be used indefinitely for the repeated administration of medications under restraint if a patient continues to lack capacity. If the period of delirium is extending into weeks, then alternative diagnoses should be considered, alongside seeking a formal psychiatry opinion. In complicated or prolonged cases where there is significant restraint and restriction (in England and Wales), the Deprivation of Liberty Safeguards (DOLS) should be used; this is a complex process which is beyond the scope of this text.

Covert medication

This is a controversial practice permissible only in the context of appropriate legislation and careful consideration of the need for its use (15). It is important that formal assessment and documentation specifically relating to the use of covert medication exists, in order to protect both the human rights of the patient and to provide legal protection for the staff administering the medications. Covert medication policies vary geographically, but key questions that they should address include

- Does the patient clearly lack capacity in relation to this medication? *e.g. a delirious man who has, when well, declined statin therapy despite high cholesterol, should not be prescribed one under a covert medication protocol. However, a delirious man who has become paranoid and is refusing to take his regular anti-epileptic medication because he believes that it to be poison could be administered these drugs covertly if other methods of administration had been explored and failed.*
- Have the prior views of the patient been established?
- Is the medication essential for the health or overall benefit to the patient?
- Is the harm of not administering the medication greater than the harm of administering it covertly?

- Is administering it covertly the least restrictive option? *e.g. careful and repeated explanation of the need for haloperidol to an agitated patient is preferable to covert administration; however, covert administration is less restrictive than repeated restraint and intramuscular
  haloperidol.*
- Have relevant others been consulted? *Consultation with the patient's next of kin, nursing
  staff and pharmacy is essential to ensure that proper documentation and procedure is followed
  when considering the use of covert medication.*

Wandering
Patients who are undistressed and easily distracted can usually be managed using
behavioural techniques by experienced nursing staff and repeated reassurance and
reorientation. This does not require legislation.

Absconding and restraint
They raise important medico-legal issues and do require legislation. Patients who lack
capacity and are repeatedly attempting to leave a ward can be restrained only in the
immediate situation against their consent under common law or the MCA. Repeated
attempts or restraint to prevent a person from leaving a ward affects their human right
to liberty; this is permissible under the Mental Capacity Act in England and Wales (but
not under the AWI Scotland, where it is required to use the Mental Health Act).

Restriction or deprivation of liberty (DOLS)
Deprivation of liberty is permissible in certain circumstances, such as when a patient
clearly lacks capacity in the context of a delirium and remaining in hospital to undergo
medical treatment is felt to be in their best interest. In England and Wales, the MCA in
combination with the DOLS can be used to manage patients appropriately in this situation, always in conjunction with input from psychiatry and social work. In Scotland,
powers to detain in hospital are provided by the Mental Health Act. Brief periods of
detention (up to 72 hours) can be authorised by any fully registered doctor after a full
and proper assessment of a patient's diagnosis, risk and capacity has been undertaken.
Longer periods of detention require assessment by a psychiatrist.

Prevention of delirium

Older patients admitted to hospital, especially those with comorbidities, are at high risk
of incident delirium: around half of delirium cases occur after admission. Studies show
that up to one-third of cases of delirium are preventable. Prevention of delirium in
high risk patients involves addressing and avoiding risk factors such as dehydration,
constipation, infections, pain, disorientation urinary catheterisation frequent changes
of environment, immobility, lack of spectacles and/or hearing aids and sleep disturbance (using non-pharmacological means, though chronic hypnotic drugs should not
be stopped abruptly). Guidelines advocate that a tailored delirium prevention plan be
put in place for high risk patients.

Take home messages

- Delirium is under-diagnosed and often poorly managed
- Delirium is a sign of a seriously unwell patient and is associated with increased morbidity and mortality
- The management of delirium is multi-faceted and multi-disciplinary
- Delirium is distressing to both patients and their relatives
- Delirious patients require regular objective reassessment of their physical and mental states
- Delirious patients require formal assessment and documentation of capacity in relation to relevant healthcare decisions
- Delirium can be effectively prevented in many cases.

References

1 Wilber ST. Altered mental status in older emergency department patients. *Emerg Med Clin North Am*. 2006;24(2):299–316.
2 Han JH, Wilber ST. Altered mental status in older patients in the emergency department. *Clin Geriatr Med*. 2013;29(1):101–136.
3 Witlox J, Eurelings LSM, de Jonghe JFM, Kalisvaart KJ, Eikelenboom P, van Gool WA. Delirium in elderly patients and the risk of postdischarge mortality, institutionalization, and dementia: a meta-analysis. *JAMA*. 2010;304(4):443–451.
4 Francis J, Kapoor WN. Prognosis after hospital discharge of older medical patients with delirium. *J Am Geriatr Soc*. 1992;40(6):601–606.
5 Stevens LE, de Moore GM, Simpson JM. Delirium in hospital: does it increase length of stay? *Aust N Z J Psychiatry*. 1998;32(6):805–808.
6 Rockwood K, Cosway S, Carver D, Jarrett P, Stadnyk K, Fisk J. The risk of dementia and death after delirium. *Age Ageing*. 1999;28(6):551–556.
7 Grover S, Shah R. Distress due to delirium experience. *Gen Hosp Psychiatry*. 2011;33(6):637–639.
8 Bruera E, Bush SH, Willey J, Paraskevopoulos T, Li Z, Palmer JL, et al. Impact of delirium and recall on the level of distress in patients with advanced cancer and their family caregivers. *Cancer*. 2009;115(9):2004–2012.
9 Matthew Cooke, David Oliver, Alistair Burns. *Quality Care for Older People with Urgent and Emergency Care Needs 'The Silver Book'*. http://britishgeriatricssociety.wordpress.com/2012/06/21/the-silver-book-guidelines-for-the-emergency-care-of-older-people/ [cited 2014 May 3].
10 Davis DHJ, Terrera GM, Keage H, Rahkonen T, Oinas M, Matthews FE, et al. Delirium is a strong risk factor for dementia in the oldest-old: a population-based cohort study. *Brain*. 2012;135(Pt 9): 2809–2816.
11 Clegg A, Young JB. Which medications to avoid in people at risk of delirium: a systematic review. *Age Ageing*. 2011;40(1):23–29.
12 Levkoff SE, Besdine RW, Wetle T. Acute confusional states (delirium) in the hospitalized elderly. *Annu Rev Gerontol Geriatr* 1986;6:1–26.
13 British Geriatrics Society (BGS). *Guidelines for the Prevention, Diagnosis and Management of Delirium in Older People in Hospital*. http://www.bgs.org.uk/index.php/clinicalguides/170-clinguidedelirium-treatment?showall=&limitstart= [cited 2013 Aug 24].
14 Scottish Delirium Association. http://www.scottishdeliriumassociation.com/
15 Haw C, Stubbs J. Covert administration of medication to older adults: a review of the literature and published studies. *J Psychiatr Ment Health Nurs*. 2010;17(9):761–768.

CHAPTER 19
Stroke and transient ischaemic attack

Introduction

The consequences of acute stroke can be devastating for a person's independence, cognitive function and quality of life. Patients aged over 80 have a higher mortality and more frequent complications, particularly pneumonia, following acute ischaemic stroke than their younger counterparts. The increased rate of complications is likely due to a more dependent pre-morbid state and more complex comorbidity.

Until recently, there has been very limited information on the benefit of specialist interventions such as thrombolysis and carotid endarterectomy in older patients; however, emerging evidence supports the proactive management of stroke and stroke risk factors in appropriately selected older patients.

This chapter is designed to help junior staff initially assess patients presenting with a stroke or transient ischaemic attack (TIA), provide information on current opinion on carotid endarterectomy and thrombolysis in older people and also provide guidance on the initiation and management of patients on newer anticoagulant agents.

Definition
Stroke
Stroke is defined as 'a clinical syndrome, of presumed vascular origin, typified by rapidly developing signs of focal or global disturbance of cerebral functions lasting more than 24 hours or leading to death' (1). 85% of strokes are ischaemic in origin, 10% are due to intracerebral haemorrhage and 5% are due to subarachnoid haemorrhage.

Transient ischaemic attack (TIA)
TIA was traditionally defined as an acute loss of focal cerebral or ocular function with symptoms lasting less than 24 hours, thought to be due to inadequate cerebral or ocular blood supply as a result of low blood flow, thrombosis or embolism associated with diseases of the blood vessels, heart or blood (2). However, owing to concerns that the arbitrary 24 hour time period may result in confusion and delays in administering time-sensitive stroke therapies, a revised *tissue-based* definition has been adopted. This definition is less dependent on any specified time periods and focuses more on the pathophysiological entity of transient rather than permanent ischaemia. This new

Geriatric Emergencies, First Edition.
Iona Murdoch, Sarah Turpin, Bree Johnston, Alasdair MacLullich and Eve Losman.
© 2015 John Wiley & Sons, Ltd. Published 2015 by John Wiley & Sons, Ltd.

approach to the condition defines TIA as *'a transient episode of neurological dysfunction caused by focal brain, spinal cord, or retinal ischemia, without acute infarction'* (3).

Background

Over 30% of acute strokes occur in patients over the age of 80, and considering the rising population of octogenarians and nonagenarians, prompt and thorough management of stroke and its risk factors in older people could confer significant reductions in morbidity and mortality (4).

A stroke or TIA is a cerebrovascular emergency and older patients can derive relatively greater benefit from early treatment compared to their younger counterparts (5). The days of the 'watch and wait' approach are gone, and further research into the treatment of acute stroke has led to thrombolysis being offered to patients aged over 80. The management of stroke in older people is an exciting and rapidly developing field.

Stroke has varied clinical presentations depending on anatomical location but is usually associated with the rapid onset of a focal neurological deficit. The classification presented in Table 19.1, based on anatomical pathophysiology, is widely used. It allows classification on clinical grounds, and the subtypes described have prognostic value.

Stroke categorisation

Symptoms which may suggest alternative pathology

- Delirium with no focal neurological signs: usually suggests global rather than focal brain dysfunction such as infection or metabolic derangement.
- Seizure: may present as a postictal state with focal neurological signs, such as Todd's paresis; remember that occasionally a seizure can be a complicating feature of stroke.
- Loss of consciousness (LOC): unless associated with significant haemorrhage and intracranial oedema. Rarely a posterior circulation stroke can present with LOC or locked-in syndrome.

Stroke mimics

Conditions which can lead to diagnostic error by mimicking acute stroke include (6):

- Seizure and post-ictal state
- Syncope
- Complex migraine or ocular migraine
- Hypoglycaemia or electrolyte disturbance
- Brain tumour
- Exacerbation of pre-existing neurological deficits by a systemic process (e.g. temporary reappearance of old stroke symptoms)
- Bell's palsy
- Vestibular disorders (however, posterior circulation stroke and vertebral artery dissection should be considered)

Initial assessment of patients with acute stroke in the ED

Rapid initial assessment is an essential part of managing acute stroke (Table 19.2), and a focused ABCDE examination should be performed to ensure that the patient is not

Table 19.1 Stroke subtypes by location, presenting symptoms and prognosis (Oxford classification).

Stroke type	Anatomical pathophysiology	Clinical features	Mortality at 30 days (%)
Lacunar infarct	Intrinsic disease of a single basal perforating artery, most commonly in the basal ganglia, internal capsule or pons	• Pure motor stroke • Pure sensory stroke • Sensori-motor stroke • Ataxic hemiparesis. Owing to the high concentration of motor fibres in the internal capsule, a small lacunar infarct in this region can cause a large motor deficit	2
Total anterior circulation infarct	Ischaemia of both the deep and superficial territories of the middle cerebral artery	Combination of: • New higher cerebral dysfunction (e.g. dysphasia, dyscalculia and visuospatial disorder) • Homonymous visual field defect • Ipsilateral motor and/or sensory deficit of at least two areas of the face, arm and leg	39
Partial anterior circulation infarcts	Occlusion of either the upper division of the MCA (therefore usually no visual field defect) or the lower division of the middle cerebral artery (usually a negligible motor/sensory component) Occlusion of the anterior cerebral artery and striatocapsular infarctions	Two of the three components of the TACI syndrome with: • higher cerebral dysfunction alone, • a motor/sensory deficit more restricted than those classified as LACI (e.g., confined to one limb, or to face and hand but not to the whole arm)	4
Posterior circulation infarcts	Infarcts associated with the brainstem, cerebellum or occipital lobes	Any of the following: • Cerebellar dysfunction without ipsilateral long-tract deficit (i.e. ataxic hemiparesis • Isolated homonymous visual field defect • Brainstem syndromes with motor and/or sensory deficit • Intranuclear ophthalmoplegia • Diplopia • Very rarely loss of consciousness	7

LACS, Lacunar infarct; TACS, total anterior circulation infarct; PACS, Partial anterior circulation infarcts; POCS, posterior circulation infarcts.
Source: Table compiled using excerpt from Bamford et al "Classification and natural history of clinically identifiable subtypes of cerebral infarction." *Lancet*. 1991 Jun 22;337(8756):1521–6. With permission from Elsevier.

Table 19.2 Recommended timescale for assessment and management of patients presenting with acute stroke.

Action	Time
Door to physician	≤10 min
Door to stroke team	≤15 min
Door to CT initiation	≤25 min
Door to CT interpretation	≤45 min
Door to drug (≥80% compliance)	≤60 min
Door to stroke unit admission	≤3 h

Source: From Jauch EC, Saver JL, Adams HP Jr, Bruno A, Connors JJ, Demaerschalk BM, Khatri P, McMullan PW Jr, Qureshi AI, Rosenfield K, Scott PA, Summers DR, Wang DZ, Wintermark M, Yonas H; Guidelines for the early management of patients with acute ischemic stroke: a guideline for healthcare professionals from the American Heart Association/American Stroke Association. *Stroke.* 2013;44:870–947. With permission from Wolters Kluwer Health.

medically unstable so that an urgent CT brain can occur within minutes of the patient's arrival in the ED. General observations and a record of conscious level using the AVPU score and capillary glucose should be performed as part of this initial assessment.

Training for paramedics and ED staff in the use of stroke screening tools is widely available and associated with increased sensitivity in initial diagnosis. The FAST test and the ROSIER score can enable the diversion of patients to appropriate stroke centres and allow appropriate triage of potential stroke patients arriving in the department.

The FAST test

This is used to aid pre-hospital recognition of stroke by the general public and emergency services providers, and can also be used in the ED to aid the rapid initial assessment of acute stroke symptoms:

Face: Ask the patient "show me your teeth" to look for facial asymmetry

Arms: "Raise both arms" to look for pronator drift over 10 seconds

Speech: "repeat after me: 'baby hippopotamus' 'British constitution'" to assess for dysarthria

Time: Establish time of onset from the patient or a witness.

KEY POINT: The assessment and management of a patient presenting with acute stroke is a time-dependent emergency. "CODE STROKE" or "THROMBOLYSIS CALL" should be put out when a patient presents to the ED with symptoms suggestive of acute stroke to facilitate an immediate assessment.

Recognition of stroke in the emergency room (ROSIER) Score

This is one of several useful screening tools developed to assist ED staff in assessing the patient presenting with symptoms of stroke.

Box 19.1 The ROSIER score (7).

1 Has there been loss of consciousness or temporary loss of consciousness due to a drop in blood pressure (syncope)? If yes score = −1, if no score = 0
2 Has there been seizure activity? If yes score = −1, if no score = 0
3 Is there a NEW onset of the following symptoms (or on waking from sleep):
- Asymmetric facial weakness? If yes score = +1, if no score = 0
- Asymmetric grip weakness? If yes score = +1, if no score = 0
- Asymmetric arm weakness? If yes score = +1, if no score = 0
- Asymmetric leg weakness? If yes score = +1, if no score = 0
- Speech disturbance? If yes score = +1, if no score = 0
- Visual field defect? If yes score = +1, if no score = 0

The total score will range between −2 and +6.

If the total score is between +1 and +6, then the stroke team should be activated and all appropriate ED personnel need to be alerted to the patient's presence in the ED.

Time of onset

This is crucial; particularly if considering thrombolysis, which is currently given up until 4.5 hours after symptom onset in patients aged under 80 and up to 3 hours after symptom onset in patients aged over 80. Some patients may be unable to provide a history; therefore, a witness account should be urgently sought. If the time of onset is unclear, it must be taken as whenever the patient was *last seen well*; if the patient awoke with the symptoms, time of onset is *when they went to bed*.

 KEY POINT: Research and guidance regarding the impact of time of onset on treatment decisions is ever-changing and it is important to consult the guidelines at your nearest Stroke Centre.

Once a rapid initial assessment has taken place and necessary scans organised, further information should be gathered as follows:

Past medical history

This should be documented, with particular focus on any previous vascular or intracerebral events. Prior neurological impairments should be recorded. Particularly relevant non-stroke conditions include epilepsy, malignancy, dementia, diabetes and risk factors such as ischaemic heart disease and atrial fibrillation.

Functional status

Functional status and pre-morbid level of independence are relevant when making decisions about thrombolysis. Factors such as nursing home residence and extreme dependence should be considered, although decisions are often made on an individual basis considering patient and family values and a review of the associated risks and benefits. Pre-morbid function is helpful when trying to predict longer term outcomes and rehabilitation goals.

Medications

Drug history should be noted with particular attention paid to warfarin use and INR (this should be checked urgently on arrival), anti-platelets, novel anticoagulants and antihypertensive medications.

Examination

General examination

Once brief initial assessment has occurred and the patient is in the CT scanner, further information can be gathered from the family, the stroke team can be involved early and the patient can undergo a more detailed neurological examination.

All patients with a suspected stroke should have a full neurological assessment, preferably incorporating the National Institute of Health Stroke Scale (NIHSS) and an assessment of coordination and higher cortical function.

Systemic examination should aim to identify precipitating causes of stroke such as atrial fibrillation, bacterial endocarditis or carotid stenosis. The patient's pulse, oxygen saturations and blood pressure should be closely monitored. Extreme hypertension or hypotension should be identified.

The national institute of health stroke scale

This is a 15-point neurological scale that aims to provide a quantitative assessment of the neurological status of patients who have suffered an acute stroke. The scale assessment takes less than 10 minutes to perform but requires specific (though simple) training before it can be carried out.

Recommended resources

There are many useful online resources that provide ED staff with information and resources to support them when managing patients with acute stroke.

- The NIHSS online training module:
  http://learn.heart.org/ihtml/application/student/interface.heart2/nihsscomputer
  .html#3
- Stroke Track app which is downloadable free from iTunes: https://itunes.apple.com/gb
  /app/stroke-track/id378682166?mt=8
- http://www.strokeassociation.org provides free online education modules.

Higher function assessment

Dysphasia

Expressive Dysphasia: is assessed by asking the patient to name familiar objects and gradually increasing the complexity of the labelling.

Example: a pen → a pen lid → a nib

Receptive Dysphasia: is assessed by asking the patient to follow commands. Start with simple commands and increase in complexity from 1 to 3 stages.

Example:

1 Stick out your tongue.
2 Close your eyes and point at the ceiling.
3 Touch your ear, close your eyes and stick out your tongue.

Sensory inattention

Touch the patient's right hand and left hand in turn and then touch both their hands simultaneously.

Patients with inattention to one side will identify touching of both right and left sides when the hands are touched separately but identify only the unaffected side as being touched when the hands are touched simultaneously.

This differs from hemisensory loss in that patients will not feel touch or note diminished sensation to touch on the affected side even when it is touched in isolation.

Visual field testing

Formal confrontational field testing can be difficult in the acute situation.

Absence of a blink or threat response from one side can suggest a homonymous hemianopia.

Visual inattention can be tested by facing the patient head on, stretching out your arms and asking the patient to identify which hand is moving. Patients with visual inattention will correctly identify individual movements but identify the unaffected side only when hands are moved simultaneously.

Neglect

Neglect can be assessed quickly using the clock drawing test: ask a patient to draw a clock with the hands pointing to ten past ten. Alternatively, ask them to copy a picture – they may copy only half of it.

Investigations

Initial investigations

All patients presenting with suspected stroke should have:

CT brain

This should occur as quickly as possible following arrival in the Emergency Department. This is essential to differentiate ischaemic stroke from intracranial haemorrhage and exclude other intracerebral pathology such as malignancy. When considering thrombolysis ideal 'door to needle' time is 60 minutes, and CT brain should be performed within 25 minutes of arrival (Table 19.2). Other indications for prompt CT (within 1 hour) include

- Anticoagulant treatment
- Known bleeding tendency
- Depressed level of consciousness (Glasgow Coma Score <13)
- Unexplained progressive or fluctuating symptoms
- Papilloedema, neck stiffness or fever
- Severe headache at onset of stroke symptoms.

Blood tests

Patients on warfarin should have a point of care INR to see if their INR is low enough for thrombolysis to be considered (<1.7). Also check full blood count, urea and electrolytes, calcium, coagulation screen, ESR, glucose and lipid profile.

ECG
This is to look for AF, other arrhythmia, or ischaemic changes.

Chest radiograph
This may identify concurrent aspiration pneumonia, lung cancer or aortic dissection.

> **KEY POINT:** A patient with a normal CT brain can still have had an ischaemic stroke. It can take hours for the CT manifestation of ischaemia to develop.

Further investigations
MRI brain
This is more accurate than CT brain in determining site and extent of ischaemic damage, particularly in small lesions and lesions in the posterior fossa. However, it is not always readily available, and in addition, some patients may be unsuitable for MRI scanning because of acute illness or the presence of a pacemaker. Scottish Intercollegiate Guidelines Network (SIGN) (8) suggests that MRI should be considered in patients who are not severely ill, where the neurological deficit is mild or the lesion thought to be in the posterior fossa, and in patients who present late (>1 week after onset of symptoms); however, practice patterns vary and some centres and countries use MRI more commonly.

Carotid Dopplers
Carotid dopplers should be performed in patients presenting with anterior circulation stroke or TIA. Patients with 50–99% stenosis (NASCET criteria) or 70–99% stenosis (ECST criteria) should be referred for consideration of carotid endarterectomy. This test is usually arranged within 24 hours of presentation.

Ambulatory ECG monitoring
A 24 hour tape or a period of cardiac telemetry should be considered in stroke patients to investigate the possibility of paroxysmal AF.

Management

General management of acute ischaemic stroke in the ED
In the case of acute ischaemic stroke, thrombolysis is an increasingly available option for older patients and the motto TIME IS BRAIN has helped to revolutionise acute stroke care in recent years.

CT brain
CT brain should be urgently arranged as discussed earlier.

Stroke team
The stroke team should be informed of the patient's presence in the Emergency Department, and involved in early decision making.

Oxygen

Oxygen should be given if the saturations are less than 95% and there are no contraindications.

Intravenous access

IV access should be established promptly and a baseline blood screen obtained.

Blood glucose

Blood glucose should be controlled to between 4 and 11 mmol/L using an insulin sliding scale if required.

Cardiac monitoring

Cardiac monitoring should be commenced.

Blood pressure

Guidelines in the UK and the US at the time of writing state that BP lowering therapies should not be initiated unless hypertension is associated with one of the following medical emergencies (9):

- hypertensive encephalopathy
- hypertensive nephropathy
- hypertensive cardiac failure/myocardial infarction
- aortic dissection
- intra-cerebral haemorrhage with systolic blood pressure over 200 mmHg.

Patients who present on established antihypertensive medication regimes should have these medications continued unless they become hypotensive or are found to have bilateral carotid stenosis in which case a systolic of between 140 and 160 mmHg should be targeted.

If a patient is being considered for thrombolysis, intravenous blood pressure lowering therapies such as intravenous GTN or labetolol 10 mg over 1–2 minutes can be used to reduce the systolic blood pressure to a target of 185/110 mmHg (10), under the guidance of senior stroke physicians.

Swallowing

Patients should have a swallow screen performed on admission and if they appear to have an unsafe swallow then they should be kept nil by mouth until a full swallowing assessment is undertaken.

Specific management considerations in the older patients
Thrombolysis in patients aged >80 years

The recently published Third International Stroke Trial revealed that the benefit of thrombolysis in the older population is similar to that seen in patients under the age of 80, and the number needed to treat (NNT) for one more older person to be alive and independent at 3 months is 17. A recently updated systematic review and meta-analysis of thrombolysis including the IST 3 trial results identified that in patients aged over 80 who received thrombolysis within 3 hours an additional 96 per 1000 individuals were alive and independent and in those aged over 80 who received thrombolysis within 6 hours an additional 38 per 100 individuals were alive and independent (4, 11).

Large observational studies and recent meta-analysis have not identified any significant age-related differences in post-thrombolysis bleeding complications (4).

 KEY POINT: Thrombolysis should not be withheld on the basis of older age alone.

Table 19.3 Inclusion and exclusion criteria for thrombolysis (12).

Inclusion criteria

    Diagnosis of ischaemic stroke causing measurable neurological deficit
    Onset of symptoms <4.5 h before beginning treatment if <80
    Onset of symptoms <3 h before beginning treatment if >80

Exclusion criteria

    Significant head trauma or prior stroke in previous 3 months
    Symptoms suggesting subarachnoid haemorrhage
    Arterial puncture at non-compressible site in previous 7 days
    History of previous intracranial haemorrhage
    Intracranial neoplasm, arteriovenous malformation or aneurysm
    Recent intracranial or intraspinal surgery
    Elevated blood pressure: systolic >185 mmHg or diastolic >110 mmHg
      Note: some centres with specialist stroke physicians on site may thrombolyse above these parameters.
    Active internal bleeding
    Acute bleeding diathesis, including but not limited to
      Platelet count <100,000/mm^3
      Heparin received within 48 h, resulting in abnormally elevated aPTT greater than the upper limit of normal
      Current use of anticoagulant with INR > 1.7 or PT > 15 s
      Current use of direct thrombin inhibitors or direct factor Xa inhibitors with elevated sensitive laboratory
        tests (such as aPTT, INR, platelet count and ECT; TT; or appropriate factor Xa activity assays)
    Blood glucose concentration <50 mg/dL (2.7 mmol/L)
    CT demonstrates multi-lobar infarction (hypodensity >1/3 cerebral hemisphere)

Relative exclusion criteria if 0–3 h from symptom onset

    Only minor or rapidly improving stroke symptoms (clearing spontaneously)
    Seizure at onset with postictal residual neurological impairments
    Major surgery or serious trauma within previous 14 days
    Recent gastrointestinal or urinary tract haemorrhage (within previous 21 days)
    Recent acute myocardial infarction (within previous 3 months)

Relative exclusion criteria if 3–4.5h from symptom onset

    Age >80 years
    Severe stroke (NIHSS>25)
    Taking an oral anticoagulant regardless of INR
    History of both diabetes and prior ischaemic stroke

Source: From Jauch EC, Saver JL, Adams HP Jr, Bruno A, Connors JJ, Demaerschalk BM, Khatri P, McMullan PW Jr, Qureshi AI, Rosenfield K, Scott PA, Summers DR, Wang DZ, Wintermark M, Yonas H; Guidelines for the early management of patients with acute ischemic stroke: a guideline for healthcare professionals from the American Heart Association/American Stroke Association. *Stroke*. 2013;44:870–947. With permission from Wolters Kluwer Health.

Decision making surrounding thrombolysis in older patients

Current guidelines state that patients over the age of 80 can be thrombolysed up to 3 hours after symptom onset (Table 19.3). The decision to administer or withhold thrombolysis in any patient with acute stroke is not to be taken lightly. For this reason, there are locally established pathways that involve seeking the input of a stroke physician early.

Inclusion and exclusion criteria exist in guidelines (Table 19.3); however, the decision is in part guided by the patient in front of you and the potential impact of their presenting symptoms on their life. A patient with mild hand weakness who is a professional musician may view a lacunar stroke with a low NIHSS as a devastating blow to their livelihood and quality of life. Older patients who are frail but living relatively independently in the community or nursing home residents presenting with devastating symptoms such as aphasia do not always fit exactly into the proposed indication/contraindication guidelines. Appropriate decision making in these patients can be difficult and should be discussed with the patient and the consultant stroke physician at the time of your initial assessment.

Consent and documentation

When discussing thrombolysis, patients should be counselled on the risks (primarily bleeding) and benefits (better functional outcome in some cases) of the treatment; see Box 19.2 for further information.

If the patient lacks decision making capacity, then effort should be made to counsel their next of kin. Full documentation of the discussion and decision should be recorded in the notes.

Box 19.2 Information to give to patients/relatives before administration of alteplase.

There has been a significant stroke caused by a blocked artery preventing blood from getting to a part of the brain, causing permanent damage. With or without treatment there may be some recovery or things could get worse. Stroke is fatal in about a third of people.

Only one treatment has been shown to prevent damage to the brain. This treatment, alteplase, dissolves the blood clot blocking the artery and allows blood to get back to the brain.

This is Only proven to work if given within 3 hours of the stroke starting and there is a risk that the treatment will cause bleeding in the brain. This occurs in 7 out of 100 patients treated and is fatal in 3 of these.

Despite this, overall the treatment is more likely to help than to cause harm. Without treatment of 100 people with a stroke, 26 will survive with minimal or no disability – with treatment of 100 people with a stroke, 40 will survive with minimal disability.

Further management of acute stroke
Stroke unit admission

This should occur as soon as possible, as specialist multi-disciplinary input in a geographically discrete location is associated with reduced mortality and better functional status at 1 year.

Intermittent pneumatic compression

This has been shown to be an effective method of reducing the risk of DVT in patients who are immobile following a stroke (13).

Anti-platelet therapy

Anti-platelet therapy should be commenced immediately (assuming no contraindications) at a dose of 300–325mg aspirin per day for 2 weeks and then changed to 75 mg clopidogrel per day thereafter (9,12).

Blood pressure control

Antihypertensives are not usually initiated until 2 weeks after a stroke, or until the time of hospital discharge, whichever comes sooner. Exceptions to this rule would be in cases where extreme hypertension is causing harm such as hypertensive encephalopathy. Target blood pressure following stroke is 130/80 mmHg unless there is severe bilateral carotid stenosis in which case a systolic blood pressure target of 130–150 mmHg is acceptable.

Nutrition and hydration

A nasogastric tube should be inserted if required for oral drug administration, nutrition and hydration. This should take place within 24 hours unless the patient has been thrombolysed, in which case ideally 24 hours should pass before attempting any potentially traumatic procedures.

Cholesterol lowering therapy

Statins confer a relative risk reduction of 20–25% over 5 years following a vascular event. The recommended first line treatment in the UK is simvastatin 40 mg once per day.

Transient ischaemic attack

Owing to the increased rate of stroke in older people, aggressive management of risk factors can result in a relatively greater benefit. Approximately 30–40% of patients with TIA will go on to have a stroke. The ABCD2 scoring system (14) helps to predict 2 day stroke risk (nearly half of all strokes occur within 2 days of a TIA) (Tables 19.4 and 19.5).

Table 19.4 The ABCD2 score (14).

Components of score	Associated points
Age >60 years	1
BP >140 mmHg systolic or >90 mmHg diastolic	1
Clinical features:	
Unilateral weakness	2
Speech disturbance	1
Duration	
>60 min	2
10–59 min	1
<10 min	0
Diabetes	1

Table 19.5 ABCD2 score recommendations (14).

ABCD2 score	2 Day % stroke risk	Management guideline
0–3	1.0	TIA clinic review within 72 h
4–5	4.1	Admit or TIA clinic review within 24 h
>5	8.1	Admit

Carotid endarterectomy in older patients

Evidence suggests that in appropriately selected cases, older patients can derive greater benefit from carotid endarterectomy than younger patients. The absolute risk reduction for stroke in the 2 years following endarterectomy in selected patients over the age of 75 is greater than in patients aged under 65 (15).

A recent large meta-analysis suggests that the benefits of carotid endarterectomy in those aged over 85 years are at least comparable to those of younger patients, although there is increased peri-procedural mortality (16, 17).

Anticoagulation in older patients

There is overwhelming evidence that anticoagulation in older patients with AF significantly reduces their annual risk of stroke. Increasing age is an important factor in stroke risk, and treatment with warfarin is superior to treatment with anti-platelet agents and decreases the relative risk of stroke by 64% (18).

Many of the factors that increase the risk of stroke also increase risk of bleeding on anticoagulation. Despite this, the risk of haemorrhage is significantly outweighed by the benefit of stroke reduction. Tools such as the CHA2DS2Vasc and HASBLED scores help to stratify the risk of stroke and risk of bleeding (Box 19.3). All patients aged over 75 are recommended to receive anticoagulation with warfarin, with the updated CHA2DS2Vasc score assigning those aged >75 two points (19).

Box 19.3 The CHA2DS2Vasc and HASBLED scores.

CHA2DS2Vasc	Points	HASBLED	Points
Congestive heart failure/LV dysfunction	1	Hypertension	1
Hypertension	1	Abnormal renal function or abnormal liver function	1 or 2
Age >75 years	2	Stroke	1
Diabetes	1	Bleeding in the past	1
Stroke/TIA/DVT	2	Labile INRs	1
Vascular event: i.e. MI, PVD	1	Elderly (>65 years)	1
Age 65–74 years	1	Drugs: anti-platelets/non-steroidals or alcohol abuse	1 or 2
Sex category: female	1		

0: No therapy is preferred option 1: Consideration of oral anticoagulation or use of aspirin depending on patient preferences (oral anticoagulation is preferred option) >2 high risk: oral anticoagulation	Rate of major haemorrhage per 100 person years: 0=1.13, 1=1.02, 2=1.88, 3=3.74, 4=8.7, 5=12.5

KEY POINT: A tendency to fall is not a justifiable contraindication to warfarin. Older patients in AF would have to fall approximately 295 times in a year before warfarin use became associated with lower Quality-adjusted life years (QALYs) than anti-platelets or no therapy (20).

Anticoagulation in the very frail

The difficulty facing clinicians every day, when assessing older patients with multiple comorbidities who present in atrial fibrillation, is that those patients who have the most to gain in terms of stroke risk reduction, also have the most to lose in terms of serious haemorrhage. The burden of repeated blood tests may also be onerous for some patients.

When both risks are high, a detailed discussion with the patient to explore their own perception of risk and personal preferences regarding stroke prevention should be considered when making a decision.

Novel anticoagulants and older patients

Anticoagulation with warfarin can be difficult in older adults due to increased sensitivity to warfarin and increased frequency of intercurrent illness and medication changes that may precipitate alterations in drug metabolism. The newer oral anticoagulants do not have these same issues, although the irreversibility of these agents raises other concerns about management in the event of haemorrhage or perioperative situations. Large trials such as the RE-LY trial which involved older patients have shown dabigatran to be non-inferior to warfarin in terms of stroke risk reduction and have not revealed any significant increase in life-threatening haemorrhage (18).

Intracranial haemorrhage

Background

Intracranial haemorrhage comprises approximately 15% of acute strokes (21). The presentation of intracranial haemorrhage is usually very similar to acute ischaemic stroke, and the two types are differentiated on CT scanning.

The commonest type of intracranial haemorrhage is intracerebral bleeding, usually caused by hypertensive bleeds from deep penetrating arteries, or 'lobar' bleeds caused by cerebral amyloid angiopathy. Cerebral amyloid angiopathy is associated with increasing age and is becoming a more frequent presentation as the population ages (3).

Subarachnoid haemorrhage is also a cause of haemorrhagic stroke and other, rarer, pathologies include arteriovenous malformation, metastatic malignancy and coagulopathy (10).

The prognosis in haemorrhagic stroke is worse than for ischaemic stroke and older patients have worse outcomes than younger patients. Mortality is 30–50% at 30 days, increased to 70% when the bleed is associated with warfarin use (22).

Management

The treatment of haemorrhagic stroke in older patients is no different than for younger patients.

Reversal of anticoagulation

Patients on anticoagulants should have the anticoagulation urgently reversed using pro-thrombin complex concentrate, intravenous vitamin K and blood product support. In the case of patients with metallic heart valves, the reversal of anticoagulation should be done in combination with input from cardiologists and haematologists to help assess the risk of life threatening thrombosis versus ongoing intracerebral haemorrhage.

Neurosurgical input

All patients with intracerebral haemorrhage should be discussed with the local neuro-surgical unit.

Blood pressure control

The guidelines for blood pressure control in haemorrhagic stroke are currently the same as for ischaemic stroke; however, the INTERACT2 trial has shown an improvement in functional outcome at 90 days following aggressive blood pressure lowering in patients with intracerebral haemorrhage (23).

Supportive care

All patients with intracerebral haemorrhage should be admitted to an acute stroke unit as soon as they are stable.

In the case of subarachnoid haemorrhage or bleeding secondary to arteriovenous malformations, cerebral angiography and coiling should be considered to reduce the risk of further bleeding.

Take home messages

- The risk of acute ischaemic stroke increases with age
- Advanced age is associated with worse outcomes following ischaemic stroke and intracranial haemorrhage
- An ageing population makes early identification and aggressive management of stroke risk factors an important part of reducing future morbidity
- Thrombolysis is an effective treatment in appropriately selected older patients with ischaemic stroke
- Carotid endarterectomy confers significant benefit in appropriately selected older patients
- Thrombolysis and carotid endarterectomy are underused in older patients
- Falls are not a contraindication to warfarinisation and the risks and benefits of anti-coagulation in patients with atrial fibrillation should be carefully assessed.

References

1 Hatano S. Experience from a multicentre stroke register: a preliminary report. *Bull World Health Organ*. 1976;54(5):541–553.
2 Hankey GJ, Warlow C. Transient Ischaemic Attacks of the Brain and Eye. London; Philadelphia: Saunders; 1994.

3 Easton JD, Saver JL, Albers GW, Alberts MJ, Chaturvedi S, Feldmann E, et al. Definition and evaluation of transient ischemic attack: a scientific statement for healthcare professionals from the American Heart Association/American Stroke Association Stroke Council; Council on Cardiovascular Surgery and Anesthesia; Council on Cardiovascular Radiology and Intervention; Council on Cardiovascular Nursing; and the Interdisciplinary Council on Peripheral Vascular Disease: The American Academy of Neurology affirms the value of this statement as an educational tool for neurologists. *Stroke*. 2009; 40(6):2276–2293.

4 Heitsch LE, Panagos PD. Treating the elderly stroke patient: complications, controversies, and best care metrics. *Clin Geriatr Med*. 2013;29(1):231–255.

5 Fairhead JF, Rothwell PM. Underinvestigation and undertreatment of carotid disease in elderly patients with transient ischaemic attack and stroke: comparative population based study. *BMJ*. 2006;333(7567):525–527.

6 Gibson LM, Whiteley W. The differential diagnosis of suspected stroke: a systematic review. *J R Coll Physicians Edinb*. 2013;43(2):114–118.

7 Nor AM, Davis J, Sen B, Shipsey D, Louw SJ, Dyker AG, et al. The recognition of stroke in the emergency room (ROSIER) scale: development and validation of a stroke recognition instrument. *Lancet Neurol*. 2005;4(11):727–734.

8 Scottish Intercollegiate Guideline Network (SIGN). *Guideline 108: Management of Patients with Stroke or TIA: Assessment, Investigation, Immediate Management and Secondary Prevention*. http://www.sign.ac.uk /guidelines/fulltext/108/index.html [cited 2014 Apr 30].

9 National Institute for Health and Care Excellence (NICE). *CG68 Stroke: Quick Reference Guide*. http://www.nice.org.uk/ [cited 2014 Feb 11].

10 Meldon S, Ma OJ, Woolard R. Geriatric Emergency Medicine. 1st ed. McGraw-Hill Medical; 2003. 585 p.

11 Wardlaw JM, Murray V, Berge E, del Zoppo G, Sandercock P, Lindley RL, et al. Recombinant tissue plasminogen activator for acute ischaemic stroke: an updated systematic review and meta-analysis. *Lancet*. 2012;379(9834):2364–2372.

12 Jauch EC, Saver JL, Adams HP, Bruno A, Connors JJ, Demaerschalk BM, et al. Guidelines for the early management of patients with acute ischemic stroke: A guideline for healthcare professionals from the American Heart Association/American Stroke Association. *Stroke*. 2013;44(3):870–947.

13 Effectiveness of intermittent pneumatic compression in reduction of risk of deep vein thrombosis in patients who have had a stroke (CLOTS 3): a multicentre randomised controlled trial. *Lancet*. 2013; 382(9891):516–524.

14 Johnston SC, Rothwell PM, Nguyen-Huynh MN, Giles MF, Elkins JS, Bernstein AL, et al. Validation and refinement of scores to predict very early stroke risk after transient ischaemic attack. *Lancet*. 2007;369(9558):283–292.

15 Alamowitch S, Eliasziw M, Algra A, Meldrum H, Barnett HJ. Risk, causes, and prevention of ischaemic stroke in elderly patients with symptomatic internal-carotid-artery stenosis. *Lancet*. 2001; 357(9263):1154–1160.

16 Antoniou GA, Georgiadis GS, Georgakarakos EI, Antoniou SA, Bessias N, Smyth JVMc, et al. Meta-analysis and meta-regression analysis of outcomes of carotid endarterectomy and stenting in the elderly. *JAMA Surg*. 2013;148(12):1140–1152.

17 Rajamani K, Kennedy KF, Ruggiero NJ, Rosenfield K, Spertus J, Chaturvedi S. Outcomes of carotid endarterectomy in the elderly: report from the National Cardiovascular Data Registry. *Stroke*. 2013;44(4):1172–1174.

18 Zarraga IGE, Kron J. Oral anticoagulation in elderly adults with atrial fibrillation: integrating new options with old concepts. *J Am Geriatr Soc*. 2013;61(1):143–150.

19 Lip GYH, Nieuwlaat R, Pisters R, Lane DA, Crijns HJGM. Refining clinical risk stratification for predicting stroke and thromboembolism in atrial fibrillation using a novel risk factor-based approach: the euro heart survey on atrial fibrillation. *CHEST J*. 2010;137(2):263–272.

20 Man-Son-Hing M, Nichol G, Lau A, Laupacis A. Choosing antithrombotic therapy for elderly patients with atrial fibrillation who are at risk for falls. *Arch Intern Med*. 1999;159(7):677–85.
21 Sudlow CLM, Warlow CP. Comparable studies of the incidence of stroke and its pathological types results from an international collaboration. *Stroke*. 1997;28(3):491–9.
22 Woodford H. Acute Medicine in the Frail Elderly. 1st ed. Radcliffe Publishing Ltd; 2013. 344 p.
23 Anderson CS, Heeley E, Huang Y, Wang J, Stapf C, Delcourt C, et al. Rapid blood-pressure lowering in patients with acute intracerebral hemorrhage. *N Engl J Med*. 2013;368(25):2355–2365.

Index

Geriatric Emergencies, First Edition.
Iona Murdoch, Sarah Turpin, Bree Johnston, Alasdair MacLullich and Eve Losman.
© 2015 John Wiley & Sons, Ltd. Published 2015 by John Wiley & Sons, Ltd.